AF609815

For the Record...

Covid-19 For The Record...

Timeline and Chronology

Jan 2020 - Apr 2020

Table of Contents

Dedication

For Shiv

Editor's Note

When the COVID Pandemic began, I remember thinking that "this is the beginning", the beginning of something much bigger than we could have anticipated, bigger than our lifetime or even our children's lifetime. It is the start of a new age where the essence of humanity starts to disintegrate, bringing epic changes to the way we live, interact, and share life.

I am not a conspiracy theorist. I am a great believer that "the facts always speak for themselves". Indeed when the COVID vaccine was first approved, I researched the vaccine thoroughly as my job required me to be vaccinated immediately and facilitate giving it to others. Ethically I was bound to make an informed choice, not a forced one. So I decided to educate myself. In doing so, the collaborative global diary was born. I am glad I had both vaccines. I do believe it was and remains the right choice. When people compare looking for a cure for cancer as the same as finding a vaccine for COVID, I laugh. I ask what research they have done that brings them to that conclusion. After all, the research and development by the scientists, in particular Katalin Kariko, who dedicated her life's work to find a solution, had been foreseen many months ago and was not born overnight.

When the time comes where vaccinations will be the norm for all generations that walk the earth, when we are served by robots, and Artificial intelligence dominates all, when facts are changed so that the story can be retold in history books, I would like to hold on to the truth of how it happened. This book serves as a reference source for what really happened and how the world really did change.

For the Record is a collection of facts put together to map the daily steps taken by World Governments, WHO, The United Nations, and various Commerce and industry organisations to illustrate how their response to the pandemic changed the world.

Future Generations will hold us accountable for the decisions we made, and both our response as a nation and the actions taken by the world will serve as a teaching. This book is intended to be a collective history of the facts, a diary of events that occurred globally, people are free to decide for themselves what lessons they learn from the past and how it is shaping the future in ways that once upon a time we could not even begin to imagine...

In The Beginning...

Health experts in Wuhan knew the wet market at the centre of the coronavirus outbreak was a pandemic risk at least five years before COVID-19 emerged, a British scientist has revealed.

In 2014 Dr Eddie Holmes, an evolutionary biologist and virologist, was taken to the Huanan seafood market by members of the Wuhan Centre for Disease Control, who used it as an example of the type of place where a virus could "spillover" from animals to humans.

Dr Holmes, who now works at the University of Sydney, said the visit was part of a wider project to hunt for new pathogens with pandemic potential in China.

"The Wuhan CDC took us there, and here's the key bit, because the discussion was: 'where could a disease emerge?' Well, here's the place – that's why I went", Dr Holmes told The Telegraph in an interview.

"I've been to a few of these markets, but this was a big one – it felt like a disease incubator, exactly the sort of place you would expect a disease to emerge".

Dr Holmes, who took pictures at the time, remembers the now-shuttered market as a sprawling network of narrow covered streets in the heart of Wuhan. It was late afternoon and not particularly crowded, but there were "crates of wildlife stacked on top of each other", including fish, snakes, rodents and racoon dogs – a fox-like animal known to be susceptible to COVID-19.

“Many of the creatures were alive”, added Dr Holmes, who remembers seeing one bludgeoned in front of him.

“An animal had got out or something, and somebody was clubbing it”, he said, mimicking the hand actions over Zoom. “I think it was a racoon dog, though I couldn’t quite see. It was pretty confronting”.

Dr Holmes added that he is unsure whether the Wuhan CDC ramped up disease surveillance or introduced new safety measures in the years preceding the pandemic, and the China CDC has not responded to The Telegraph.

The Huanan market gained global notoriety when the first cases of COVID-19 (initially reported as a “mystery pneumonia” on 31 December 2019) were found in people who worked and shopped there.

Of the initial 41 people hospitalised with pneumonia who were officially identified as having COVID, two-thirds were exposed to the market, which was closed and sealed off by the Wuhan authorities on 1 January 2020.

The UK government called on the World Health Organisation to “explore all possible theories” around the origin of the coronavirus pandemic following reports that researchers at Wuhan’s virology laboratory received hospital treatment in November 2019.

The leaked US intelligence report said three researchers from the Wuhan Institute of Virology (WIV) were so ill that they sought hospital care a month before China said the first patient was discovered in the central Chinese city with what became known as COVID-19.

The intelligence report, first leaked to the *Wall Street Journal*, has fuelled further debate about the origins of the coronavirus pandemic.

Asked about the report, the Prime Minister's official spokesman said: "The WHO investigation into the origins of the virus is ongoing, and we have been clear throughout that it must be robust, transparent and independent.

"The investigation needs to explore all possible theories on how COVID-19 made that jump from animals to humans and how it spread, and that's vital to ensure we learn lessons from this crisis and prevent another global pandemic".

Jen Psaki, the White House press secretary, said the Biden administration hoped the WHO could move into a more transparent investigation of the origins of the coronavirus pandemic.

However, she said the government could not confirm the intelligence report leaked to the *Wall Street Journal*: "We don't have enough data and information to come to a conclusion at this point in time".

The US intelligence report about the researchers' illness goes beyond the details released in a State Department fact sheet issued in the final days of Donald Trump's presidency.

The factsheet, released on 19 January, stated that three researchers at the WIV, a lab for the research of coronaviruses and other pathogens, fell ill in the autumn of 2019 and had symptoms “consistent with both Covid-19 and other seasonal illnesses”.

The leaked US intelligence report does not contain any further information on what illness the three researchers had.

The documents differ from a report filed by the Chinese government to the World Health Organisation, which stated the first patient with Covid-like symptoms was discovered in Wuhan on 8 December 2019.

The new details came as Dr Anthony Fauci, America’s top infectious disease expert and the lead figure in the government’s coronavirus response, said he was “not convinced” the virus developed naturally.

“I think we should continue to investigate what went on in China until we continue to find out to the best of our ability what happened”, he said.

According to the *Wall Street Journal*, officials familiar with the US intelligence had varying opinions on the strength of the information.

One individual told the newspaper that the report was provided by an international partner and needed further investigation. Another said the information “from various sources was of exquisite quality”.

Authorities in China have strongly denied that the virus leaked from one of its labs.

"The US continues to hype the lab leak theory," China's foreign ministry said in response to The Wall Street Journal. "Is it actually concerned about tracing the source or trying to divert attention"?

"I've read it, it's a complete lie", said Yuan Zhiming, director of the Wuhan Institute of Virology, in response to the US report. "Those claims are groundless. The lab has not been aware of this situation, and I don't even know where such information came from".

A spokesperson at the virology lab said in response to a comment from The Telegraph: "Is there any necessary connection? It's also very normal for people to go to the hospital".

The Biden administration has declined to comment, stating all theories on the origin of the pandemic should be investigated by the World Health Organisation.

Last year, a WHO team travelled to Wuhan, the original epicentre, to investigate the origins of the virus.

In a joint report with Chinese experts, they concluded that the virus was most likely to have spread from bats to humans through another unknown animal and that a laboratory leak was "extremely unlikely".

At the time, experts revealed that while the first known case was detected on 8 December, the virus was likely to have started spreading earlier.

On the same day the report was released, WHO chief Tedro Adhanom Ghebreyesus said that the team did not thoroughly examine the possibility of a lab leak.

China did not grant investigators access to raw data, original lab reports and other records at the Wuhan Institute of Virology.

Timeline of

The Covid-19 Global Pandemic

According to information reported by the South China Morning Post on 13 20 March20, in a retrospective study, Chinese authorities identified 266 people who had been infected before the beginning of 2020.

According to the Chinese state-sponsored Xinhua News, the Huanan Seafood Market was closed on 1 January 2020 for “remediation”. In the Consortium’s report of 24 January 2020, it was stated that the Huanan Seafood Market had been closed on 1 January 2020 for “cleaning and disinfection. However, the virus could only stay on surfaces for so long, so this was useless”.

US CDC Director Robert Redfield was briefed about the severity of the virus from his Chinese counterparts George F. Gao when he was on vacation with his family – according to reports, what he heard “rattled him”.

WHO, in its Newsroom: Emergencies preparedness, the response said “the causal agent has not yet been identified or confirmed” and has requested further information from the Chinese authorities to assess the risk.

Pandemic Chronology January 2020

1 January

- Huanan Seafood Wholesale Market, the source of the initial pneumonia cases, was closed on 1 January 2020 for cleaning and disinfection. On the same day, Chinese state news reported that Wuhan police interviewed eight residents for spreading "misinformation," referring to the new infection as another SARS and "exaggerating" the danger. However, CNA reported on the same date that Wuhan police said they had punished eight people for "publishing or forwarding false information on the internet without verification."
- On 1 January 2020, a genetic sequencing company was notified by the Wuhan Municipal Health Committee that further sequencing of novel coronavirus samples were no longer allowed, existing samples must be destroyed, and all data must be kept secret.

2 January

- On 2 January, 41 admitted hospital patients in Wuhan, China, were confirmed to have contracted (laboratory-confirmed) the 2019-nCoV (novel coronavirus); 27 (66%) patients had direct exposure to Huanan Seafood Wholesale Market. All 41 patients were subsequently relocated from the hospital they had originally been diagnosed into the Jinyintan Hospital in Wuhan, China.
- On 2 January 2020, Central Hospital of Wuhan banned its staff from discussing the disease publicly or recording them

using text or image that can be used as evidence; the situation of individual patients can only be mentioned verbally when doctors change shifts.

3 January

- China's National Health Commission (NHC) ordered institutions to not publish any information related to the disease and ordered labs to either transfer all samples to designated testing institutions or destroy them. The order did not list any designated testing institutions.
- Li Wenliang, a Wuhan ophthalmologist, was summoned to the Wuhan Public Security Bureau, where he was told to sign an official confession and admonition letter promising to cease spreading "false" "rumors" regarding the coronavirus. In the letter, he was reprimanded for "making false comments by announcing the confirmation of 7 cases of SARS at the Huanan Seafood Wholesale Market" that had "severely disturbed the social order". The letter stated, "We solemnly warn you: If you keep being stubborn, with such impertinence, and continue this illegal activity, you will be brought to justice—is that understood?" Li signed the confession writing: "Yes, I understand".
- The Chinese government formally notified the US of the outbreak. At a White House briefing on 20 March, Health and Human Services Secretary Alex Azar said officials had been alerted to the initial reports of the virus by discussions between CDC director Robert Redfield and Chinese CDC Director Gao on 3 January. Mr Azar also told his chief of staff to make sure that the National Security Council was

aware that "this (the outbreak) is a very big deal" The BBC ran its first story on the outbreak.

- Health authorities in Wuhan reported 44 cases, a big jump from the 27 reported on Tuesday. Eleven of the 44 were seriously ill, the Wuhan Municipal Health Commission said, although there had been no reported deaths to date. The health of the 121 close contacts of the cases was being monitored.
- Chinese scientists at the National Institute of Viral Disease Control and Prevention (IVDC) ruled out the possibilities for 26 common respiratory pathogens, including influenza A and B virus, parainfluenza virus, adenovirus, respiratory syncytial virus metapneumovirus rhinovirus, enterovirus, and other common respiratory viruses. They determined the genetic sequence of the novel β-genus coronaviruses (naming it '2019-nCoV') from specimens collected from patients in Wuhan, China, and three distinct strains were established.
- On 3 January 2020, China's National Health Committee Office published an announcement classifying the novel coronavirus as a highly pathogenic microorganism (type 2) and request all the samples to be handed to provincial or higher level health authorities, other organisation or person with the virus sample should either destroy or transfer them and keep the log, and emphasise that all data must be kept secret and prior approval from the authority will be needed before any results can be published.
- Thailand began screening passengers arriving from Wuhan at four different airports.
- Singapore has also begun screening passengers at Changi Airport.

4 January

- The head of the University of Hong Kong's Centre for Infection, Ho Pak-Leung, warned that the city should implement the strictest possible monitoring system for a mystery new viral pneumonia that infected dozens of people on the mainland, as it was highly possible that the illness was spreading from human to human. The microbiologist also warned that there could be a surge in cases during the upcoming Chinese New Year. Ho said he hoped the mainland would release more details as soon as possible about the patients infected with the disease, such as their medical history, to help experts analyse the illness and to allow for more effective preventive measures to be put in place.
- The Singapore Ministry of Health said on Saturday, 4 January that it had been notified of the first suspected case of the "mystery Wuhan virus" in Singapore, involving a three-year-old girl from China who had pneumonia and a travel history to the Chinese city of Wuhan. On 5 January, the Singapore Ministry of Health released a press statement stating that the earlier suspected case was not linked to the pneumonia cluster in Wuhan and was also tested negative for the SARS and MERS-CoV.
- Chinese officials were criticised for failing to disclose any information about the "mysterious virus" that machine translations of official reports suggested may be caused by a new coronavirus.
- The WHO waited for China to release information about the "mysterious new pneumonia virus". The United Nations agency activated its incident-management system at the

country, regional and global level and was standing ready to launch a broader response if it was needed. The WHO's regional office in Manila said in Twitter posts Saturday: "#China has reported to WHO regarding a cluster of pneumonia cases in Wuhan, Hubei Province. The Govt has also met with our country office and updated @WHO on the situation. Govt actions to control the incident have been instituted, and investigations into the cause are ongoing".

- The Wuhan Institute of Virology did not respond to an emailed request for comment on the infectious source.
- The US CDC Director Redfield, following up the previous day's contact, emailed the Chinese CDC Director, Gao, formally offering to send US experts to China to investigate the outbreak.

5 January

- The number of suspected cases reached 59, with seven in a critical condition. All were quarantined, and local medical officials commenced the monitoring of 163 of their contacts. At this time, there had been no reported cases of human-to-human transmission or presentations in healthcare workers.
- Department of Zoonoses (National Institute of Communicable Disease Control and Prevention, Chinese Center for Disease Control and Prevention) submitted the complete genome of Wuhan seafood market pneumonia virus isolate Wuhan-Hu-1 (published 12 January 2020).
- Early investigations into the cause of pneumonia ruled out seasonal flu, SARS, MERS and bird flu.

6 January

- The US Centres for Disease and Prevention (USCDC) offers to send a US team to assist Chinese experts in their research in regard to transmissibility, severity, and incubation period of the disease.
- Hong Kong began screening passengers arriving on trains stopped at Wuhan.
- Monday, 6 January, the Wuhan health authorities announced they continued seeking the cause but had so far ruled out influenza, avian influenza, adenovirus, and coronaviruses SARS and MERS as the respiratory pathogen that had infected 59 people as of 5 January. The New York Times ran its first story on the outbreak.

7 January

- In a closed meeting of the Central Politburo of the Communist Party of China, Xi Jinping "made requests for the prevention and control work of the coronavirus outbreak" and issued instructions to similar ends. This meeting occurred 13 days before Xi's first public comments on the outbreak on 20 January.
- Scientists of the National Institute of Viral Disease Control and Prevention (IVDC) confirmed the novel coronavirus isolated on 3 January was the pathogenic cause of the viral pneumonia of unknown aetiology (VPUE) cluster, and the disease has been designated novel coronavirus-infected pneumonia (NCIP).
- Scientists in China announced the discovery of a new coronavirus.

- Since the outburst of social media discussion of the mysterious pneumonia outbreak in Wuhan, China, Chinese authorities censored the hashtag #WuhanSARS and were now investigating anyone who was allegedly spreading misleading information about the outbreak on social media.
- The world continued to wait for China to disclose more information about what had triggered an unexplained pneumonia outbreak in Wuhan, China's tenth-largest city.
- The U.S. Centers for Disease Control and Prevention (CDC) created an "incident management system" and issued a travel notice Monday for travellers to Wuhan, Hubei province, China due to the cluster of cases of pneumonia of an unknown aetiology..."
- According to prof. Mikhail Shchelkanov (FEFU Scientists' Council on 17 20 March20) he knew the sequence of the novel coronavirus genome by 7 January ("we – world scientists' circles").
- On 7 January 2020, Chinese Paramount leader and Party general secretary Xi Jinping raised demand on the prevention and control of the pneumonia epidemic caused by novel coronavirus in Wuhan in a Politburo Standing Committee of the Communist Party of China meeting, according to an article published by himself in February.

8 January

- South Korea announced the first possible case of the virus coming from China. South Korea put a 36-year-old Chinese woman under isolated treatment amid concerns that she had brought back a form of viral pneumonia that had sickened dozens in mainland China and Hong Kong in the previous weeks. The unidentified woman, who worked for a South Korean company near capital Seoul, had experienced cough and fever since returning from a five-day trip to China on 30 December, the KCDC said in a press release. The woman had spent time in Wuhan, China, but had not visited the Huanan Seafood Market.

9 January

- The first death from the virus occurred in a 61-year-old man who was a regular customer at the market. He had several significant medical conditions, including chronic liver disease, and died from heart failure and pneumonia. The incident was reported in China by the health commission via Chinese state media on 11 January.
- The WHO confirmed that the novel coronavirus had been isolated from one person who had been hospitalised. On the same day, the European Centre for Disease Prevention and Control posted its first risk assessment. The WHO also reported that Chinese authorities had acted swiftly, identifying the novel coronavirus within weeks of the onset of the outbreak, with the total number of positively tested people being 41.
- Chinese scientists reported on Chinese state broadcaster CCTV that they had found a new "coronavirus in 15 of 57 patients with the illness in the central city of Wuhan, saying it has been preliminarily identified as the pathogen for the outbreak". The scientists announced that the current 'Wuhan Virus', a coronavirus, appears to not be as lethal as SARS. They reported that the new viral outbreak was first detected in the city of Wuhan on 12 December 2019. Additionally, a

total of 59 people have been identified as contracting the illness, seven patients had been in a critical condition at some stage, and no healthcare workers were reported as having been infected.

10 January

- The gene sequencing data of the isolated 2019-nCoV, a virus from the same family as the SARS coronavirus, was posted on Virological.org by researchers from Fudan University, Shanghai. A further three sequences from the Chinese Center for Disease Control and Prevention, one from the Chinese Academy of Medical Sciences, and one from Jinyintan Hospital in Wuhan were posted to the Global Initiative on Sharing All Influenza Data (GISAID) portal. The same day, Public Health England issued its guidance.
- On 10 January 2020, Li Wenliang, a Chinese ophthalmologist and coronavirus whistleblower, started having symptoms of a dry cough. On 12 January 2020, Wenliang started having a fever. He was admitted to the hospital on 14 January 2020. His parents also contracted the coronavirus (presumably from Wenliang) and were admitted to the hospital with him. Wenliang tested negative several times for the coronavirus until finally testing positive on 30 January 2020. He died on 7 February 2020.
- First two patients in Shenzhen, Guangdong, China, attend University of Hong Kong-Shenzhen Hospital.
- The gene sequencing data of the isolated 2019-nCoV, a virus from the same family as the SARS coronavirus, was posted on Virological.org by researchers from Shanghai Public Health Clinical Center and Fudan University,

Shanghai. A further three sequences from the Chinese Center for Disease Control and Prevention, one from the Chinese Academy of Medical Sciences, and one from Jinyintan Hospital in Wuhan were posted to the Global Initiative on Sharing All Influenza Data (GISAID) portal. The same day, Public Health England issued its guidance.

- Beginning of the 2020 Chunyun travel season in China.

11 January

- The first two patients in Shenzhen city transferred into a negative pressure room in Third People's Hospital of Shenzhen City due to matching lab test results, symptoms, and epidemiology and are being listed as suspected cases. The cases were not confirmed at the time because the requirement from the Chinese government at the time was that the first case in each city needs to be submitted to the provincial CDC, verified by the national CDC, and then evaluated and confirmed by a specific diagnostic team in national CDC.
- The first viral genome sequence was shared to GENBANK and Virological.org by Professor Zhang Yongzhen of the Shanghai Public Health Clinical Centre through the auspices of the Wuhan Institute of Virology, which was before the government's official disclosure of the same to WHO, which occurred on the following day when the National Health Commission released several viral sequences to GISAID.
- In China, more than 700 close contacts of the 41 confirmed cases, including more than 400 healthcare workers, had been monitored, with no new cases reported in China since 5 January. The WHO published initial guidance on travel

advice, testing in the laboratory and medical investigation. WHO is saying that "The Chinese government reports that there is no clear evidence that the virus passes easily from person to person".

12 January

- Hubei's provincial representatives from all over the province met in Wuhan until 18 January.
- Shanghai Public Health Clinical Center, the facility that published the first genome sequence of the virus, was closed without reason.

13 January

- The USCDC announced that the genome had been posted on the NIH genetic sequence database, GenBank. On the same day, Thailand witnessed the first confirmed case of 2019-nCoV, first outside China. The affected 61-year-old Chinese woman, who is a resident of Wuhan, had not visited the Huanan Seafood Wholesale Market but was noted to have been to other markets. She had arrived in Bangkok on 8 January. In response, the WHO urged China to continue searching for the source of the new virus.

14 January

- WHO sent a tweet which said, "preliminary investigations conducted by the Chinese authorities have found no clear evidence of human-to-human transmission of the novel coronavirus (2019-nCoV) identified in Wuhan, China". According to Reuters in Geneva, WHO said there may have been limited human-to-human transmission of a new coronavirus in China within families, and it is possible there could be a wider outbreak.

- On 14 January, The Wuhan Municipal Health Committee published a Q&A regarding the coronavirus, stating: “current investigation hasn’t found clear evidence of human to human transmission, however, the possibility of human to human transmission cannot be ruled out”.
- On 14 January, two of the 41 confirmed cases in Wuhan were reported to include a married couple, raising the possibility of human-to-human transmission.
- On 14 January, Maria Van Kerkhove, acting head of WHO’s emerging diseases unit, said that there had been limited human-to-human transmission of the coronavirus, mainly small clusters in families, adding that “it is very clear right now that we have no sustained human-to-human transmission”.
- In a confidential government teleconference on 15 January, between Ma Xiaowei, the head of the National Health Commission and the provincial health authorities, the government internally acknowledged the threat of a pandemic due to the reporting of the Thailand viral infection a day earlier and the public health threat that New Year holiday travel presented for the further spread of the virus.
- Reporters from Hong Kong being taken to the police station after trying to film the situation within Wuhan hospital.

15 January

- A second death occurred in a 69-year-old man in China on 15 January.
- The first known travel-related case of 2019 novel coronavirus entered the United States: "The patient from Washington with confirmed 2019-nCoV infection returned to the United States from Wuhan on 15 January 2020. The patient sought care at a medical facility in the state of Washington, where the patient was treated for the illness. Based on the patient's travel history and symptoms, healthcare professionals suspected this new coronavirus. A clinical specimen was collected and sent to CDC overnight, where laboratory testing yesterday confirmed the diagnosis via CDC's Real-time Reverse Transcription-Polymerase Chain Reaction (rRT-PCR) test."
- US Embassy in China issued a Health Alert Watch Level 1 for an outbreak of pneumonia in Wuhan, preliminarily identified to be caused by a novel coronavirus.

27 January

- The Health Secretary, Matt Hancock, tells the House of Commons that 200 British citizens trapped in Wuhan, China, will be offered repatriation to the UK in light of the coronavirus outbreak there.

28 January

- The Foreign and Commonwealth Office updates its travel advisory, advising against all but essential travel to the rest of Mainland China.

- British Airways suspends all flights to and from mainland China with immediate effect due to the ongoing coronavirus threat.
- Wanda Group waives all rent and property fees for all merchants from 24 January to 25 February, amounting to an estimated fee reduction of ¥3–4 billion (US$432–577 million).
- Sasseur REIT shuts four malls temporarily, with another seven outlet malls shut to slow the outbreak.
- Dasin Retail Trust shortens hours for its five malls and temporarily closed crowded places.
- ComfortDelGro Corporation, a Singapore transport company, was told by authorities to shut the Nanjing Comfort Delgro Xixia Driving Centre as a precautionary measure against the coronavirus. Other centres were unaffected.

29 January

- Tibet reported its first suspected case identified on the previous day and declared a level 1 health emergency in the evening, the last mainland provincial division to do so. Suspected cases have now been reported in all 31 mainland provincial divisions.
- Companies in Hubei are required not to resume services before 13 February, and schools in Hubei are to postpone the reopening of schools.
- Chinese police drop their case against eight people, accused on 1 January of spreading "false rumours" about a "new SARS-like virus"; they have been referred to as "the eight brave (八勇士)" on some Chinese social media.

- CapitaLand temporarily shuts all four malls in Wuhan and both malls in Xian after instructions from local authorities, with supermarkets still open. The company's remaining 45 malls will operate for shorter periods. It has also set up a 10 million Yuan fund to fight the coronavirus.
- The government of Papua New Guinea banned all travellers from Asian countries and closed its border with Indonesia. The order takes effect from 30 January.
- Palau and Vanuatu temporarily suspended flights from mainland China, Macau, and Hong Kong until the end of February and restricted diplomatic work in those countries. The Federated States of Micronesia is considering the same measures.
- The government of Kazakhstan suspended visa issuances to Chinese citizens. In addition, all transport links from and to China have been halted; accordingly, movement by train will stop on 1 February and will stop by aeroplane from 3 February. Georgia temporarily suspended all direct flights with China.
- Rasuwa Fort, which is a border crossing between Rasuwa District (Nepal) and Tibet (China), will be sealed for 15 days starting 29 January. The decision was preceded by a meeting between security and immigration authorities of two countries earlier that day.
- The WHO announces that its director-general has decided to reconvene their international health regulations emergency committee on 30 January to reconsider declaring a global health emergency, technically a "public health emergency of international concern" (PHEIC). The reconvening is due "mainly on the evidence of an increasing number of cases,

human-to-human transmission outside of China, and the further development of transmission." The committee meeting is planned to start at 13:30 Geneva time. Further, the WHO announces their having set up "The Pandemic Supply Chain Network (PSCN)" in collaboration with the World Economic Forum.

- The Government of Canada issued a travel advisory to avoid non-essential travel to China due to the novel coronavirus outbreak. The Government of Canada also issued a regional travel advisory to avoid all travel to the Province of Hubei—including the cities of Wuhan, Huanggang and Ezhou—due to the imposition of heavy travel restrictions to limit the spread of the novel coronavirus. On the same day, the Minister of Foreign Affairs François-Philippe Champagne announced that an aircraft would be sent to repatriate Canadians from the areas affected by the novel coronavirus in China. As a result of the travel advisories issued by the Canadian government, Air Canada suspended all direct flights to China until at least 29 February.
- The Ministry of Popular Power for Health announced that the Rafael Rangel National Institute of Hygiene (Spanish: Instituto Nacional de Higiene Rafael Rangel) in Caracas will perform the detection of other respiratory viruses based on non-influenza types, including coronaviruses in humans. It is also the only health institute in the country with the installed capacity for the diagnosis of respiratory viruses in Venezuela and is able to carry out logistics in the 23 states, the Capital District and Federal Dependencies.
- British Airways and Lufthansa cancelled all flights to and from mainland China.

- Singapore expanded temperature screening to cover all incoming flights with additional checks on flights from China and passengers from Hubei.

- The Panama Canal began to require all ships to report if they had any contact with coronavirus-infected countries. The Panamanian health ministry also established an isolation ward for coronavirus patients.
- The Philippines and Sri Lanka suspended issuance of visas-on-arrival to Chinese nationals.
- Singapore announced a suspension from 29 January, 12 pm of entry or transit for all new visitors with a recent travel history to Hubei within the last 14 days, or holders of China passports issued in Hubei.
- Hong Kong temporarily closes four of the eleven ports with the mainland. Carrie Lam, the Chief Executive, stated the high-speed rail service between Hong Kong and mainland China would be suspended starting 30 January, and all cross-border ferry services would also be suspended in a bid to stop the spread of coronavirus. Additionally, flights from mainland China would be cut in half, cross-border bus services reduced, and the Hong Kong government is asking all its employees (except those providing essential or emergency services) to work from home. In a later press conference, Carrie Lam said that the Man Kam To and Sha Tau Kok border checkpoints would be closed.
- Thailand starts scanning all travellers from China with immediate effect.

- The UK's Foreign Office warns Britons not to travel to mainland China unless their journey is essential. Existing advice against all travel to Hubei Province remains in place.
- The USCDC stated it was boosting staffing at 20 US airports that have quarantine facilities.
- Singer Miriam Yeung postponed a concert in Singapore, which was scheduled for 8 February. This comes after the virus situation in China worsened, with most of the logistics coming from there.
- Tibet reported its first suspected case identified on the previous day and declared a level 1 health emergency in the evening, the last mainland provincial division to do so. Suspected cases have now been reported in all 31 mainland provincial divisions.
- Companies in Hubei are required not to resume services before 13 February, and schools in Hubei are to postpone the reopening of schools.
- The UAE confirms its first case. Shortly afterwards, an Emirates' news agency confirmed four people from a Chinese family to be infected. Finland reports its first case of the virus in Lapland, found in a Chinese tourist who left Wuhan before Wuhan was locked down. Singapore confirms three more cases of the virus, bringing the total infected to 10. Malaysia confirms three additional cases, bringing its total to seven. Japan reports four additional cases, including a tour bus guide that was on the same bus as one of the cases confirmed on 28 January and three evacuated from Wuhan. France confirmed a fifth case, the daughter of the patient in the fourth case.

- Two Chinese nationals were placed in isolation wards in Armenia amid the first suspected case of coronavirus in the country. The Chinese nationals were tourists travelling to Armenia from neighbouring Georgia. Liana Torosyan, the head of the Department of Infectious Diseases, advised that samples will be sent to European labs, as Armenia does not have the capacity to test for the novel coronavirus. Brazil reports a total of 9 suspected cases in six states of the country.
- Air Canada is halting all direct flights to China following the federal government's advisory to avoid non-essential travel to the mainland due to the coronavirus epidemic. The suspension is effective Thursday and is slated to last until 29 February.
- Trump administration trade advisor Peter Navarro issued a memo warning that coronavirus could "evolve into a full-blown pandemic, imperilling the lives of millions of Americans" and that the "risk of a worst-case pandemic scenario should not be overlooked". A critic of the Chinese government before the pandemic, Navarro argued for restrictions on travel from China.
- The Wuhan police clarified that Li Wenliang was not arrested nor fined but was warned as he had spread that "there had been seven confirmed cases of SARS", which was not true.
- The WHO confirmed over 6,000 confirmed cases in China to date.

30 January

- As of 30 January, inter-provincial charter cars in mainland China and inter-provincial passenger routes to Hubei have all been suspended. Passenger transport on roads in ten provinces and municipalities, including Hubei and Beijing, has been suspended, inter-provincial passenger trains have been suspended in 16 provinces, urban bus routes have been suspended or partially suspended in multiple cities in 28 provinces, and urban rail transportation has been suspended in 5 cities including Wuhan.
- The Huanggang Communist Party committee announced the dismissal of its health chief, Tang Zhihong.
- Micro-Mechanics temporarily shuts its Suzhou factory after instructions from the authorities there due to the coronavirus, with operations to resume on 10 February.
- The WHO director-general declares the coronavirus outbreak a "Public Health Emergency of International Concern" (PHEIC), reversing two previous decisions after emergency committee meetings in the last week. WHO also issued a warning that "all countries should be prepared for containment, including active surveillance, early detection, isolation and case management, contact tracing and prevention of onward spread" of the virus.
- Vietnam shuts down air traffic with China. The Ministry of Public Security temporarily ceased issuing visas to Chinese citizens within the epidemic areas. Additionally, crossing at gateways, airports, seaports are put under higher supervision, with strict monitoring and medical check-ups (applied to both humans and items; prohibited against wildlife animals and derivatives). Later that day, after

confirmation of the virus for the first three Vietnamese patients, the Prime Minister ordered for further visa restrictions apart from diplomatic work, suspension of activities at border gates (with China) which are still active, evacuation for citizens when necessary, and an emergency alert being considered.

- The Liaison Office between the two Koreas in the border town of Kaesong was shut down for an unspecified time regarding infection concerns. The decision was made after negotiations between the representatives of both countries early in the morning on 30 January, informed by the Unification Ministry of South Korea.
- North Korea's news agency KCNA declared a "state emergency" and reported the establishment of anti-epidemic headquarters around the country.
- Singapore announced that every household was to receive four masks starting from 1 February.
- Russia announces restrictions on railway travel with China, such that only a direct train between Moscow and Beijing remains.
- Italian Prime Minister Giuseppe Conte stated in a press conference that Italy had closed all air traffic to and from China. It is believed that Conte has also called a cabinet meeting for Friday to discuss further actions. Six thousand people are briefly quarantined on board an Italian cruise ship as tests are carried out on two Chinese passengers suspected of having coronavirus, a spokesman for the Costa Crociere cruise company said. On the same day, all passengers are released as it is found that the ill individual has the flu, not coronavirus.

- The US State Department issued an updated travel advisory as "Level 4: Do Not Travel to China." Its website stated that "Those currently in China should consider departing" and warning that "Travelers should be prepared for travel restrictions to be put into effect with little or no advance notice". Additionally, it authorised American diplomatic staff and their families to evacuate China. The State of Washington in the US declared a Level 1 Emergency and activated its Emergency Response Center for dealing with the now global coronavirus outbreak.
- British foreign secretary Dominic Raab disclosed that the emergency flight containing about 120 Britons from Wuhan that was delayed by 24 hours was due to land at RAF Brize Norton on Friday morning, where the passengers will be taken to Wirral for a fortnight's quarantine.
- Trinidad and Tobago's health minister, Terrance Deyalsingh, announced that Trinidad and Tobago had decided to implement restrictions on persons travelling from China. Persons who are living or who have visited China will be barred from entering Trinidad and Tobago unless they had already been out of China 14 days prior to attempting to travel to Trinidad and Tobago.
- Air France and KLM cancel all flights to mainland China until 9 February.
- Two K-pop concerts in Singapore by Taeyeon and NCT Group respectively were postponed after the virus situation worsened.
- The National Library of Medicine began a collection of websites and social media reporting of the virus outbreak as part of its Global Health Events archiving.

31 January

- China National Railway Group announced that starting 1 February, rail ticket purchases must provide the traveller's mobile phone number (email address for foreign nationals).
- Russian authorities announced the border closure with China would be extended to at least 1 March.
- Authorities in Guangxi (China) and Lạng Sơn (Vietnam) announced the temporary suspension of nine auxiliary border gates (namely in pair: Tân Thanh – 浦寨, Chi Ma – 爱店, Cốc Nam – 弄怀, Bình Nghi – 平宜, Pò Nhùng – 油隘, Bản Chắt – 板烂, Co Sâu – 北山, Na Hình, and Nà Nưa) and border markets starting 31 January until 8 February, and prohibited all travel over cross-border trails.
- Singapore closed borders to all visitors arriving from mainland China (including passengers transiting through Singapore) except Singaporeans, Singapore residents and long-term visa holders. The measure took effect on 1 February at 11.59 pm.
- Macau announced it would postpone schools indefinitely and that schools should contact students to arrange for assignments to be done online. Hong Kong extends the public holiday to 2 March and also requests all visitors who have been in Hubei in the past 14 days to be quarantined. All government employees may work from home until 9 February.
- Italy declared a state of emergency, the first EU country to do so, and allocates an initial 5 million Euros to tackle the virus.

- The United States government declares a Public Health Emergency due to the coronavirus and is closing its borders to all foreign nationals "who pose a threat of transmitting the virus from entering the country and would quarantine US citizens returning from Hubei province in China, the epicentre of the outbreak, for up to 14 days", starting Sunday, 2 February at 5 pm. The 195 Americans on the Air Force base in California who were recently evacuated from Wuhan recently will also be quarantined.
- Jamaica's health minister, Christopher Tufton, announced a government decision to ban travel between China and Jamaica. All persons entering Jamaica from China will be subject to immediate quarantine for at least 14 days, and anyone who was allowed to land and shows symptoms of the virus will be put in immediate isolation. In keeping with the new policy, 19 Chinese nationals who arrived at the Norman Manley International Airport on the evening of 31 January were denied entry, quarantined and put on a flight back to China on 1 February.
- The Ecuadorian Ministry of Health, Catalina Andramuño, announced that the country now possesses reagents for testing new cases locally, becoming the first in South America.
- LOT Polish Airlines cancels all flights to Beijing until 9 February. Delta Airlines suspends all China flights, and American Airlines pilots sue for the same action. Later, American Airlines ceased flights to China as well. Later still, United Airlines halts all flights to China, excepting San Francisco to Hong Kong.

- Basra International Airport in Iraq has declared that passengers of any nationality travelling from China will be denied entry.
- Turkish Airlines halted all flights to China until 9 February.
- K-pop band Got7's concert in Singapore, scheduled for 22 February, was postponed due to the virus.
- WHO declared the virus was a Public Health Emergency of International Concern and advised: "all countries should be prepared for containment, including active surveillance, early detection, isolation and case management, contact tracing and prevention of the onward spread of 2019-nCoV infection, and to share full data with WHO."
- Tibet confirms its first case, which was previously suspected. Cases have now been confirmed in all 31 provincial divisions of mainland China. India confirms its first case of coronavirus in a student who had returned from Wuhan University to the Indian state of Kerala. The Philippines confirms its first case of coronavirus in a female Chinese national who arrived in Manila via Hong Kong on 21 January. Japan confirms three more cases, bringing the total to 14. Malaysia confirms one more case, bringing the total to eight. Singapore confirms three more cases, bringing the total to 13. South Korea confirms two more cases, with one of them being the first human-to-human transmission there, bringing the total to six. Vietnam confirms three new cases, bringing the total to five. France confirms its sixth case. Italy confirms its first two cases in a press conference by the Prime Minister, Giuseppe Conte. Germany confirms its fifth case, an employee of the company where the four previously known cases are also employed.

- The United States confirmed its sixth case, the spouse of another patient in Chicago. This is the first confirmed case of human to human transmission within the United States. Azar, Redfield and Anthony S. Fauci agreed that a ban on travel from the epidemic's centre could buy some time to put into place prevention and testing measures. Redfield said in an interview that "there was so much we didn't know about this virus. We were rapidly understanding it was much more transmissible, that it had a great ability to go global".
- The United Kingdom and Russia confirmed their first coronavirus infections. The first Swedish and Spanish cases were confirmed. The seventh confirmed case in the US is in Santa Clara County, California. A fourth case of coronavirus in Canada has been confirmed in London, Ontario. Thailand confirmed five more cases with the first human-to-human virus transmission inside the country of a local taxi driver, bringing the total to 19. Singapore confirmed three more cases, including the first Singaporean patient, bringing the total to 16. South Korea confirmed five more cases, bringing the total to 11. Chinese health experts warn the public that coronavirus patients can become re-infected. China starts repatriating citizens to Wuhan.
- A senior leader at the US Department of Health and Human Services said staff members were sent to Travis Air Force Base and March Air Reserve Base in late January and early February and were ordered to enter quarantined areas were not provided with proper safety-protocol training or equipment, with at least one person staying in a nearby hotel and leaving California on a commercial flight. The US bans the entry of foreign nationals who had been to China in the previous 14 days.

- The first two cases of coronavirus (2019-nCoV) in the United Kingdom are confirmed.

Pandemic Chronology February 2020

1 February

- Import duties and US-specific tariffs were exempted on imported materials donated for epidemic prevention and control, including VAT and sales tax; the duties and tariffs previously levied were to be refunded.
- The Ministry of Ecology and Environment issued a notice late in the evening to deploy medical wastewater and urban sewage supervision, regulate emergency medical wastewater treatment, sterilisation and disinfection requirements in order to prevent the spread of new coronavirus through faeces and sewage after the faeces of a patient was tested positive for the virus in Shenzhen.
- The Department of Civil Affairs of Hubei Province suspends all marriage registrations starting on 3 February 2020.
- Huanggang, Hubei implements a much stricter control, allowing only one person from each household every two days to be on the street for purchases, unless for medically-related reasons, required for epidemic control, or as shop workers.
- Alibaba Group announced free taxi service for health professionals in Wuhan.
- Hunan government required companies in the province not to resume business before 24:00 on 9 February; the new semester is not to start earlier than 17 February for primary and secondary schools and kindergartens, and 24 February for post-secondary institutions. Tianjin government issued a

notice to postpone business resumption and the start of the new semester.

- Huanggang, Hubei converted Dabie Mountain Regional Medical Centre to an emergency treatment hospital, adding 1000 new beds. Huoshenshan Hospital was fully electrified on 23:49.
- China Securities Regulatory Commission waived the 2020 annual listing fee that listed companies in Hubei are required to pay to the stock exchange.
- China Federation of Radio and Television Associations issued a notice to pause the filming of all films and TV dramas in mainland China during the epidemic.
- 310 Hubei citizens were repatriated from Thailand, Malaysia, and Japan.
- Apple Inc. temporarily closed all Apple Stores in mainland China until 24:00 on 9 February.
- China's National Health Commission (NHC) announced new regulations Saturday requiring that all who lose their lives to the coronavirus must be cremated at the nearest facility. "No farewell ceremonies or other funeral activities involving the corpse shall be held", according to the new ruling.
- The Badminton World Federation announced it has postponed the 2020 Lingshui China Masters tournament, originally scheduled to be held from 25 February to 1 March.
- Australia reported another three cases, including the first two cases in South Australia, bringing their total to 12.
- Japan reported three more cases, increasing their total to 20.
- Singapore confirms two more cases, bringing the total to 18.

- South Korea confirmed the twelfth case of the coronavirus: a 49-year-old Chinese man who works as Japanese tour guide in western Seoul.
- Spain confirmed its first case of the virus on La Gomera in the Canaries.
- The United States of America reported its eighth case, a man from Boston who recently returned to college after travelling to Wuhan.
- Vietnam confirmed its sixth case in Khánh Hòa Province, another domestic transmission in direct contact.
- Australia's Department of Health issued directives, going into effect from 1 February. Accordingly, travel advisory was increased to level 4: do not travel to all of mainland China. All travellers arriving out of mainland China were asked to self-isolate for a period of 14 days from the time of leaving. Additional border measures were implemented to deny entry of people who have arrived from mainland China, with the exception of Australian citizens, permanent residents and their immediate family and aircrews who have been using appropriate personal protective equipment.
- International border gates Móng Cái (Quảng Ninh Province, Vietnam) - Dongxing (Guangxi, China) ceased functioning on 1 February for an unspecified time; border gates Hoành Mô and Bắc Phong Sinh experienced a 24-hour closure, awaiting further measurements from authorities. Taiwan barred nationals from Guangdong (mainland China), and travellers who recently visited the area will be subject to a mandatory 14-day quarantine from entry beginning 1 February.

- With the sixth case being another domestic transmission, Vietnamese Prime Minister Nguyễn Xuân Phúc signed an epidemic declaration. Aviation permits which already had been granted for flights between Vietnam and China Mainland-Hong Kong-Macau were all revoked, effective immediately from 13:00 (UTC+7, 1 February) for an unspecified time. It perhaps lasts until 1 May, according to the United States Federal Aviation Administration.
- India banned the export of N-95 masks with immediate effect.
- The Government of Japan barred: entry of foreign nationals infected with the virus and entry of Chinese citizens with passports issued in Hubei province.
- 102 German citizens and 26 relatives, all of whom were symptom-free on departure, were evacuated from the Wuhan region to Frankfurt am Main by the Executive Transport Wing of the German Air Force. After their return, they were placed in quarantine in a military barrack in Rhineland-Palatinate for 14 days. The coronavirus was found in two passengers on 2 February. On the outward flight, the Bundeswehr aircraft had 10,000 protective suits on board, which were handed over to the Chinese authorities.
- Trinidad and Tobago's travel restrictions on persons arriving from China goes into full effect. Persons now have to wait 14 days after leaving China before being able to enter Trinidad & Tobago. Additionally, persons who may already be at a port of entry and who were in China or are showing symptoms will be subject to quarantine measures. Thermal screening is also being conducted on passengers arriving from Canada, Panama, the United Kingdom and the United

States. Testing will also be done by the Caribbean Public Health Agency (CARPHA) on 3 February.

- Qatar Airways has suspended flights to mainland China from 3 February until further notice. It is the first air carrier in the Middle East to do so.
- Princess Cruises announces restrictions on crew members and guests who have recently travelled within mainland China. Guests who have travelled through or in mainland China 14 days prior to the scheduled departure of their cruise will not be allowed to board. Crew members from mainland China are prohibited from getting on any ship until further notice from the company. Crew members scheduled on connecting flights to China have been rerouted. Two cruises in June have been cancelled, and two cruises have been rerouted to arrive or depart in Tokyo instead of Shanghai.
- Wuhan's Epidemic Prevention and Control Headquarters arranged for Jointown Pharmaceutical to overtake the warehouse management of Wuhan Red Cross after days of scandals and controversies regarding the Red Cross' incompetence, extreme delays in allocating donation resources, and unexplained apparent misallocation of crucial medical supplies.
- On the same day, the Prevention and Control HQ issued a set of traditional Chinese medicine (TCM) prescriptions "to help treat the infection". This move follows the 22 January recommendation from the National Health Commission to use TCM to treat the disease. The same official file that contains the prescription also demands that all patients in Wuhan be treated by TCM.

- Wenzhou, Zhejiang announces implementing the same measure as Huanggang, where every household may send one person every two days outside for purchases, from 00:00 on 2 February to 24:00 on 8 February.
- Huoshenshan Hospital completed construction in the morning and was transferred to the military half a day earlier than scheduled.
- Hubei allows imported and re-imported masks that are unlisted in China to be sold in the provincial market.
- The Ministry of Transport extended the cut-off time for the toll-free minibus period of the 2020 spring.
- Festival to 24:00 on 8 February 2020.
- Meituan starts an initiative to disinfect all shared bikes in eight mainland cities regardless of the brand.
- With immediate effect, Wuhan's government announced the quarantining of "all suspected patients and those known to have been in close contact with a confirmed case." It stated, "Patients shall cooperate. Whoever refuses to cooperate will be subject to enforcement by the police".
- Chinese Premier Li Keqiang has asked the European Union to facilitate the sale of medical supplies "through commercial channels". According to a Chinese government statement, the President of the European Commission, Ursula von der Leyen, said the European Union will try its best and coordinate all necessary resources to provide assistance to China.
- India announced its second case.
- The Philippines saw the first confirmed death from Covid-19 outside mainland China announced. The case was that of a 44-year-old male who was the companion of the first

confirmed case in the country; both are Chinese nationals from Wuhan who had arrived in the country via Hong Kong on 21 January. He had been in stable condition prior to his death on 1 February.

- South Korea reported three more cases, bringing their total to 15.
- The United Arab Emirates reported its fifth case.
- The United States of America confirmed three more cases, all in California, bringing the total to 11.
- Two Germans aboard the evacuation flight from Wuhan tested positive for the virus, bringing the number of cases there up to twelve.
- Vietnam announced its seventh case of Covid-19, a Vietnamese-American who had had a two-hour layover at Wuhan Airport.

2 February

- New Zealand has temporarily banned all foreign nationals travelling from or transiting through mainland China after 2 February to assist the containment of the coronavirus into New Zealand and the Pacific Islands. Foreign travellers in transit to New Zealand on 2 February will be subject to enhanced scanning, but pending clearance will be allowed into New Zealand. New Zealand citizens and permanent residents, and their immediate family members, will be allowed to enter New Zealand but must self-isolate for 14 days. The ban will last for 14 days but will be reviewed every 48 hours.
- The Philippines has temporarily banned foreigners arriving from China and its territories, including those who visited

such areas within the past 14 days, from entering the country; Filipino citizens and permanent residents of the Philippines arriving from such would have to undergo quarantine for 14 days. Travel from the Philippines to China and its territories have been temporarily banned as well.

- According to a diplomatic note distributed to foreign residents in North Korea, North Korean authorities have suspended the flight route between Pyongyang and Vladivostok performed by Air Koryo's. According to the same note, "During the month of February, events, ceremonial visits and meetings shall not proceed, and essential meetings shall be conducted via telephone"... all diplomats or international organization staff going to North Korea will now be subjected to a mandatory 15-day quarantine process at their "place of residence" from the day of arrival". Those subject to quarantine by North Korean authorities will not be allowed to come into contact with other persons and must not enter public places. KCNA reported all people who entered the country after 13 January to have been placed under "medical supervision".
- South Korean Prime Minister Chung Sye-kyun announced to the public the entry barring of all foreign nationals, who have been to Hubei Province since 21 January, will go into effect starting 4 February for an unspecified time. Also, the visa-free policy for Chinese citizens to visit Jeju Island is to be temporarily nullified.
- Indonesia banned all flights from and to Mainland China starting from 5 February. The government also stopped giving free visas and visas on arrival for Chinese nationals. They banned those who live or stay in Mainland China for at

least 14 days before entering or transiting Indonesia. Indonesians are discouraged from travelling to China.

- The Vietnamese Ministry of Labors, Invalids and Social Affairs issued directive on temporary suspension to Chinese labours returning to work after public holidays.
- Numerous landmark buildings in the United Arab Emirates lit up a Sunday night, showing support for Wuhan and Chinese communities around the world over pain and horror by the novel coronavirus, namely: the Burj Khalifa, ADNOC Headquarters, the Capital Gate, Abu Dhabi Global Market, Emirates Palace, Sheikh Zayed Bridge, Burj Al Arab, Hazza bin Zayed Stadium, etc.
- Air Asia Philippines, Philippine Airlines and Cebu Pacific have suspended flights to and from mainland China, Macau and Hong Kong.
- Group of Seven countries are seeking a unified approach to combat the spread.
- US Health and Human Services imposed restrictions on travellers entering the US, which went into effect at 5 pm ET. The plan included temporarily denying entry to foreign nationals who visited China in the 14 days prior to their arrival to the US, US citizen returning to the US who has been in Hubei Province in the previous 14 days will be subject to up to 14 days of mandatory quarantine and US citizens returning from the rest of mainland China in the 14 days prior will undergo health screenings at selected ports of entry and face up to 14 days of self-monitored quarantine. President Trump said, "We pretty much shut it down coming in from China". Wall Street Journal in its Opinion page called "China Is the Real Sick Man of Asia which enraged China ".

Florida Governor DeSantis said, “Coronavirus may have spread at Super Bowl in Miami”.

- The Government of Maldives denies entry to passengers arriving from China.
- Hong Kong announced further tightening of the border with the mainland. Beginning 00:00 on 4 February, the special administrative region closed most of its border crossings, except the Hong Kong International Airport, the Shenzhen Bay Port and the Hong Kong-Zhuhai-Macau Bridge.
- Indonesia set to ban live animal imports from China as coronavirus fears grow.
- The Japanese authorities denied entry to any foreign nationals who have been to Hubei province in the past 14 days, even if there are no symptoms of the virus. Japanese officials quarantined a cruise ship, carrying approximately 3,500 people, off the port of Yokohama due to a former passenger on the ship having contracted the virus.
- The Venezuelan government announced that the country has imposed epidemiological surveillance, restrictions and diagnostic system to detect possible coronavirus patients at the Simón Bolívar International Airport in Maiquetía, Venezuela’s main international airport, and that Venezuela will receive a diagnostic kit for the virus strain from the Pan American Health Organization (PAHO).
- Lunar New Year holidays was extended for one week to all k-through-12 students in Ho Chi Minh City; public schools will resume on 10 February. The city authorities ordered to build two speciality emergency hospitals designed to treat people with the 2019 novel coronavirus. With 500-bed accommodation in total, master plans for construction are

due 15 February. The capital city Hanoi is considering taking the same measures.

- The global Cruise Lines International Association bans trips to mainland China and says that it "will deny boarding to any individual, whether guest or crew, who has travelled from or through mainland China within the previous 14 days".
- Boise State University suspends travel to and from China.
- At a news briefing, The Centers for Disease Control and Prevention plan to distribute testing kits to speed up the diagnosis of the coronavirus. The CDC states that this measure will help speed up the testing and diagnosis of the coronavirus after cases in the US reached 11. The Food and Drug Administration first has to approve the test for wider distribution, the CDC said.
- India invalidated all e-visas given to Chinese passport holders since 15 January. It also has stopped giving out new e-visas to Chinese passport holders. India also gave a travel advisory to not travel to China. The travel advisory also stated that anyone who comes to knowledge that had visited China since 15 January could get quarantined.
- Several exhibitors and South Korea's Black Eagles have decided to pull out of the Singapore Airshow. This comes as the virus situation worsens.
- K-pop band Winner cancelled its concert in Singapore, supposed to be held on 8 February. Several Huayi events in Esplanade were cancelled owing to travel restrictions. In addition, a Stage Club play was postponed.

3 February

- The Chinese New Year holiday period ended after having been extended for a week. Mainland stock exchanges reopened, Shanghai Stock Exchange falling by 7.72% and Shenzhen Stock Exchange by 8.45%, with a total of 3,177 shares triggering the limit down to 10%. The RMB to USD exchange rate fell through 7.00, opening at 6.9249 and closing at 7.0257.
- In Wuhan, the People's Liberation Army Ground Force takes over medical supplies delivery. "The Beijing leadership realised that almost all the donation points in Hubei and Wuhan have had delivery problems, that there are some opportunists using this crisis to make money", according to a military source.
- 4,000 passengers on the World Dream cruise ship were quarantined, after four among them positive to the coronavirus.
- India confirmed its third case in Kerala.
- Vietnam announced its eighth Covid-19 case, a Vietnamese woman who had been on the same flight with three other positive cases.

4 February

- Belgium confirmed its first case, bringing the total in the European Union to 24.
- Hong Kong confirmed its first death from a 39-year-old patient, the thirteenth confirmed case in the city.
- Malaysia confirmed two more Covid-19 cases, which included a Malaysian citizen, bringing the total to 10 cases.

- Singapore confirmed six more cases, including the first locally transmitted cases involving four, bringing the total to 24. Two others came from an evacuation plane from Wuhan.
- South Korea confirmed its 16th case after a tourist returned from Thailand, the first to have been infected there.
- Thailand confirmed six more cases, bringing the total to 25.
- Vietnam announced its ninth and tenth Covid-19 case, including a Vietnamese man who had been on the same flight with four other positive cases.
- The President of Federated States of Micronesia, David Panuelo, declared a state of emergency. Accordingly, Micronesian citizens are banned from visiting mainland China. Anyone who had been in mainland China from 6 January was barred from entering the country.
- Iran bans exports of facial masks to reduce shortages as domestic use increases significantly.
- The Nanning–Hanoi through train shall cease service as per agreement between the two national operators. Accordingly, the last train from Nanning railway station departed at 18:05 4 February and the last from Gia Lâm railway station at 21:20 5 February.
- The city government of Macau ordered a shutdown of all casinos for at least 15 days.
- The United Kingdom directed its citizens to leave China if possible. Foreign Secretary Dominic Raab said, "We now advise British Nationals in China to leave the country if they can, to minimise their risk of exposure to the virus".
- The Knesset in Israel is forming a special committee to deal with coronavirus.

- Cathay Pacific Airways, the flag carrier of Hong Kong, announces that it is ceasing 90% of its flights to mainland China.
- Royal Caribbean Cruises cancels more ships and adds Hong Kong to the No-Board list. This goes beyond what the Cruise Lines International Association had done the day before.
- Princess Cruises confirmed quarantine of the Diamond Princess carrying about 3,700 people after one of its passengers tested positive in a Hong Kong hospital and at least 20 more infected by the ship's return to Japan.
- Hyundai, blaming a parts shortage due to the effects of coronavirus infection, announces it will shut down some production. Nike has also temporarily shut down half of all their stores in China due to the virus epidemic.
- Air India announces that starting from 8 February, they will temporarily suspend flights to Hong Kong.
- An aviation conference during the Singapore Airshow is cancelled to allow leaders to deal with the coronavirus. This comes after 16 exhibitors pulled out of the Airshow. High at the global level.
- The United Nations Secretary-General announced that the WHO was taking rapid action to tackle a coronavirus 'infodemic', including that the virus could be airborne and stigmatisation, mainly of Chinese.
- The People's Bank of China provided an additional 500 billion yuan (roughly US$71 billion) of liquidity into the country's financial system on Tuesday, following 1.2 trillion yuan (over US$170 billion) the previous day.

- Chinese state-backed importers of liquefied natural gas (LNG) are investigating the invocation of force majeure to halt existing LNG contracts, as the coronavirus outbreak depresses energy demand.

5 February

- The National Health Commission releases the fifth diagnostic criteria. For Hubei, CT scan results are no longer required for declaring suspected cases, and "clinical diagnoses" may now be made using "imaging features of the pneumonia", without nucleic acid testing required. For suspected cases, "respiratory symptoms" are now admitted as part of the criteria nationwide.
- Hubei released an additional ¥200 million (US$28.56 million) as special subsidies for the construction of treatment sites.
- The first shelter hospital is put into use. Designated hospitals in Wuhan will now accept only serious cases (confirmed or suspected); other existing and future patients would be redirected to shelter hospitals or community quarantine points.
- The Wuhan Institute of Virology applied for a patent of Gilead's antiviral drug, remdesivir, as applied toward 2019-nCoV, in China. The granting of a patent by Chinese authorities was not certain, but a patent would provide China with leverage in negotiating license fees with Gilead. The institute said that it made the patent application "out of national interest, and won't exercise its patent rights if foreign pharmaceutical firms work together with China to curb the contagion". Seeking a patent instead of a "compulsory license" option does demonstrate some

sensitivity on China's part toward honouring Gilead's intellectual property rights. Gilead is working with China on Phase III clinical trials there.

- Wuhan, China, now reported 10,117 cases in total, exceeding 10,000. Tianjin, reported its first death. Chinese experts said that nucleic acid testing was only able to identify 30%-50% positive cases.
- Hong Kong confirmed three more cases, bringing the total to 21.
- Japan confirmed 10 new cases from the quarantined cruise ship Diamond Princess, near Yokohama, bringing the total number up to 35 cases. There were more than 3,500 onboard to be tested.
- Malaysia announced two more cases, bringing the total cases to 12.
- The Philippines confirmed its third positive case, a 60-year-old woman from Wuhan, China.
- Singapore confirmed four more cases, including a six-month-old Singaporean, bringing the total cases to 28.
- South Korea confirmed two more cases of Covid-19, including a patient who returned from Singapore, bringing the total cases to 18. Another case was later reported, bringing the total cases to 19.
- The United States of America saw Health officials in the state of Wisconsin announce the first case in that state.
- United Airlines and American Airlines suspended US flights to and from Hong Kong. Cathay Pacific asked all of its 27,000 employees to take three weeks of unpaid leave in order to preserve cash during the virus epidemic.

- Hundreds more Americans were evacuated by two planes from Wuhan to the United States, landing in this case at Travis Air Force Base near Sacramento, California. One of the planes would continue on to Marine Corps Air Station Miramar in San Diego. All evacuees would undergo a two-week quarantine. "Inbound evacuation flights to Wuhan were using their cargo space to deliver donated medical supplies for coronavirus relief efforts". A 12th US case of coronavirus was confirmed in Dane County, Wisconsin".
- Hong Kong announced the beginning of mandatory two-week quarantine for all visitors from mainland China or Macau from 8 February.
- Taiwan banned entry of non-citizens who have been to mainland China, Hong Kong or Macau within the past 14 days.
- With the US CDC's endorsement, Colombia INS confirmed it to be the first country in Latin America that might detect the novel coronavirus without sending samples to foreign centres.
- Canadian Minister of Foreign Affairs François-Philippe Champagne advised all Canadians in China but outside the quarantine zone to leave the country "via commercial means".
- India starts scanning passengers in flights coming from Singapore and Thailand, along with further travel restrictions on China to prevent the spread of the virus.
- The Bill & Melinda Gates Foundation committed over $100 Million for better detection, isolation, and treatment research for the virus.

- Yum China Holdings temporarily closed 30% of all Pizza Huts and KFCs that they operate in China due to the virus epidemic.
- Tesla stated that due to the virus epidemic, there would be a delay in the shipment of their Tesla Model 3 car, as they are produced and assembled in a new plant in Shanghai. Production at the plant will restart on 10 February 2020.
- World Health Organization (WHO) stated that there had been a large surge in new cases in the 24 hour period, of an amount that had not been seen in any day since the start of the epidemic. The number 3,100 new patients confirmed within China. Via its contingency fund for emergencies, the WHO has allocated $9 million.
- Countering rumours in the media, the WHO stated that there are no known therapeutics, drugs, or treatments that are effective for the virus yet. At least one news source attributed the stock market and oil price rise to these rumours. [excessive citations]
- The WHO appealed for $675 million to boost international measures to counter the epidemic, as deaths neared 500.

6 February

- Dali City apologises for intercepting and requisitioning 300 thousand masks designated as emergency supplies for Chongqing and promises to “return” all of them.
- The start of the new semester is postponed to at least the end of February in Zhejiang, Jiangsu, Chongqing, and Shanghai.
- Sichuan and Guangdong rolled out measures to help small and medium-sized enterprises in response to the epidemic.

- Tencent news issued a statement saying screenshots of its Epidemic Tracker circulating on the Internet showing substantially higher numbers are doctored.
- China announces that they will halve the tariff on US$75 billion goods imported from America, and Chinese official media Global Times commented that China is considering the use of disaster provision in the US-China Phase One trade deal, which was signed in the previous month.
- Canada announced 2 presumptive cases in British Columbia.
- China, In Zhejiang, over 1,000 cases were confirmed, the first such province besides Hubei. Doctor Li Wenliang, who notified his class colleagues in a private chatroom on social media of the coronavirus, died of the infection.
- Germany confirmed its thirteenth case, and Italy confirmed its third, bringing the total number of confirmed cases in Europe to 31.
- Hong Kong confirmed three more cases, bringing the total to 24.
- Japan confirmed another 10 new cases from Diamond Princess, quarantined in Yokohama, bringing the total to 45.
- Malaysia confirmed two more cases, bringing the total to 14. One of the cases was locally transmitted, the first in Malaysia.
- Singapore confirmed two more cases, bringing the total to 30.
- South Korea confirmed four more cases, bringing the total to 23.
- Taiwan announced three more cases, bringing the total to 16.

- The United Kingdom saw the third case confirmed, with the patient having visited Singapore.
- A patient in San Jose, California, became the first Covid-19 death in the United States discovered by April 2020. She died at home without any known recent foreign travel, after being unusually sick from flu in late January, then recovering, working from home, and suddenly dying on 6 February. A 7 February autopsy was completed in April (after virus tests on tissue samples) and attributed the death to Transmural Myocardial Ischemia (Infarction) with a Minor Component of Myocarditis due to Covid-19 Infection. Her case indicates that community transmission was happening undetected in the US, most likely since December.
- Vietnam confirmed two more cases, bringing the total to 12.
- Virgin Australia announced the permanent cancellation of its Hong Kong routes, citing the coronavirus outbreak and anti-government protests.
- Taiwan suspended visas for Hong Kong and Macau citizens.
- The Singapore government stated that a 14-day leave of absence would be mandatory for all workers who return from China.
- A business meeting held in mid-January 2020 at the Grand Hyatt in Singapore of an unnamed international sales company resulted in the infection of four persons in attendance: one from Malaysia, one from Korea and two from Singapore.
- Panic buying of consumer goods was reported in Hong Kong due to rumours of an impending quarantine.

- Virgin, KLM, Air France, American Airlines (not including the Hong Kong route), and Iberia extended their current flight suspensions till sometime in March.
- Volvo stated that two plants in China were still not reopened and will reopen after a few more weeks.
- Shinzo Abe stated that the 2020 Summer Olympics would not be postponed.
- Canada started the evacuation of its citizens from Wuhan. The aircraft would land on 7 February.
- The Better Business Bureau warned about face mask scams that attempt to use the ongoing fears and make false claims. The scams will either give low-quality or incorrect masks or will send no mask at all when paid.
- The Pentagon was asked by the Department of Health and Human Services (HHS) to provide military installations near 11 major airports that could each house up to 220 US citizens in support of coronavirus quarantines.
- Professor Neil Ferguson, director of the MRC Centre for Global Infectious Disease Analysis at Imperial College London is summarised in a news report as saying "that the true scale of the coronavirus isn't being reported by Chinese officials and claims that around 50,000 new cases are emerging in the country daily".
- Welsh singer Novo Amor postponed a concert in Singapore to July.
- Results of later autopsies in Santa Clara County, California, found that the first known death due to coronavirus in the United States occurred on 6 February.

7 February

- Li Wenliang dies. Wenliang was a 34-year-old ophthalmologist at Wuhan Central Hospital and one of eight doctors who tried to share information about the coronavirus when it was first emerging, only to be reprimanded by Wuhan police. He likely became infected by the coronavirus while treating patients during January. His death from complications of the infection is declared at 2:58 am local time.
- Another 41 tested positive for the coronavirus on Diamond Princess, bringing the total number of cases in Japan to 86.
- On 7 February, the Joint Defence and Control Mechanism of the State Council introduced a scheme of "one province for one city", where 16 provinces would provide medical force support for every city in Hubei except Wuhan.
- Hangzhou imposed a temporary ban on retail pharmacies selling fever and cough medicines, asking citizens with the symptoms to see a doctor instead.
- Germany announced its fourteenth case.
- Hong Kong confirmed 2 more cases, bringing the total number to 26.
- Malaysia confirmed one more case from a tourist entering from Singapore, bringing the total to 15.
- Singapore confirmed three more cases, bringing the total to 33. Most of these cases were initially of unknown origin, causing the Disease Outbreak Response System Condition (DORSCON) level to increase to Orange.
- South Korea confirmed one more case, bringing the total to 24.

- Vietnam confirmed one additional case, bringing the total to 13.
- The White House asked scientists in the US to investigate the origins of the virus. One of the reasons for this was because of the large amount of misinformation that is available about the virus online. The Washington Post also reported that some U.S. senators have been frustrated with the lack of information provided by the federal government to the states they represent. Vice President Mike Pence in an interview with CNBC said "China has shown 'unprecedented' transparency on coronavirus" and "the threat (of the virus) here in US remains fairly low".
- The WHO announced that the sudden demand for face masks had created "a shortfall for those in real need".
- Many colleges across the world were starting to reconsider and look into reviewing current student plans for Study Abroad programs to and/or from China. This was due to the health safety for the students. Colby College isolated students who showed no signs of the virus, after they returned from China.
- The third British citizen who contracted coronavirus did so through travel to Singapore. "The government is now telling travellers arriving in the UK from a total of nine Asian countries and territories to check for symptoms. They are advised to stay at home and call the NHS if they are ill and have flown home in the past 14 days." The countries and territories are Thailand, Japan, South Korea, Taiwan, Singapore, Malaysia, Hong Kong, and Macau.
- Singapore raises the Disease Outbreak Response System Condition (DORSCON) (its contagion threat level) to Orange

as the virus is spreading there from unknown origins. This is only the second time Singapore has activated Code Orange; the first was for the swine flu (H1N1) pandemic of 2009. Similar to reactions in Hong Kong the previous day, panic buying of groceries and consumer goods ensued.

- Two Hong Kong jewellery trade fairs, hosted by the Hong Kong Trade Development Council, got rescheduled due to the virus epidemic. Art Basel Hong Kong international art fair that was being held in March also gets cancelled due to the virus epidemic.
- The Canadian evacuation plane landed in British Columbia for refuelling. The plane was also carrying Chinese nationals and citizens who have valid visas for Canada, these were for escorting Canadian minors. The plane's final destination is CFB Trenton.
- Continuing the evacuation of American citizens from Wuhan, a rescue plane is landing in Omaha, Nebraska today. Others are landing near San Diego, California and San Antonio, Texas today; two passengers are stated as having symptoms of the virus.
- Royal Caribbean cruise lines bans Chinese, Hong Kong and Macau passport holders, as well as travellers who have been in those locales within the last 14 days.
- The United States announced aid of up to $100 million for China and other nations affected by the new coronavirus.
- The first Canadian evacuation plane lands at its final destination.
- Honda shuts down 3 of its plants around the Wuhan region area till 13 February.

- The Federal Reserve Bank warns that the virus is a potential threat to the growth of the US economy.
- VF Corporation announces that its subsidiary Vans has temporarily closed 60% of all its stores in China.
- Burberry temporarily closes a third of their stores in China.
- India offers to test samples for other Southeast Asian countries.
- Nvidia withdraws from the Barcelona Mobile World Congress by informing the GSMA, due to the threat of the virus.
- 98 Degrees postponed its Singapore concert due to the coronavirus, which was supposed to be held on 20 February.
- Performances of First Fleet, a Mandarin play originally planned from 14 to 23 February, were rescheduled to 20 March21.
- Lockheed Martin and Raytheon decided to pull out of the Singapore Airshow as coronavirus fears have caused event turnout to drop. Meanwhile, the United States Department of Defense reduced the size of its delegation for the Airshow.

8 February

- Wuhan confirmed 63 more deaths, bringing its total to 608; this now includes a Japanese citizen and a US citizen dying on this day.
- Henan became the third province besides Hubei to report over 1,000 cases. Nationally, the number of cases outside Hubei exceeded 10,000.
- Aerosol was confirmed as a medium of transmission for the first time.
- Beijing reported a first type of case involving a patient, who tested positive after three negative test results, and Qingtian,

Zhejiang reported a case where the patient tested positive only after being tested for the fifth time.

- France confirmed five cases involving British nationals, bringing the total number to 11.
- Japan, three more cases tested positive on Diamond Princess, bringing the total number of cases in Japan to 89.
- Malaysia confirmed 1 more case, bringing the total to 16.
- Singapore confirmed seven more cases, bringing the total to 40.
- Thailand confirmed seven additional cases, bringing the total to 32.
- United Arab Emirates confirmed two more cases, bringing the total to seven.
- The school break in Vietnam was extended in all 63 first-level subdivisions, with the majority to 16 February and five to an unspecified time.
- Apple extends the shutdown period of its stores and corporate offices in China. They will reopen at some time during the week of 10 February which is the week after the originally stated week Apple said they will reopen.
- Norwegian Cruise Line bans Chinese, Hong Kong, and Macau passport holders, or anyone who visited these regions in the past 30 days.
- Hyundai has shut down its largest factory due to lack of wiring that connects the electronic systems in its cars.
- Indonesia advised travellers to take precautions and be alert while in Singapore, with the government raising the travel alert to Yellow, the second out of three tiers.

9 February

- Israel has advised travellers to delay travel to countries and territories hit by the coronavirus. In the mention are Singapore, Thailand, South Korea, Japan, Taiwan, Macau and Hong Kong.
- The Kuwaiti Embassy in Singapore called its citizens to delay their travel plans after the Singaporean government raised the coronavirus alert level to Code Orange. The Embassy of the State of Qatar has since followed suit.
- Malaysia expands their Chinese traveller ban to include the provinces of Zhejiang and Jiangsu.
- Families in the French village Les Contamines-Montjoie get lined up to get tested for the virus.
- China (Mainland) now confirmed a total of 40,213 cases, exceeding 40,000, of which 29,631 were in Hubei. The coronavirus death toll in China rose to 811, surpassing the toll from the SARS epidemic from 2002 to 2003.
- Hong Kong confirmed ten more cases, with nine from the same family, bringing the total number to 36.
- Malaysia confirmed 1 more case, bringing the total number to 17.
- Singapore confirmed three more cases, bringing the total number to 43.
- South Korea reported three new cases of the virus, bringing the country's total to 27.
- Spain confirmed the second case in the country in Palma de Mallorca.
- Taiwan confirmed its eighteenth case.
- United Kingdom confirmed its fourth case.

- Vietnam confirmed its fourteenth case, a 55-year-old woman in Vĩnh Phúc.
- Six more cases were confirmed aboard Diamond Princess, bringing the total number of cases on the ship to 70, with Japan having 96 cases.

10 February

- Business has now resumed in all 30 mainland province-level divisions, apart from Hubei.
- Food prices in China have risen in the month of January. According to the consumer price index (CPI) the price of pork rose 8.5%, while the CPI came in at 5.4%. The reason may be due to food hoarding, besides the disruptions of supply chains due to transportation, lockdown measures and holiday demand. The CPI is the highest since October 2011.
- Chinese Communist Party general secretary Xi Jinping has appeared in public wearing a protective mask and his temperature was checked while visiting the Anhuali Community in Chaoyang District of Beijing.
- The Director-General of the WHO, in response to increasing infections, announced that containment was the main priority.
- Amazon, and Sony, Ericsson states that they will not partake in the Barcelona Mobile World Congress due to the virus. The virus daily death toll reaches a new record of 97 people dead from the virus in a single day.
- Asian stock markets fell and went into red due to investor fears relating to the virus impact on the economy.
- HSBC Women's World Championship, LPGA Tour Championship, and LPGA cancelled two more events overall

within Singapore and Thailand due to the virus. Thus meaning only two more events remain uncancelled.

- The United Kingdom included Singapore in a list of countries where travellers returning are advised to self-isolate if they have symptoms as a precautionary measure.
- Sarawak imposed a 14-day quarantine for travellers coming from Singapore in a bid to slow down the spread of the coronavirus. This comes after Singapore's DORSCON was raised to Orange on 7 February.
- Over 70 exhibitors have decided to withdraw or not take part in the Singapore Airshow due to the virus. Lockheed Martin, Bombardier Inc., and De Havilland Canada, are some of the many well-known exhibitors or companies that withdrew from the airshow.
- President Trump told supporters at a rally in New Hampshire that the virus will be gone by April, claiming that when temperatures rise, "the virus" will "miraculously" go away.
- Hong Kong confirmed six more cases, bringing the total number to 42.
- Japan confirmed 65 more cases on Diamond Princess, bringing the total to 135.
- Malaysia confirmed one more case involving a citizen, bringing the total to 18.
- Singapore confirmed another two cases including a Certis officer who served Quarantine Orders, bringing the total to 45.
- United Arab Emirates confirmed its eighth case, an Indian national.

- United Kingdom saw four additional cases were confirmed, bringing the total to eight. The transmission in these cases is believed to have occurred in France.
- United States of America confirmed its thirteenth case in San Diego, a patient who had been evacuated from Wuhan.

11 February

- Shenzhen University announced the successful development of a new coronavirus antibody detection kit capable of obtaining a result in 22 minutes and reducing the risk of infection of medical staff.
- The Ministry of Human Resources and Social Security expanded existing relief measures for micro, small, and medium size enterprises. The NDRC announced its intention to "strictly curb the practice of restricting the resumption of production and production by simple and crude methods such as via approval." The Ministry of Transport (MoT) introduced measures to for the transportation security of both citizens, especially migrant workers, and animal feed. The State Taxation Administration allowed enterprises affected by the epidemic to carry forward losses up to 8 years. The Ministry of Commerce issued a notice to ensure security of living materials in key cities.
- Guangdong passed an emergency legislation banning the trading and overeating of wildlife and devolves emergency legislative powers to county-level governments. The provincial government authorised Guangzhou and Shenzhen governments with the power of the emergency requisitioning of houses, facilities, and materials for emergency epidemic response. This was the first time a government was

authorised with the power of requisitioning private property since the 1978 Chinese economic reform and since the passage of Property Law in 2007.

- China Banking Regulatory Commission proposed to extend Hubei automobile insurance coverage by one month. Shanghai Stock Exchange announced the full exemption of the bill service fees charged to Hubei legal persons in Hubei from February to December 2020.
- Shanghai introduced measures to support tech companies and exempt the rent of SMSEs due to nationalised enterprises. Jiangsu's bank and government branches introduced financial measures including liquidity support and credit placement. Zhejiang implemented a one-time subsidy for key acquisition and processing enterprises of poultry and fresh milk in the province.
- Cainiao released measures to aid the supply chain and logistics industry. Tmall reduced costs for vendors for the first half of 2020.
- A man in Chengdu was under police investigation for interference with the prevention and control of the epidemic.
- The first batch of central reserve frozen pork arrived at Wuhan.
- Apple extended its device warranty to provide a one-time exception.
- The total number of cases in the UK reaches eight as four further cases are confirmed in people linked to an affected man from Brighton.
- A ninth case is confirmed in London.
- The WHO confirmed over 1,000 deaths from the virus as its 'Research and Innovation Forum on novel coronavirus

2019', attended by over 300 scientists and officials, met in Geneva; the possibility of a vaccine being available in 18 months was mooted.

- The Global Grain Conference that was going to take place in Singapore, has been postponed to sometime in June and/or July, due to the virus.
- Authorities in Hong Kong evacuate a Tsing Yi Estate apartment building, after two residents who lived separately got diagnosed with the virus.
- The virus is lowering crude prices worldwide, as China's demand for crude oil decreases due to shutdowns, lockdowns, fears, and other measures. Oil prices have just reached a 1-year low again, and have been falling for 5 weeks.
- South Korea has advised travellers to delay travel to countries and territories hit by the coronavirus; mentioned are Singapore, Malaysia, Thailand, Vietnam, Japan, and Taiwan in addition to mainland China.
- Taiwan urged travellers to take precautions when travelling to Singapore or Thailand, and to avoid Hong Kong or Macau unless absolutely necessary.
- Singapore and Malaysia will form a joint working group to prevent and control the coronavirus infection.
- The Thailand public health minister does not allow a Holland America cruise ship, MS Westerdam to disembark in the country. The reason cited by the public health minister is that there are 32 cases in Thailand.
- During a live broadcast on the Fox Business Network, anchor Maria Bartiromo suggests China developed Covid-19 as a biological weapon of mass destruction and deliberately

attempted to infect United States diplomats at the White House and in Davos, Switzerland.

- Germany confirmed two more cases, bringing the total number to 16.
- Hong Kong confirmed seven more cases, bringing the total to 49.
- Singapore confirmed another two cases, bringing the total to 47.
- South Korea confirmed one more case, a 30-year-old Chinese woman, bringing the total number to 28.
- Thailand confirmed 1 new case, bringing the total in the country to 33.
- Vietnam confirmed its fifteenth case, a three-month-old baby infected by her grandmother.
- WHO gives the disease the new name COVID-19. Additionally, the virus itself is named SARS-CoV-2.

12 February

- Hong Kong confirmed one more case, bringing the total number to 50.
- Japan confirmed 39 more cases on Diamond Princess, including one quarantine officer, bringing the total to 174. Another case was reported in Japan itself, bringing the total number to 29.
- Singapore confirmed three more cases, bringing the total to 50. Earlier, 300 employees of DBS Bank were asked to evacuate from the office at Marina Bay Financial Centre Tower 3 due to a confirmed case there.
- United Kingdom - The first case in London was confirmed, bringing the country's total to 9.

- United States of America confirmed one more case, bringing the total number to 14.
- American Airlines extend their flight suspensions to Hong Kong and China through some point in late April.
- The WHO announced it was developing a COVID-19 virus treatment master plan. The WHO stated that a coronavirus vaccine could be ready in approximately 18 months.
- The United States Postal Service, Singapore Post, PostNord Sverige, and Austrian postal services will temporarily stop sending mail or other postal services to China, and/or Hong Kong as well as Macau. This is due to the available flight shortages and flight suspensions, which is making it hard to send mail to China, Hong Kong, and Macau.
- Bulgari CEO states that half of its stores in the greater China region have been temporarily closed due to the virus.
- The Formula 1 Chinese Grand Prix 2020 which was set to be held in April, was postponed to a later date due to the outbreak.
- The Dalai Lama announced he stopped all public engagement due to the outbreak.
- The Mobile World Congress (MWC), due to start on 24 February, is cancelled.
- CDC announces that a diagnostic kit it developed does not work. This kit was made available to certified laboratories in the United States besides being shared with more than thirty countries. Due to a possible problem with one of the reagents some results could be made inconclusive (neither positive nor negative).
- According to the Deutsche Bank, the outbreak of COVID-19 may contribute to a recession in Germany.

- Three people escape from a quarantine facility in Russia. They did this because according to them, the conditions and officials of the quarantine were not good.
- Cancellations in hotel bookings in the Greek island of Santorini have climbed up to 60-70% in the months of February and March, while there are fears of 100% cancellations for April.
- A State Council executive meeting in China was convened, which emphasised efforts to restore the economy to normal activity and asked local governments to implement measures. The MoT and NHC issued a joint Notice to forbid quarantining of material security providers and drivers if they have not entered Wuhan, provided temperature checks are passed and necessary protection measures are being taken.
- China National Railway Group stopped selling seatless tickets and initiated measures to control train occupancy. Tencent announced free cloud service for SMSEs.
- Jiangsu rolled out measures to help economic development during the epidemic. Zhejiang decreased the price of enterprise utilities until 30 April. Shanghai decreased enterprise gas price and waived residential gas arrear penalties.
- Yunnan now required QR code scanning for entering all public spaces. Airbnb suspended booking in Beijing until 30 April. Foshan, Guangdong was to require advance declaration for vehicles to enter the city starting 13 Feb.
- Chinese Communist Party general secretary Xi Jinping ordered a tax cut to invigorate the economy. Many organizations were ordered to keep rents low and banks to keep interest low. A stimulus package is expected.

- Honghu, Hubei began an official investigation into a controversial fine of ¥42630 (US$6110.54) on a local pharmacy for selling 44,000 single-use masks stocked at ¥0.6 (US$0.086) each for ¥1 (US$0.143) each, as it violated a province-wide ban on selling medical items related to the epidemic 15% above the stocking price during the epidemic. The move came after heavy criticism online after the fining became known.

13 February

- Japan confirmed four more cases, bringing the total to 33. At the same time, 44 new cases were confirmed on the Diamond Princess, bringing the total to 218. Later on, Japan confirmed its first death from the virus.
- Hong Kong confirmed three more cases, bringing the total number to 53.
- Malaysia confirmed one more case, bringing the total number to 19.
- Singapore confirmed eight more cases, bringing the total number to 58. A school in National University of Singapore will conduct e-learning from 14 to 21 February as a precaution after one of the cases involved a professor.
- United States of America, the CDC confirmed the 15th US coronavirus case, a Wuhan evacuee quarantined at a military base in Texas.
- Vietnam confirmed its 16th case.
- Hubei released 1.3 million masks for civil use, providing pharmacies at ¥1 each and requiring them to sell at the "affordable price" of ¥2 (US$0.287) each.

- In Hubei, The Zhangjiawan District of Shiyan entered wartime control starting 00:00, as well as Dawu County in Xiaogan.
- Hubei postponed business resumption and start of new semester across the province; businesses were not to resume before 24:00 on 20 Feb. Guangxi prohibited the start of new semester before 1 March.
- Wuhan enacts a new rule prohibiting people from leaving their neighbourhoods for non-medical reasons, updating the curfew to a full lockdown.
- The WHO suggested that the coronavirus 'iceberg' outside China might not be "as big as feared" and that the slowdown in the number of new infections should be taken cautiously as the situation can change in any direction. The WHO also stated that it is too early to predict the outbreaks' end.
- A lockdown on Sơn Lôi Commune (Vĩnh Phúc Province, Vietnam) was implemented by the authorities after five investigated cases had been infected by a cluster. This would last until 3 March.
- Japan announced that a woman in her eighties outside of Tokyo has died. Two taxi drivers also were tested positive.
- A solo traveller from China was quarantined at Lackland Air Force Base in Texas. This is the 15th case in the U.S. excessive citations
- Champalimaud Foundation, a Portuguese private biomedical research foundation, announced the cancellation of a conference that was programmed to happen on 12 to 13 March.
- European Union ministers of health held a meeting in Brussels.

- The ship MS Westerdam was allowed to dock in Sihanoukville, Cambodia.
- Hong Kong will extend school closures until 16 March instead of 2 March, with an exam for primary school students cancelled. Kindergartens will receive subsidies for cleaning works. In addition, civil servants will work from home for another week until 23 February.

14 February

- The central districts of Yunmeng County in Xiaogan, Hubei entered wartime control. Huanggang, Hubei escalated control starting 00:00, prohibiting non-essential persons or vehicles from entering and exiting communities and initiating the organised distribution of basic necessities.
- A new test kit was developed by a team led by Zhong Nanshan, able to yield a result in fifteen minutes with a very high sensitivity and expected to raise the positive detection rate.
- Huanggang decided to convert another hospital as a secondary medical institution for COVID-19, after Dabie Mountain Regional Medical Centre. Xiantao, Hubei implemented mask ex-factory price control, requiring the ex-factory price of single use medical masks not to exceed ¥1.20 (US$0.172) each and non-medical ones ¥1.00 (US$0.143) each.
- Beijing required all persons returning to the city to self-quarantine for 14 days.
- Shenzhen Metro would start using real-name system starting 16 Feb for epidemic tracing, with passengers able to self-

register the carriages they ride in by scanning the QR code in the train.

- The Office of the State Council Education Steering Committee prohibited all after-school training institutions from conducting offline training in any form.
- All mainland IELTS exams in March were cancelled.
- Canada confirmed British Columbia's fifth presumptive case, bringing the total number in the country to 8.
- Egypt confirmed its first case, a foreigner of undisclosed nationality. This was the first case on the African continent.
- Hong Kong confirmed three more infections, bringing the total number to 56.
- Japan confirmed four more cases, bringing the total number to 37.
- Singapore confirmed nine more cases, bringing the total number to 67.
- The WHO stated that investing in preparedness was the smartest way to make sure that the coronavirus and other outbreaks are "identified and stopped quickly" and that solidarity should triumph over stigma.
- Portugal announced one more suspected case of a child of unspecified age that had returned from China. All previous six suspected cases were revealed to be negative after clinical analysis.
- In Bragança, Portugal, two Chinese college students agreed to stay on a voluntary quarantine when they return to Bragança. Although they did not show symptoms and neither had they been in contact with infected persons as far it was known, the reason for the quarantine was a recent holiday travel to China.

- In the United Kingdom, two Members of Parliament, Lilian Greenwood and Alex Sobel, self-quarantined after learning that they had attended a conference on 6 February where a confirmed case had also been in attendance.
- A German citizen in Palma de Mallorca was released from hospital quarantine after he had been tested negative twice. Previously, he had tested positive for SARS-CoV-2 and was always asymptomatic.
- The first case of coronavirus infection on the African continent was reported in Egypt.
- Grab started GrabCare for healthcare workers in Singapore. This came after reports of increased discrimination due to the COVID-19 situation, making it difficult for healthcare workers to get rides.
- The Catholic Church of Singapore will suspend masses indefinitely from noon of 15 February in view of the coronavirus.
- The 2020 ASEAN Para Games will be suspended indefinitely. The event was supposed to be held from 20 to 28 March in Manila.

15 February

- Honghu, Hubei entered wartime control at 00:00, the decision announced in the evening of 13 Feb.
- Jingmen, Hubei escalated control, prohibiting outside vehicles and persons from entering its central districts except for medical and living supplies, and shutting down all business except approved pharmacies, supermarkets, and hotels.

- The MoT announced that all toll roads country-wide would be toll-free from 00:00 17 Feb to the end of the epidemic response. The Ministry of Science and Technology introduced measures to strengthen the biosafety management of SARS-CoV-2 high-level virus microbiology laboratories.
- Hubei's Provincial Party Committee issued another ¥100 million (US$14.3 million) to local authorities for epidemic control.
- The Central Bank of China required cash from outbreak areas to be stored for at least 14 days before entering market, 7 days for other areas. PBC branches reporting to its Guangzhou branch would destroy all cash retrieved from hospitals, agricultural markets, and public transit.
- France saw the first death outside Asia being confirmed, an 80 year old Chinese tourist in France. The country also confirmed its 12th case.
- Japan confirmed nine additional confirmed cases not aboard Diamond Princess. Japan also confirmed 67 additional cases aboard the cruise ship Diamond Princess, bringing the total number of cases from the ship to 285.
- Malaysia confirmed three more cases, including an American passenger from the cruise ship MS Westerdam flying from Cambodia, bringing the total number to 22.
- Singapore confirmed five more cases, bringing the total number to 72.
- Thailand confirmed one more case, bringing the total number to 34.
- The WHO Director-General cautioned against panic over COVID-19 but also urged governments to improve their

preparedness, stating, “It’s impossible to predict which direction this epidemic will take.”

- The United States announced it would evacuate Americans currently aboard the cruise ship Diamond Princess.

16 February

- Hong Kong confirmed 1 new coronavirus case, bringing the total to 57.
- Japan also confirmed six new cases, bringing the total of infected people not aboard Diamond Princess to 59. 70 additional cases were confirmed on Diamond Princess, increasing the tally to 355.
- Singapore confirmed three more cases, bringing the total number to 75.
- South Korea confirmed one more case, bringing the total number to 29.
- Taiwan confirmed its first death from COVID-19, a man in his 60s. Moreover, two new cases were confirmed, bringing the total number to 20.
- United Arab Emirates confirmed one more case, a 37-year-old Chinese citizen, bringing the total number to 9.
- Hubei implements “hard quarantine” in units of natural villages; no outsiders are to be allowed in and each household is allowed one person every three days to go out for provisions and urgent agricultural material, on designated routes and in limited time. All nonessential public spaces in Hubei are to be closed and all gatherings forbidden.
- Following its decision on the previous day, the city of Wuxue in Huanggang now bans residents and vehicles without medical or epidemic control reasons from the streets.

Anyone in violation is to be sent to a stadium for "centralised compulsory study" about the laws and epidemic response, and any such cars would be seized. All communities in Dongcheng District, Beijing are required to implement closed management.

- Guizhou resumes normal traffic, removing all temporary quarantine checkpoints.
- The first two autopsies of patients killed by SARS-CoV-2 were carried out in Jinyintan Hospital; its pathology was obtained and submitted for testing. A vaccine of the virus developed by national institutions began its animal experiment stage; clinical trials are expected in April at the earliest.
- The NHC urges for the reduction of the workload of grassroots workers, asking for all legally unnecessary procedures to be halted. The General Administration of Customs has introduced 10 measures to support foreign trade enterprises to resume production. Instructed by the Office of the State Council, Alipay is now developing a national unified system of "Health Code" first used in Hangzhou on 11 Feb, a digital health evaluation certificate for the safe resumption of business. Wuhan released a partial list of hospitals accepting patients not with COVID-19.
- The first internet hospitals open in Hunan. Yunnan expedites the approval processes for medical supplies. All secondary and tertiary hospitals in Beijing would start operating on an appointment basis by 25 and 20 Feb respectively for all non-emergency departments.
- Nanjing and Suzhou implements real-name system for public transit, following Shenzhen.

- Huanggang announced that any person with fever or cough taking the initiative to see a doctor would receive a financial reward of ¥500 (US$71.6).
- In response to allegations that patient zero was its research student, Wuhan Institute of Virology released a statement saying no members of the institute were infected and that the student had been working in other provinces for years.
- WHO-China Joint Mission on Coronavirus Disease with 25 member led by Dr. Bruce Aylward and Dr Wannian Liang and consisted of experts from China, Germany, Japan, Korea, Nigeria, Russia, Singapore, USA and WHO started an investigation.

17 February

- Hong Kong confirmed three more cases, bringing the total number to 60.
- Japan confirmed seven new cases, bringing the total of infected people not aboard Diamond Princess to 66. Diamond Princess in Japan confirmed 99 new coronavirus cases, bringing the total number of infected people on the cruise ship to 454.
- Singapore confirmed two more cases, bringing the total number to 77.
- South Korea confirmed one more case, bringing the total number to 30.
- Taiwan confirmed two more cases, bringing the total number to 22.
- Thailand confirmed one more case, bringing the total number to 35.

- The United States had its second known death from COVID-19, from unknown (community) transmission to a 69-year-old man in Santa Clara County, California. This death was attributed to COVID-19 in April by a delayed autopsy. February
- American passengers evacuate the Diamond Princess and will return to the US. They will be held in quarantine for 14 days.
- Singapore will enforce Stay-Home Notices for all Singapore residents and long-term pass holders returning from China taking effect from 18 February. They will not be allowed to leave home during the next 14 days.
- Following the confirmation of infection aboard the MS Westerdam, the Malaysian authorities barred passengers who had travelled on the luxury cruise ship from entry. Singapore follows suit, only allowing citizens to enter with quarantine imposed.
- Japanese Emperor Naruhito's birthday ceremony and greetings to the public on 23 February will be cancelled.
- The Israeli Ministry of Health requested people returning from Asian countries and territories to self-quarantine. In the mention are mainland China, Taiwan, Macau, Hong Kong, Singapore, Thailand, South Korea and Japan.
- The Tokyo Marathon, due to take place on 1 March, will be restricted to elite runners and wheelchair athletes. Initially, it was expected that 38,000 people would take part but with this change the number will be reduced to 206 participants.
- The seventh episode of A Certain Scientific Railgun T, "Auribus oculi fideliores sunt. (The eyes are more trustworthy

than the ears)", is replaced by a rerun of the sixth episode due to production delays associated with the virus outbreak.

- Following its announcement the previous night, Xiaogan now bans all its urban residents from leaving home, all its rural residents from wandering, visiting neighbours, and gathering, and all vehicles from roads. Exceptions are made for medical reasons, medical staff, providers of medical and living provision, pregnancies, deaths, essential vehicles, and others granted permissions. Violators would be subject to up to 10 days of detention and put on the dishonest list.
- Following rumours that a researcher named Huang Yanling at The Wuhan Institute of Virology was patient zero, the Institute first denied that there was ever a researcher working there by that name; only after being informed that the researcher's name was still on their Internet page, although her photograph and background were blank, did the Institute acknowledge that a person by that name had worked there, and had since "left the office," current whereabouts unknown.

18 February

- Hong Kong confirmed two more cases, bringing the total number to 62.
- Japan confirmed eight more cases across the nation, bringing the total to 74. At the same time, 88 additional cases aboard Diamond Princess were confirmed, bringing the total on the ship to 542.
- Singapore confirmed four more cases, bringing the total number to 81.

- South Korea confirmed one more case, bringing the total number to 31.
- The WHO Director-General announced that, as the coronavirus continued to spread, there was still a chance to prevent a broader global crisis, while it shipped personal protective equipment and coronavirus testing kits to countries.
- Getty Images confirmed that it was protecting the identity of photojournalists in China "due to worries about their safety".
- Bushiroad, a Japanese entertainment company best known for creating the BanG Dream! and Revue Starlight multimedia franchises, announced that they would postpone and cancel several events up to 19 March due to the outbreak, and that they would offer refunds. The seventh episode of Infinite Dendrogram, "The Dueling Cities", is replaced with a rerun of the first episode due to production delays stemming from the virus outbreak. The 14th Seiyu Awards will have no after-party celebrations, and only winners, presenters, and journalists will allowed to attend the award ceremony on 7 March.
- Singapore's Deputy Prime Minister and Finance Minister Heng Swee Keat announced S$6.4 billion in reliefs to help businesses and citizens tide through the crisis. Of these, a S$4 billion Stabilisation and Support Package will be given to hard-hit businesses as well as for retraining workers, with a S$1.6 billion Care and Support Package to help household expenses. An additional S$800 million will be set aside, especially for healthcare efforts. A planned Goods and Services Tax hike to 9% will not take place in 2021 owing to the economic impact, with a $6 billion Assurance Package should the hike take effect.

- The State Council introduced exemptions of enterprise social security and housing fund contributions. The State Taxation Administration (STA) extended the February taxation filing deadline outside Hubei to 28 February. The State Council and Ministry of Finance (MoF) announced allocating more budget this year to areas heavily affected by the epidemic.
- Wuhan passes its strictest control measures. Tianjin now requires QR code scanning for entering public spaces and transport services.
- Yiwu International Trade City reopened for business.
- Shanghai requires educational institutions to conduct online education when the new semester starts on 2 March, so that student will not go to school.

19 February

- Hong Kong confirmed its second death from the coronavirus. In addition, three new cases were confirmed, bringing the total number in Hong Kong to 65.
- Iran confirmed its first two cases resulting in deaths.
- Singapore confirmed three more cases, bringing the total number to 84.
- South Korea confirmed 20 more cases, bringing the total number to 51 with the majority of these transmissions happening in a church in Daegu.
- Taiwan confirmed one more case, bringing the total number to 23.
- Passengers started to disembark from Diamond Princess, one of the cruise ships in the outbreak. The sheer number of passengers infected has led to questions over the effectiveness of quarantine measures. 79 more cases are

confirmed on the cruise ship, bringing the total number to 621. Japan also reported 10 new cases.

- The WHO Director-General stated that COVID-19 was not yet a pandemic.
- The Nipponbashi Street Festa in Osaka, a cosplay event described as the biggest of its kind, was cancelled due to concerns with the virus outbreak.
- Mediacorp, Singapore's main broadcaster, postponed its Star Awards ceremony to the second half of 2020, initially scheduled for 26 April due to concerns over the ongoing outbreak.
- The NHC published the sixth pilot version of Diagnostic and Treatment Plan of the Novel Coronavirus Pneumonia, which removed the category of clinical diagnosis introduced in the previous edition for Hubei, as well as adjusted several descriptions, criteria, and treatment guidelines of COVID-19,.
- Following its announcement on the previous day, Zhejiang now requires declaration for vehicles entering the province. Meanwhile, public transport across the province apart from Wenzhou will now resume normal service.
- Wuhan bans all vehicles from roads apart from essential vehicles.
- Hunan introduced measures to support businesses. Chengdu adjusted its epidemic control procedures and business resumption would no longer require approval.

20 February

- Hubei requires businesses in the province not to resume before 10 March, except for essential industries.
- Wenzhou removed all checkpoints except in Yueqing and reopened highways.
- Wuhan requires residents to measure their temperature twice daily and report any measurements exceeding 37.3 °C (99.1 °F).
- The Ministry of Human Resources and Social Security authorises provinces to exempt certain social security contributions from SMSEs starting February for up to five months.
- Macau reopened all casinos after a 15-day closure. However, all patrons and service staff would be required to wear masks as part of enhanced measures to reduce the virus spread.
- Israel banned passengers who have been to China, Hong Kong, Thailand or Singapore in the previous 14 days.
- In Novi Sanzhary, Ukraine, the buses carrying the evacuees from China were attacked by a mob hurling stones and engaging in violent clashes with the police.
- Iraq halted travel to and from Iran after the number of cases spiked there. At the same time, travellers from Iran will not be allowed entry.
- Hong Kong confirmed four more cases, bringing the total number to 69.
- Iran confirmed three more cases, bringing the total number to five.

- Japan confirmed ten more domestic cases, bringing the total number to 94.
- Singapore confirmed one more case, bringing the total number to 85.
- South Korea confirmed 53 more cases, bringing the total number to 104. The first death from the virus was also confirmed.
- Taiwan confirmed one more case, bringing the total number to 24.
- The United States confirmed one more case in California, bringing the total number to 16.
- Two deaths were confirmed aboard the cruise ship Diamond Princess along with 13 more cases, bringing the total number to 634.

21 February

- More than 500 cases has been confirmed in five prisons in Hubei, Shandong, and Zhejiang. Following the news of the outbreak, the responsible officials in Shandong and Hubei were sacked.
- Henan and Shandong removed all road quarantine measures.
- Gansu adjusts its emergency response level for COVID-19 from level 1 to level 3.
- Following some public confusion with the data released, Hubei prohibited the subtracting of clinically diagnosed cases. A corrected province-wide statistical report was available late in the evening.
- Wuhan finished the testing of all existing suspected patients, patients with fever, and people with close contact.

- Australia confirmed four more cases involving evacuees from the cruise ship Diamond Princess, bringing the total number to 19.
- Canada confirms one more case, a woman who had recently visited Iran, bringing the total number to nine.
- Israel also confirmed its first case, an evacuee from Diamond Princess.
- Italy confirmed 17 cases, bringing the total number to 20. Authorities also reported the first death, a 78-year-old man.
- Iran announces 13 new cases, bringing the total to 18. Two more deaths were also confirmed.
- Japan confirmed 15 more cases, bringing the total number to 109.
- Lebanon confirmed its first case.
- Singapore confirmed one more case, bringing the total number to 86.
- South Korea confirmed 100 more cases, bringing the total number to 204. The country also reported its second death.
- Taiwan confirmed two more cases, bringing the total number to 26.
- United Arab Emirates confirmed two more cases, bringing the total number to 11.
- The United States confirmed 20 more cases, bringing the total number to 35. Furthermore, the Association of Public Health Laboratories (APHL) announced that only three states were capable of testing for the coronavirus: California, Nebraska, and Illinois.
- In addition, the first known case of COVID-19 occurred in New Zealand, and was retroactively reported on September 23.

22 February

- Kuwait halts flights to and from Iran, and imposed a ban on travellers arriving from Iran as a precaution. Any Kuwaiti returning will be isolated. In addition, authorities there advised against travel to Iran.
- Samsung shut its phone factory in Gumi until 24 February, with the floor the infected employee worked shut until 25 February. This comes after a cases was confirmed involving a worker there.
- Australia announced an easing of travel restrictions for Chinese students in Year 11 or 12 except for those in Hubei, which will be considered on a case-by-case basis. The students will need to get approval from states and territories, as well as the schools involved. Similar exemptions for Chinese university students are being considered.
- Hubei introduced measures to reduce business cost.
- Liaoning adjusted its COVID-19 emergency response level from level 1 to level 3.
- Australia confirmed three more cases, bringing the total number to 22.
- Hong Kong confirmed one more case, bringing the total number to 70.
- Iran confirmed 10 more cases, bringing the total number to 28. A fifth death was also confirmed.
- Italy confirmed 59 more cases spread across three different administrative regions, bringing the total number to 79, making Italy the European country with the biggest number of cases of coronavirus infections. The second death was also confirmed, an Italian woman from Lombardy.

- Japan confirmed 26 more cases, bringing the total number to 135.
- Singapore confirmed three more cases, bringing the total number to 89.
- South Korea confirmed 229 more cases, bringing the total number to 433. Concerns are raised that 9 tourists from South Korea may have caused a widespread exposure in Israel.
- The United Arab Emirates confirmed two more cases, bringing the total number to 13.
- The urine sample of a patient tested positive.
- A genome analysis indicated that the virus in Huanan Seafood Market originated from outside.
- Wuhan requires a 14-day quarantine for patients discharged from COVID-19.

23 February

- Turkey shut down its border with Iran and banned all incoming flights as a precaution for stopping the spread of disease after Iran had reported 43 cases. Pakistan also closed its border with Iran, Afghanistan suspends travel to and from Iran and Jordan bans citizens from China, Iran, and South Korea. Georgia imposes restriction on inbound air flights with Iran, allowing passengers only in one direction.
- Italy introduces strict measures which place almost 50,000 people in lockdown in an attempt to control the virus. Fines are imposed on those caught entering or leaving outbreak areas. Carnival of Venice and Carnival of Ivrea are cancelled.

- South Korea raises its disease alert to the highest level, coming after the number of cases had continued to increase sharply.
- Singapore expanded its health advisory to Daegu and Cheongdo in South Korea, advising travellers to "avoid non-essential travel". At the same time, the definition of suspect cases was expanded to include travellers arriving from these two cities.
- Kuwait banned ships coming from Iran to stopping at its ports due to the coronavirus.
- Israel extended its travel ban to Japan and South Korea taking effect the following day, following a previous travel ban that included Taiwan, Italy, Australia, and Macau.
- Taiwan banned its healthcare professionals in hospital from travelling out to manage the shortage of workers amid the outbreak. Those who need to attend important meetings overseas have to seek permission. This comes after three local governments banned travel by public servants. In addition, military personnel are advised to avoid places affected by COVID-19, with quarantine imposed should they return from these places.
- Guizhou adjusted its emergency response level for COVID-19 from level 1 to level 3, and Shanxi to level 2.
- China Global Television Network, a state-owned television broadcaster, issued a report entitled, "Rumors Stop With The Wise", declaring that the Weibo user claiming to be Chen Quanjiao, a researcher at the Wuhan Institute of Virology, who had reported to the public on 17 February that the Director of the institute was responsible for leaking the novel

coronavirus, had committed identity fraud and was not in fact Chen Quanjiao.

- Canada confirmed one more presumptive case in Ontario. The samples had been sent to the National Microbiology Lab for further testing. Later, the cases was confirmed positive, bringing the total number to 10.
- Hong Kong confirmed four more cases, bringing the total number to 74.
- Iran confirmed 15 more cases and two more deaths, bringing the total number to 43 and 8 respectively.
- Israel confirmed one more case, who was a passenger on the cruise ship, bringing the total number to 2.
- Italy confirmed 73 new cases, bringing the total to 152 spread across five different administrative regions. The third death was also reported. Italy is now the third country in the world by number of cases, after China and South Korea.
- South Korea confirmed 169 more cases, bringing the total number to 602. Four more deaths were also confirmed, bringing the total to 6.
- Taiwan confirmed two more cases, bringing the total number to 28.
- The United Kingdom confirmed four new cases, all involving evacuees from the Diamond Princess Cruise ship, bringing the total number to 13.
- There were 57 more cases aboard Diamond Princess, bringing the total number to 691. One death associated to the cruise ship was also confirmed, bringing the total number to 3.

24 February

- Oman halted flights to and from Iran with immediate effect. This comes after its first confirmed case there.
- In Germany the Light + Building Trade Fair in Frankfurt was postponed until September.
- In Najaf, Iraq, mid-year exams which had already started will be cancelled until further notice to protect the health of students.
- UAE banned citizens from travelling to Iran and Thailand as a precaution against the coronavirus. Oman also banned citizens from travelling to Iran.
- Hong Kong bans travellers arriving from South Korea starting from 25 February at 6 am. This comes after the number of cases there increased sharply. Authorities there have also advised against trips there, with a quarantine of 14 days imposed should Hong Kong residents arrive from Daegu and Cheongdo. Several tour groups have since cancelled trips there.
- Six countries have since banned travellers from South Korea from entering their countries. They include Israel, Bahrain, Jordan, Kiribati, Samoa and American Samoa. Nine others have since placed restrictions.
- Mongolia will ban flights to South Korea starting from 25 February to 2 March. The flight ban has since included Japan, with the ban on both countries to last until 11 March.
- Taiwan revises rules to require approval for healthcare professionals in hospital to travel to Level 1 and 2 countries, with a ban on travel to Level 3 countries.

- Rock lobster deliveries from the US to China are on hold, and wedding dress orders in the US are not able to be fulfilled due to shortage of them as 80% of wedding dresses used in the US are made in China.
- The United States Department of State advised Americans to reconsider cruise travel to or within Asia due to the evolving situation.
- Afghanistan confirmed its first case involving a person who recently returned from the Iranian city of Qom.
- Bahrain confirmed its first case involving a Bahraini citizen who travelled to Iran.
- Canada confirmed one more case in British Columbia, bringing the total number to 11.
- Hong Kong confirmed seven more cases, bringing the total number to 81.
- Iran confirmed 18 more cases, bringing the total number to 61. Four more deaths were also reported in the country, bringing the total number to 12.
- Iraq confirmed its first case involving an Iranian student.
- Italy confirmed 74 new cases, bringing the total to 229 spread across six different administrative regions. Four more deaths were also confirmed, bringing the total number to 7.
- Kuwait announced their first cases involving five people arriving from the Iranian city of Mashhad.
- Oman confirmed its first cases involving two Omani women who had come from Iran.
- Singapore confirmed one more case, bringing the total number to 90.
- South Korea confirmed 231 more cases, bringing the total number to 833. The seventh death was also confirmed.

- Spain confirmed its third positive case, an Italian man, in Tenerife, Canary Islands.
- Taiwan confirmed two more cases, bringing the total number to 30.
- The United States confirmed 18 more cases including evacuated passengers from the cruise ship, bringing the total number to 53.
- A patient in Sichuan province tested positive only on her 9th test.
- WHO-China Joint Mission on Covid-19 held a press conference in Beijing releasing the main findings of the mission report. The major findings were in five aspects including the knowledge about the virus itself, the epidemic situation, the characteristics of the epidemic (or the kinetics of transmission), the severity of the disease, and the strategies and measures taken by the Chinese government.
- Quarantine measures in Wuhan were eased slightly, with non-residents allowed to leave the city under certain conditions. The notice was declared null and void hours later as it was published without the proper authorisation. Several officials behind the order were reprimanded as a result.
- Yunnan adjusted its emergency response level from level 1 to level 3, and Guangdong and Jiangsu to level 2. Jiangxi adjusted its levels to level 3 or level 2 depending on the risk of the county.
- Draft legislation was introduced to the Standing Committee of the National People's Congress with a comprehensive ban of the trading and overeating of wildlife.
- The Third Session of the 13th CPPCC National Committee originally scheduled for 3 March was postponed.

25 February

- Algeria reported its first case, an Italian man who arrived on 17 February.
- Austria reported its first two cases, two Italians living in Tyrol tested positive for the coronavirus. One of the couple was a receptionist at a hotel and as a result the hotel in the Alpine tourist hub of Innsbruck was sealed off in an effort to contain the outbreak.
- Bahrain confirmed its second case, a Bahraini woman who had travelled from Iran through Dubai International Airport. This later increased to eight confirmed cases with the addition of two Bahraini men and four Saudi Arabian women. Later on the same day, Bahrain updated the number of cases to 17, with all infected people travelling from Iran. This total later rose again to 23 cases, again all having travelled from Iran.
- Brazil Ministry of Health reported the first positive case of coronavirus in the country and South America, a 61-year-old man from São Paulo, who travelled to Lombardy, Italy, between 9 and 21 February. He was showing mild symptoms and quarantined at home, the confirmation test was also positive.
- Croatia announced its first case of the virus, with a patient hospitalised in the capital, Zagreb, who had travelled to Italy and stayed in Milan.
- France saw two additional cases: one was a French man returning from a trip in the Lombardy region of Italy; the other was a young Chinese woman returning to France from a trip to China. This took the total number of cases in the country to 14.

- Germany saw a case identified in the state of North Rhine-Westphalia of a person recently returned from Italy, taking the country's cases to 17. Another man was later confirmed to be positive, bringing the total number to 18.
- Hong Kong confirmed three more cases, bringing the total number to 84.
- Iranian officials confirmed the death toll officially at 16. There were 34 more cases, bringing the total number to 95. The same day, Iranian MP Mahmoud Sadeghi confirmed he had tested positive for the virus, along with Iraj Harirchi, the Deputy Minister for Health, who had the previous day been part of a press conference about Iran's handling of the virus.
- Iraq confirmed five more cases - an Iranian student and a family of four who had arrived from Iran, taking the total number of cases to 6.
- Italy confirmed 94 new cases, bringing the total to 323 spread across nine different administrative regions. Three more deaths were also confirmed, bringing the total number to 10. This later in the day rose to four deaths, bringing the total to 11.
- Kuwait confirmed four additional cases, all of them people who had returned from Iran, taking their total to 9 cases.
- Oman confirmed two additional cases, taking its total to four cases. Both the additional cases were linked to travel to Iran.
- Singapore confirmed one more case, bringing the total number to 91.
- South Korea confirmed 144 more cases, bringing the total number to 977. Four more deaths were also confirmed, bringing the total to 11. Among those infected included a Korean Air crew member.

- Spain, Canary Islands: on the island of Tenerife two Italian hotel guests tested positive for the virus. This resulted in hundreds of guests at the H10 Costa Adeje Palace hotel being isolated to facilitate further testing and to halt the spread of the disease. Later in the day, the first case was reported in mainland Spain, with a woman from Catalonia, who had recently returned from Italy, diagnosed in Barcelona. A seventh case was confirmed in the late evening by the Madrid regional government.
- Switzerland's government announced the first infection in the country.
- Taiwan confirmed one more case, an 11-year-old boy, bringing the total number to 31.
- Thailand reported two more cases, taking its total to 37. The two new cases, both Thai nationals, were people who were being monitored due to the travel history of others who had travelled to countries with infection risks.
- The fourth death associated with Diamond Princess was confirmed.
- In response the epidemic situation in South Korea and an apparent significant surge of demand for flight tickets from South Korea to Shandong cities, Qingdao will now quarantine all persons entering with a travel history of areas with the epidemic, Weihai will now quarantine all persons entering from Japan and South Korea for 14 days, Shenyang will now test the temperature of all passengers entering from the city, and Dalian will now include all foreigners into its epidemic control mechanism.
- The State Council introduced an exemption of the VAT of small-scale taxpayers in Hubei for three months, as well as

aid measures for individual businesses and stimulus measures for migrant workers and university graduates.

- Inner Mongolia adjusted its emergency response level to level 3.
- Guangzhou will now test all inpatients for SARS-CoV-2.
- Shenzhen introduced a legislation draft for public comment, intending to ban the consumption of all non-aquatic animals except for nine enumerated.

26 February

- The WHO Director-General, Tedros Adhanom, noted that "...14 countries that have had cases have not reported a case for more than a week, and even more importantly, 9 countries have not reported a case for more than two weeks: Belgium, Cambodia, Finland, India, Nepal, Philippines, the Russian Federation, Sri Lanka and Sweden."
- Australia confirmed one more case, bringing the total number to 23.
- Bahrain confirmed three additional cases, bringing its total to 26. Later in the evening it confirmed another 7 cases, taking the total to 33.
- Canada confirmed a new case in Toronto of a woman with travel history to Iran. This took the country's total to 12.
- Croatia confirmed its second and third cases, the second being the twin brother of the first patient and the third being a man who works in Parma, Italy.
- Finland reported its second case.
- France confirmed three new cases, taking it to 17 cases. It also announced its second death from the disease, a 60-

year-old French man who had been diagnosed the night before. An eighteenth case was later declared.

- Georgia reported its first case in the country, a Georgian native travelling from Iran.
- Germany reported five additional cases. By the end of the day the overall total number of cases in the country had risen to 27.
- Greece confirmed its first case, a 38-year-old woman who had recently travelled to Italy.
- Hong Kong reported six new cases, including a 16-year-old boy and his 21-year-old sister who were both aboard Diamond Princess, bringing the total to 91 cases.
- Italy confirmed 51 additional cases, bringing its total to 374. It also confirmed the twelfth death from the virus. In the evening they declared 27 new cases followed by an additional 54 cases, with two earlier cases declared false positives.
- Iran confirmed four more deaths, taking the total to 19. Another 44 cases were confirmed, bringing the total number to 139.
- Japan confirmed its second death from the virus. It also reported 5 new confirmed cases in Nagoya. A third death was later confirmed.
- Kuwait confirmed that their total of confirmed cases had risen to 12 with one new case. Later that day they confirmed the overall total had risen to 25.
- Lebanon confirmed its second case.
- North Macedonia confirmed its first case, a woman who had recently returned home from Italy.

- Norway confirmed its first case, a person who had returned from China.
- Pakistan confirmed its first case, a 22-year-old man from Sindh province who had travelled to Iran, and also confirmed a second case with no further details.
- Romania confirmed its first case.
- Russia confirmed three more cases, who were passengers on the cruise ship Diamond Princess, bringing the total number to 5.
- Singapore confirmed two more cases, bringing the total number to 93.
- Spain confirmed five more cases including a man who was hospitalised in Seville after testing positive, bringing the total number to 12. This was the first confirmed case in the southern region of Andalusia. Another case was later confirmed in the Canary Islands.
- South Korea confirmed 169 more cases, bringing the total number to 1,146. It also recorded an additional death, increasing its total to 12. In the afternoon, the country reported 115 more infections, bringing the total number to 1,261.
- Sweden reported a new case, the second in the country.
- Taiwan confirmed an additional case, bringing its total to 32.
- Thailand confirmed three additional cases, bringing its total to 40 cases.
- The United States confirmed three new cases - one being a domestic case in California with no travel history, and the other two being former passengers aboard Diamond Princess - bringing the total number to 60.

- Diamond Princess saw 14 new confirmed cases, taking it to 705 cases aboard the ship. It is estimated that more passengers on the ship could be infected than previously thought.
- For the first time, a case was re-imported back to China from another country; the patient travelled from Iran.
- Beijing required foreign travellers arriving from areas affected by COVID-19 to be quarantined for 14 days.
- National measures were introduced to aid business resumption, clamp down on malicious disruptors of traffic and logistics, and prohibit the excessive raising of essential medical supplies or disruption of market order.
- Jilin adjusted its emergency response level to level 2, and Hainan to level 3. Fujian adjusted its level to level 2 or 3 based on the risk of the region.
- Yantai, Shandong will now test all persons entering China from the city for SARS-CoV-2 for free.

27 February

- Austria reported its third case, the first in Vienna.
- Canada confirmed the first human-to-human transmission in Toronto, the husband of the woman who had travelled to Iran, bringing the total cases in the country to 13.
- The country later reported a presumptive case in Quebec. The patient had travel history to Iran. This presumptive case was the first case in Quebec, bringing the total number to 14.
- China reported through the National Health Commission 433 new cases and 29 new deaths across the mainland. Of those, 409 cases and 26 deaths were in Hubei province.

- Denmark confirmed its first case, a person who had recently returned from Italy.
- Estonia reported its first case, an Iranian man who had recently returned from Iran.
- France reported 20 new cases, raising the number of cases in the country to 38.
- Germany saw another case reported in North Rhine-Westphalia. In the evening it was reported that there were 14 new cases in the same state, bringing Germany's total to 40 cases. The cases rose to 45 by the end of the day.
- Greece confirmed two more cases, the first patient's daughter and another woman in Athens, bringing the total to 3 cases.
- Hong Kong reported two additional cases, both women infected after visiting a Hong Kong temple at the centre of a COVID-19 cluster. This took the total number of cases to 93.
- Iran reported that 22 people had now died amid 141 people infected by the virus. The chairman of Iran's National Security Committee, Mojtaba Zolnour, announced he had been infected. Iran later announced an increase to 26 deaths and 245 cases. The country's vice president for Women and Family Affairs Masoumeh Ebtekar also tested positive.
- Iraq reported a new case associated with travelling to Iran, the sixth in the country and the first in Baghdad. A seventh case was confirmed in Kirkuk later in the day.
- Israel reported an additional case, a person who had travelled to Italy, bringing the total number to 3.
- Italy reported that two more people had died, bringing the death toll to 14. The Civil Protection agency reported the number of confirmed cases had risen from 420 to 528. Later

in the day it was announced that three more people had died, taking the death toll to 17, and the total confirmed cases had risen to 650. At the end of the day, the total cases rose to 655. Mayor Pietro Mazzocchi of Borgonovo Val Tidone was diagnosed with the virus.

- Japan reported 17 new cases. It confirmed a case involving a recovered patient being reinfected with COVID-19. The total number of local cases had increased to 186. An eighth person died, a Japanese man in his 80s, who lived in the northernmost island of Hokkaido. Additionally, Prime Minister Shinzo Abe asked that all elementary, middle, and high schools shall be closed until late March.
- Kuwait confirmed the total cases in the country were 43, with all having recently travelled to Iran.
- Lebanon reported a third case with the person having travelled from Iran.
- Malaysia confirmed an additional case, a woman who had recently travelled to Japan, bringing the total to 23. That made it the first case to be imported from Japan.
- The Netherlands reported its first case, a person who had been skiing in Italy.
- Nigeria confirmed its first case, an Italian citizen who worked in Nigeria and returned from Milan. It was the first case of coronavirus in sub-Saharan Africa.
- Norway confirmed three additional cases, two in Oslo and one in Bærum, taking the total to four cases. Two returned from Italy and one from Iran.
- Oman reported an additional case, raising the country's total to 5. An additional case was confirmed later that day, who had travelled from Iran.

- San Marino confirmed its first case.
- Singapore confirmed three more cases, bringing the total number to 96.
- South Korea reported 334 new cases, bringing the total number to 1,595. 171 additional cases were later confirmed, taking the total number to 1,766.
- Spain saw a new case reported in Valencia and two more in Madrid. A further case was reported in Barcelona. By the early evening, the total number of confirmed cases had risen to 22. In the evening six additional cases were declared in Valencia.
- Sweden had five new cases confirmed, one in the Uppsala region, three people in Västra Götaland, and one in the Stockholm region.
- Switzerland reported more cases, with a total of six confirmed cases across five cantons. By the end of the day, a total of eight cases had been detected.
- The United Arab Emirates reported the recovery of two patients, and six new cases, bringing the total number to 19. It also saw two suspected cases attached to the UAE Tour, a cycling event, which resulted in the cancellation of the event.
- The United Kingdom confirmed two more cases, contracted in Italy and Tenerife, taking the total to 15 cases. In the evening, a sixteenth case was confirmed, and the first case in Northern Ireland, someone who had come from Italy via Dublin.

28 February

- Australia confirmed one additional case, a former Diamond Princess passenger now in Western Australia, bringing the total number to 24.
- Azerbaijan confirmed its first case, a Russian national who recently returned from Iran.
- Bahrain announced three new cases, raising the total to 36. An additional two cases were later confirmed, both having recently travelled from Iran, one being a Saudi Arabian national.
- Belarus confirmed its first case, a student from Iran.
- Canada reported two positive cases in Ontario. One of them had travel history to Iran, while the other had visited Egypt. The total number of cases rose to 16.
- China confirmed an additional 327 new confirmed cases, of which 318 were in the province of Hubei. There were 44 deaths of which 41 were in Hubei, one in Xinjiang and two in Beijing.
- Croatia confirmed two new cases, one being the girlfriend of the first patient and the other the wife of the third patient, bringing the total number to 5.
- Denmark confirmed an additional case, bringing the total number to 2.
- Finland confirmed an additional case, taking it to 3 confirmed cases.
- France announced two new cases, bringing the total number to 40. The total number of cases later rose to 57.

- Georgia confirmed a second case, a citizen who had returned from Italy. More than 18 people were reported to be in quarantine.
- Germany reported cases totalling "almost 60", according to a Health Ministry official.
- Greece confirmed an additional case, who had recently travelled to Italy. This was the country's fourth case.
- Hong Kong confirmed an additional case, a patient from Diamond Princess, bringing the total number to 94.
- Iceland confirmed its first case, a person who had returned from Italy.
- Iran confirmed 143 new cases and 6 more deaths, with a total of 388 cases and 32 deaths. Four MP's had tested positive, an increase from the two who had already announced their cases.
- Iraq confirmed an eighth case, a woman who recently came back from Iran.
- Israel confirmed an additional case, the second in the country - the wife of the previous person diagnosed. Five additional cases were later confirmed, taking the total to 7. One of the new cases was an Israeli who had recovered in Japan, who was diagnosed again after returning.
- Italy reported that four more people had died, bringing the death toll to 21. The number of confirmed cases had risen from 650 (the day before) to 888.
- Japan announced an additional death, bringing the total to 5. They also confirmed 12 new cases in Hokkaido. Japan also later confirmed another death regarding a British native on board Diamond Princess, marking the first foreign victim on the cruise ship.

- Kuwait announced two additional cases, taking its total to 45.
- Lebanon confirmed its fourth case, a Syrian man, the first case of local transmission.
- Lithuania confirmed its first case, a woman who returned from Italy.
- Malaysia confirmed two more cases, bringing the total number to 25.

- Mexico confirmed its first two cases, one in Mexico City and one in Culiacán. Both cases were individuals who recently returned from a trip to Bergamo, Italy.
- Monaco saw the government confirm the first case in the principality.
- New Zealand confirmed its first case, an individual who had returned from Iran to Auckland earlier in the week.
- The Netherlands confirmed its second case.
- Norway confirmed two other cases, with the second having serious implications. First it was confirmed that a person from Bergen, who returned from Italy, tested positive. Later it was confirmed that a person working at Ullevaal Hospital in Oslo also tested positive, after having returned from Italy. According to standard recommendation he was told to go to work, since he had no symptoms, and he had worked with a significant number of patients for a couple of days before testing positive. Norway now has 6 confirmed cases.
- Romania confirmed two new cases, both having recently returned from Italy.
- Singapore confirmed two more cases, bringing the total number to 98.

- Spain confirmed more cases, taking it to 32 cases with 5 in Madrid, 8 in Comunidad Valenciana, 6 in the Canary Islands, 6 in Catalonia, 1 in the Balearic Islands, 6 in Andalucía, 1 in Aragón and 2 in Castilla y León.
- South Korea confirmed 256 new cases, bringing the total number of infected in the country to 2,022. 182 of the new cases were in Daegu. There were three new deaths, raising the number to 16. Later, the number of cases there shot up by 315, bringing the total number to 2,337.
- Sweden confirmed four more cases, raising the country's total to 11.
- Switzerland's cases increased to 15.
- Taiwan confirmed two additional cases, taking its total to 34.
- Thailand confirmed an additional case, taking the overall number to 41.
- The United Kingdom reported its 17th and 18th cases, in people who had travelled from Iran, and its 19th case and the first in Wales, being someone who had travelled from Northern Italy. In the evening, the 20th case was confirmed, the first case of being passed on in the UK from an unknown source.
- The United States confirmed 4 more cases, including 2 former passengers of Diamond Princess. Washington state authorities later confirmed two additional presumptive cases, bringing its total to 66. One had recently returned from South Korea, and the other case was unrelated and locally acquired.
- SARS-CoV-2 was detected for the first time in tears and conjunctival secretions (pink eye) of a patient. This was only detected in 1 out of the 30 patients that were tested. The

excerpt from the study stated, “In the study of this small sample, we used conjunctival test paper to obtain tears and conjunctival secretions of 30 patients for standard RT-PCR assay. Only one patient with conjunctivitis found viral RNA in his tear fluid and conjunctival secretion twice.”

29 February

- Australia confirmed one more case, bringing the total number to 25.
- Austria confirmed four new cases, bringing the total to 10.
- Azerbaijan reported two new cases, both recently returned from Iran.
- Bahrain confirmed three additional cases, all who had travelled to Iran, bringing the total number to 41.
- Brazil confirmed the second case, a 32-year-old man who arrived from Milan, Italy.
- Canada confirmed four new cases, three in Ontario and one in British Columbia, bringing the total to 20.
- China confirmed 427 new cases - 423 of which were in Hubei province - bringing the total number to 79,251. Deaths increased by 47, to a total of 2,835.
- Croatia confirmed its sixth case, a close relative of the third and fifth patients.
- Denmark confirmed its third case, a person recently returned from a trip to Munich, Germany, where he came into contact with someone who was later determined to have the virus.
- Ecuador confirmed its first case, a woman who recently returned from a trip to Spain.

- France confirmed 16 additional cases, bringing the total number to 73. Additional cases were confirmed, taking the number to 100.
- Georgia confirmed one new case, taking the total number to 3.
- Germany's confirmed cases increased to 66.
- Greece confirmed three new cases, two of which were close contacts of a previous confirmed case, the other had travelled to Italy.
- Iran confirmed 205 new cases, and 9 new deaths, bringing the total to 593 infected and 43 dead.
- Iraq confirmed 5 new cases, bringing the total number to 13. Four of them are in Baghdad and the fifth is in Babil province.
- Ireland confirmed its first case, associated with travel to northern Italy.
- Italy confirmed 239 new cases and 8 new deaths, bringing it to 1,128 cases and 29 deaths.
- Lebanon confirmed three more cases, bringing the total number of cases to seven.
- Luxembourg confirmed its first case.
- Mexico confirmed two more cases, one man in the State of Mexico who participated in the same trip to Bergamo, Italy, that the first two infected made, and a woman in Coahuila who travelled to Milan, Italy, between January and February, bringing the total to 4.
- The Netherlands confirmed four additional cases, bringing the total to 6. A seventh case was later confirmed.
- Norway confirmed nine new cases, bringing the total to 15.

- Pakistan confirmed two more cases, bringing its total to 4. One is a person from Karachi who had recently travelled to Iran, and the other case was in the Federal Area.
- Qatar confirmed its first case, a Qatari national who had recently returned from Iran.
- Singapore confirmed four more cases, bringing the total number to 102.
- South Korea confirmed 594 more cases, bringing the total number to 2,931. This later increased with another 219 cases declared, bringing the total number to 3,150. Another death was confirmed, bringing the total to 17. The first reinfection case was also confirmed.
- Spain confirmed 26 more cases, bringing the total number to 58.
- Sweden reported two new cases, taking the total to 13.
- Switzerland confirmed 3 more cases, bringing the total number to 18.
- Taiwan confirmed five more cases, bringing the total number to 39.
- Thailand confirmed one more case, bringing the total number to 42.
- The United Kingdom confirmed three additional cases, taking the total to 23.
- The United States confirmed its first death, a man from Washington near the Seattle area. The country also reported two more cases, bringing the total number to 68.

Pandemic Chronology March 2020

1 March

- Armenia confirmed its first case, a 29-year-old man returning from Iran.
- Australia confirmed the first death in the country, a 78-year-old man from the cruise ship Diamond Princess. 1 additional case was confirmed, bringing the total number to 26.
- Austria confirmed 4 more cases, bringing the total number to 14.
- Bahrain confirmed 6 more cases, bringing the total number to 47.
- Canada confirmed 4 new cases in Ontario, bringing the total number to 24. All 4 had travel history to Iran or Egypt.
- China confirmed 573 new cases; 570 of which were in Hubei province, bringing the total number to 79,824. Deaths increased by 35 to a total of 2,870.
- Czech Republic confirmed the first 3 cases in the country, individuals that had travelled from Northern Italy.
- Dominican Republic confirmed its first case, a 62-year-old Italian tourist.
- Ecuador confirmed 5 more cases, bringing the total to 6.
- Egypt confirmed 1 more case, bringing the total number to 2.
- Finland confirmed 2 more cases related to woman diagnosed on 27 February, bringing the total number to 6.
- France confirmed 30 more cases, bringing the total number to 130.

- Germany confirmed 63 more cases, bringing the total number to 129.
- Hong Kong confirmed 3 more cases, bringing the total number to 98.
- Iran confirmed 385 new cases with 11 more deaths, bringing the total number to 978 and 54 respectively. A total of 23 members of Parliament of Iran, about 8%, had tested positive for the virus.
- Iraq confirmed 6 more cases, bringing the total number to 19.
- Israel confirmed 3 more cases, bringing the total number to 10.
- Italy confirmed 566 new cases and 5 deaths, bringing the total number to 1,694 and 34 respectively.
- Japan confirmed another death from the coronavirus, bringing the total to 6.
- Malaysia confirmed 4 more cases, bringing the total number to 29.
- Mexico confirmed 1 additional case, bringing the total number to 5.
- The Netherlands confirmed 3 more cases, bringing the total number to 10.
- Saint Barthélemy confirmed its first case.
- Saint Martin confirmed its first case.
- San Marino confirmed 7 more cases, bringing the total number to 8. The first death was also confirmed.
- Scotland confirmed its first case.
- Singapore confirmed 4 more cases, bringing the total number to 106.

- South Korea confirmed 376 more cases, bringing the total number to 3,526. Another 210 cases were later confirmed with the 18th death reported, bringing the total number to 3,736.
- Spain confirmed 26 more cases, bringing the total number to 84.
- Spain also confirmed its first death due to the outbreak, in Valencia.
- Sweden confirmed 1 more case, bringing the total number to 14.
- Thailand confirmed its first death from the coronavirus, a 35-year-old retail worker who also had dengue fever.
- The United Kingdom further reported 13 additional cases of the virus, including. Greater Manchester was added to the list of areas affected bringing the total to 36, 3 of which are believed to be contacts of a case in Surrey who had no history of travel abroad.
- The United States reported the second confirmed death in Washington State. The first cases in Rhode Island, Florida, and New York were confirmed. The authorities confirmed 21 more cases in total, bringing the number to 89.
- The United Nations released $15 million from the UN's Central Emergency Fund emergency funds to help vulnerable countries fight coronavirus COVID-19.
- Authorities in South Korea advised people to stay indoors and not attend any events. The school break was extended by one week across the country, and three weeks in Daegu.
- Seoul authorities have filed a complaint to prosecutors, asking them to charge the leader of Shincheonji Church of

Jesus, Lee Man-hee and 11 others for murder and obstructing efforts to contain the coronavirus.

- In the United States, the American Physical Society cancelled its annual meeting, which was to be held in Denver, Colorado from 2 to 6 March.
- In Japan, one of Sharp Corporation's LCD panel factories will turn some of its production capacity to surgical masks by April. They will produce 150,000 masks a day, eventually rising to 500,000 a day. Other Japanese mask makers have increased their production 5-fold, rising from 20 million, to 100 million masks per week, combined.

2 March

- Andorra confirmed its first case.
- Australia confirmed 4 new cases, bringing the total number to 30, including its first human-to-human transmission.
- Bahrain confirmed 2 more cases, bringing the total number to 49.
- Canada confirmed 3 more cases, all in Ontario, bringing the total number to 27.
- China confirmed 202 new cases, bringing the total number to 80,026. Deaths increased by 42 to a total of 2,912.
- France confirmed 61 more cases, bringing the total number to 191. The third death was also reported.
- Germany confirmed 21 more cases, bringing the total number to 150.
- India reported its first cases since the initial outbreak. 1 case was detected in New Delhi, while the other was from Telangana. Another confirmed case was later detected in Jaipur, bringing the total number to 6.

- Indonesian president Joko Widodo announced the first 2 confirmed cases in the country. The 2 people contracted the virus from a Japanese in Depok, who later tested positive in Malaysia. The mother and daughter are now hospitalised in North Jakarta.
- Iran's total cases rose to 1,501 with 66 deaths.
- Iraq confirmed 2 more cases, bringing the total number to 21.
- Ireland Tourism authorities announced that one of the largest annual events, the 2020 Dublin St Patrick's Day Parade, was cancelled.
- Israel confirmed 2 more cases, bringing the total number to 12.
- Italy confirmed 342 new cases and 18 deaths, bringing the total number to 2,064 and 52, respectively.
- Jordan confirmed its first case.
- Kuwait confirmed 10 more cases, bringing the total number to 56.
- Latvia confirmed its first case, a woman who had flown from Milan to Riga through Munich.
- Morocco confirmed its first case.
- The Netherlands confirmed 8 new cases, bringing the total number to 18.
- Portugal confirmed its first 2 cases, one of whom had returned from Italy, the other from Spain.
- Qatar confirmed 4 new cases, taking their total to 7.
- Russia confirmed 1 additional case, bringing the total to 6 cases.
- Saudi Arabia confirmed their first case in a citizen who had travelled to Iran and returned to Saudi Arabia via Bahrain.

- Senegal confirmed its first case, where the person had recently travelled from France.
- Singapore confirmed 2 more cases, bringing the total number to 108.
- South Korea confirmed 476 more cases, bringing the total number to 4,212. 4 more deaths were confirmed, bringing the total to 22. Another 123 cases were later confirmed, bringing the total number to 4,335.
- Spain confirmed 36 more cases, bringing the total number to 120.
- Sweden confirmed 1 more case, bringing the total number to 15.
- Taiwan confirmed 1 additional case, bringing the total to 41 cases.
- Thailand confirmed 1 more case, bringing the total number to 43.
- Tunisia confirmed its first case.
- The United Kingdom confirmed 3 additional cases, taking the total to 39. An original fourth diagnosis of positive of a person was confirmed later as negative.
- The UK government holds a COBRA meeting to discuss its preparations and response to the virus, as the number of UK cases jumps to 36.
- The United States confirmed 13 more cases, bringing the total number to 102. 5 more deaths were also confirmed, bringing the total number to 6.
- The WHO Director-General announced that containment of the virus must still be the international top priority.

- Wuhan closed its first makeshift hospital, 1 of the 16 built to contain the epidemic after the last person was discharged. This came as the number of new cases declined.
- The European Centre for Disease Prevention and Control announced that it has increased the risk level from moderate to high for people in the European Union.
- In the United States, several schools were closed in the state of Washington due to the rise of coronavirus cases.
- The United Kingdom calls an emergency meeting on the virus, as cases there increased by 12.
- The Lower House of the Polish Parliament passed a bill on special measures regarding the spread of the new coronavirus.
- The leader of Shincheonji Church of Jesus, Lee Man-hee, apologised for its role in the outbreak.
- New Zealand extended travel restrictions on Iran and China by seven days. Travellers arriving from northern Italy and South Korea will be required to self-isolate for 14 days.
- The Badminton World Federation announced it has postponed the Portugal International tournament, originally scheduled to be held from 5 to 8 March.

3 March

- South Korean president Moon Jae-in declared war on the epidemic, with more hospital beds and face masks to be made available. More than 30 trillion won will be injected into the economy for support, and government agencies will operate round the clock.

- South Korean CDC officials approve the first test completed by a Korean life science company and approve another test the following day.
- Indonesia plans to build a hospital in Galang Island to treat people with the coronavirus .
- Singapore will ban visitors arriving from South Korea, Iran and northern Italy from 4 March, with Singapore citizens, permanent residents and long-term pass holders returning from these places to be issued Stay-Home Notices (SHN) lasting 14 days. All travellers entering Singapore with fever or signs of respiratory illness will be required to undergo swab tests, with penalties for refusal. The travel advisory is expanded to include Iran, northern Italy, Japan and South Korea.
- India suspended all visas belonging to citizens of Italy, Iran, South Korea and Japan immediately, along with travellers who went to these places. Authorities advised against non-essential travel to China, Iran, Italy and South Korea, along with medical screening for travellers arriving from 14 places.
- Iran has temporarily released more than 54,000 prisoners due to the spread of the new coronavirus in crowded jails. Iran has also announced plans to mobilise 300,000 soldiers and volunteers against the outbreak.
- Hong Kong arranged four chartered flights to evacuate 533 Hong Kong residents stuck in Hubei province.
- The World Health Organization (WHO) Director-General stated that the latest global death rate of the new coronavirus outbreak was far higher than seasonal flu, 3.4% and much less than 1% respectively. The WHO also announced a severe shortage of personal protective

equipment due to panic buying and hoarding, which was endangering medical workers. In addition, with Ebola on the wane, UN officials announced they were preparing to combat coronavirus in the Democratic Republic of the Congo.

- France has closed about 120 schools in virus-hit areas having the highest number of infections, with more expected to shut in the coming days. Schools in Oise will remain shut until further notice, while schools in Morbihan will remain shut until 14 March.
- Australia will use a little-known biosecurity law (the Biosecurity Act 2015) to restrict the movements of those suspected to have the coronavirus, which since its enactment had only been used for agricultural purposes. This came after cases of community transmission were confirmed there.
- Italy announced that it may set up quarantine red zones to contain the spread of the virus. As a result of the outbreak, a wine fair has been cancelled.
- Shanghai and Guangdong province will quarantine travellers arriving from coronavirus-hit countries for 14 days.
- Argentina confirmed its first case, a person who had recently returned from Italy.
- Australia confirmed 8 more cases, bringing the total number to 38.
- Canada confirmed 6 more cases, 2 in Ontario and 4 in British Columbia, bringing the total to 33.
- Chile confirmed its first case.

- China confirmed 125 new cases, the lowest number of new cases since January, bringing the total number to 80,151. 31 new deaths were also confirmed, bringing the total to 2,943.
- Ecuador confirmed 3 more cases, bringing the total number to 10.
- France confirmed 21 more cases, bringing the total number to 212. The fourth death was also reported.
- Germany confirmed 38 more cases, bringing the total number to 188.
- Gibraltar confirmed its first case, a person who had travelled back from Northern Italy via Malaga airport.
- Iran confirmed that 23 MPs were diagnosed with the virus. The country confirmed 835 more cases with 11 more deaths, bringing the total number to 2,336 and 77, respectively.
- Ireland confirmed 1 more case, bringing the total number to 2.
- Italy confirmed 466 new cases and 28 deaths, bringing the total number to 2,502 and 80, respectively.
- Liechtenstein confirmed its first case.
- Malaysia confirmed 7 more cases, bringing the total number to 36.
- San Marino confirmed 2 new cases, bringing the total number to 10.
- Singapore confirmed 2 more cases, bringing the total number to 110.
- South Korea confirmed 600 more cases, bringing the total number to 4,812. 12 more deaths were also confirmed, bringing the total to 34. 377 more cases were confirmed in the afternoon, along with 2 more deaths, taking total to 5,186 cases and 36 deaths.

- Spain confirmed the first death in the country, a person who died on 13 February, making him the earliest recorded death in Europe. The country reported 31 more cases, bringing the total number to 151.
- Sweden confirmed 15 more cases, bringing the total number to 30.
- Ukraine confirmed its first case, a person having travelled from Italy via Romania.
- The United Kingdom confirmed 12 new cases, bringing the total number to 51.
- The UK government publishes its action plan for dealing with coronavirus. This includes scenarios ranging from a milder pandemic to a "severe prolonged pandemic as experienced in 1918" and warns that a fifth of the national workforce could be absent from work during the infection's peak.
- The United States confirmed 3 more deaths, bringing the total to 9. The first case of coronavirus in North Carolina was reported, coming from the nursing home in Washington State responsible for the first deaths from the virus. Another case in Florida was presumptively confirmed positive, bringing the total number of Floridian cases to 3. The number of cases stood at 126, increasing by 24 from 102.

4 March

- Brazil confirmed 2 more cases, bringing the total number to 4.
- Canada confirmed 1 more case in British Columbia, bringing the total number to 34.

- China confirmed 119 new cases, bringing the total number to 80,270. 38 new deaths were also confirmed, bringing the total to 2,981.
- Faroe Islands confirmed its first case.
- France confirmed 73 more cases, bringing the total number to 285.
- Germany confirmed 52 more cases, bringing the total number to 240.
- Hong Kong confirmed a case of human-to-animal transmission involving a pet dog.
- Hungary confirmed its first cases, 2 Iranian students who were asymptomatic.
- India confirmed 23 more cases, including 15 Italian tourists, bringing the total number to 29.
- Iraq confirmed its first death from the coronavirus.
- Italy confirmed 28 more deaths, bringing the total to 107. This made it the highest jump in a single day. The country confirmed 587 new cases, bringing the total number to 3,089.
- Cases in Japan had topped the 1,000 mark (including 706 cases on the cruise ship Diamond Princess which the World Health Organization classifies as being located "on an international conveyance" and not in Japan) with the first confirmed case in Yamaguchi prefecture.
- Malaysia confirmed 14 more cases, bringing the total number to 50.
- New Zealand confirmed its second case of the coronavirus. The infected individual had returned the previous week from Italy with her family on an Air New Zealand flight from Singapore to Auckland.

- Poland confirmed its first case.
- San Marino confirmed 5 more cases, bringing the total number to 15.
- Singapore confirmed 2 more cases, bringing the total number to 112.
- Slovenia confirmed its first case, a person who had travelled through Italy.
- South Korea confirmed 516 more cases, bringing the total number to 5,328. Another 293 cases were confirmed in the afternoon, bringing the total number to 5,621.
- Sweden confirmed 22 more cases, bringing the total number to 52.
- The United Kingdom confirmed 34 new cases, then Northern Ireland confirmed an additional 2, bringing the total number to 87.
- The United States confirmed 11 total deaths, with the first death outside of Washington state in California. California's total of infections has jumped to 51. The country confirmed 33 new cases, bringing the total number to 159.
- United Nations economists at the UN Conference on Trade and Development, World Bank and IMF announced a likely $50 billion drop in worldwide manufacturing exports in February, together with an IMF pledge of support for vulnerable countries. The UN's top economist, Pamela Coke-Hamilton of UNCTAD, warned against panic.
- Canadian Prime Minister Justin Trudeau announced the creation of a new cabinet committee to manage "the federal response to the coronavirus disease."

- The Malaysian state of Sarawak bans entry by travellers who had visited Italy, Iran, South Korea, and China in the last 14 days.
- The Portuguese Parliament is due to discuss the outbreak on 4 March, as the Portuguese Prime Minister António Costa will open the biweekly debate on the theme of "the prevention and containment of the COVID-19 epidemic".
- Thailand has advised travellers arriving from 9 countries to self-quarantine and register their addresses. They are Singapore, China (including Hong Kong and Macau), Japan, South Korea, Taiwan, Germany, France, Italy, and Iran. The authorities later clarified that quarantine is not compulsory until a high-risk list of countries is finalized.
- Iraq has since shut schools, universities, cinemas, cafes and other public places, which will reopen on 7 March. Authorities have banned mass prayers including on Fridays until further notice.
- French cycling team Cofidis are placed under quarantine in the UAE, lasting until 14 March. This comes after several staff members tested positive for the coronavirus, leading to the cancellation of the UAE Tour.
- The Tokyo government urged residents to refrain from joining in cherry blossom parties in parks in view of the coronavirus.
- Russia banned exports of hazmat suits, masks, and respirators among a list of 17 items to ensure that medics can access these items to treat people. The decree, which was published today, started two days ago and will expire on 1st June. The ban does not cover exports for humanitarian and personal purposes.

- The Australian Football League has moved a game between St Kilda Saints and Port Adelaide Power, originally scheduled on 31 May in Jiangwan Stadium in Shanghai, China to Docklands Stadium in Melbourne, Australia, to be played on 7 June instead.
- The Louvre, a museum in France, reopened after a three-day strike by staff concerned over the coronavirus.
- Italy will close schools and universities until 15 March to contain the virus, with crowd control measures instituted. At the same time, Serie A matches could be played without spectators in a bid to stop the virus.
- Workers in the UK who self-isolate will get statutory sick pay from the first day since being off work.
- UK-based regional airline Flybe collapsed at 10pm GMT and was sent into administration, risking the possible closure of several local airports throughout the UK.
- Saudi Arabia suspended the umrah pilgrimage temporarily for citizens and residents there owing to the coronavirus. It also disallowed visits to the mosque in Medina.
- Japan said that the torch relay for the 2020 Olympics could be adjusted to prevent the spread of the virus.
- Malaysia suspended all autogate and e-gates systems at all checkpoints to deal with the virus.
- In Hong Kong, small business owners started a petition for the government to provide them with HK$6 billion in aid, as they had trouble staying open. The government began to use female prison inmates to produce 180,000 surgical masks per month.
- Emirates removed its charges for changing flight bookings.

5 March

- Algeria confirmed 9 additional cases, bringing the total number to 17.
- Belgium confirmed 27 new cases, bringing the total number to 50.
- Brazil confirmed 3 new cases, bringing the total to 8.
- Bosnia and Herzegovina confirmed the first 2 cases in the country.
- Canada confirmed 11 new cases in Ontario, and the first one in Alberta, bringing the total to 45.
- China confirmed 139 new cases, bringing the total number to 80,409. 31 new deaths were also confirmed (all in Hubei), bringing the total to 3,012.
- Ecuador confirmed 3 more cases, bringing the total number to 13.
- Egypt confirmed the first case in an Egyptian national, who had recently travelled from Serbia via France.
- France registered 92 new confirmed cases, taking the total number of cases to 377. It also saw deaths rise from 4 to 6. This then rose to 423 total cases and 7 deaths. Jean-Luc Reitzer, was the first Assembly member to be diagnosed with the virus.
- Georgia confirmed 5 new cases, all of whom had recently returned from Italy.
- Germany confirmed 87 new cases, taking it to a total of 349.
- Greece confirmed its tenth case. It later confirmed an additional 21 cases, taking it to a total of 31.
- India confirmed 1 more case, bringing the total number to 30.

- Iran saw its largest daily increase in cases, with 591 new cases, taking it to a total of 3,513 confirmed cases. It also saw 15 new deaths, increasing its total to 107. Hossein Sheikholeslam, a diplomat and a former Member of Parliament and Iran's former ambassador to Syria died from the virus.
- Ireland confirmed 6 new cases, bringing the total number to 13.
- Israel confirmed 2 new cases, bringing the total to 17. And of these was a bus driver from East Jerusalem who drove a group of Greek tourists in Israel and the West Bank, the other having recently returned from Italy.
- Italy reported 769 new cases and 41 new deaths, bringing the total number to 3,850 and 148 respectively.
- Malaysia confirmed 5 more cases, bringing the total number to 55.
- Martinique confirmed its first 2 cases.
- The Netherlands confirmed 44 new cases, bringing the total number to 82.
- New Zealand confirmed its third case, an Auckland man who had contracted the virus after family members had returned from a trip to Iran. Relatives of the man at two Auckland schools, Auckland Grammar School and Ormiston Junior College, had also been placed into isolation.
- Norway confirmed 6 new cases, bringing the total number to 66.
- Pakistan confirmed a sixth case, a 69-year-old man in Karachi.
- Palestine reported its first cases in the West Bank city of Bethlehem. Seven staff at a hotel were reported to be

infected by visiting tourists from Greece. These tourists were the same ones who the Israeli bus driver was infected from.

- Russia confirmed 1 more case, bringing the total number to 7.
- Saudi Arabia confirmed 3 additional cases, bringing the total number to 5.
- Scotland confirmed 3 more cases, bringing the total to 6.
- Singapore confirmed 5 more cases, bringing the total number to 117.
- South Africa records its first case in the KwaZulu-Natal province.
- South Korea confirmed 145 more cases, bringing the total number to 5,766. The death toll had reached 35. Another 322 more cases and 6 more deaths are confirmed later in the afternoon, bringing the total to 6088 cases and 41 deaths respectively.
- Spain had confirmed that the total number of cases had risen to 234.
- Sweden confirmed 42 more cases, bringing the total number to 94.
- Switzerland reported its first death from the virus.
- Thailand confirmed 4 new cases, bringing the total to 47.
- The first death from coronavirus in the UK is confirmed, as the number of cases exceeds 100, with a total of 115 having tested positive. England's Chief Medical Officer, Chris Whitty, tells MPs that the UK has now moved to the second stage of dealing with COVID-19 – from 'containment' to the 'delay' phase.
- The United Kingdom's total increased to 90. The UK also later confirmed the total number of cases had increased

further up to 116, as well as recording the first death in the country, an older person with underlying health conditions.

- 1 additional death in Washington state brought the U.S. total to 12. The United States saw a significant increase in cases, with 31 new cases in Washington state. In New York state, cases doubled to 22. Colorado's first 2 cases were confirmed. In total, the US confirmed 69 more cases, bringing the total number to 228.
- Dr. Tedros Ghebreyesus, WHO Director-General, stated, "This is not a drill…This is a time for pulling out all the stops", while UN education agency UNESCO announced that 290 million students globally were now stuck at home.
- South Korea extends a daycare closure across the whole country for two more weeks. On the same day, a new 'special care zone' was declared in Gyeongsan after a spike in cases there.
- Australia banned travelers arriving from South Korea, as well as from mainland China and Iran. Enhanced screening will be conducted on travelers arriving from Italy.
- The Rome Marathon, scheduled for 29 March, was cancelled.
- The Paris Marathon, scheduled for 5 April, was postponed until October 2020.
- Indonesia will ban travellers arriving from the worst-affected regions of Iran, Italy and South Korea from 8 March. Indonesians who arrive from these places will undergo a health examination.
- The Catholic Church of Singapore will resume services on 14 March with precautions in place.

- Japan announced voluntary self-quarantine up to two weeks at designated facilities for travellers arriving from China and South Korea from 9 March. This measure would last until 31 March for now. Visas for these travellers are also cancelled too.

6 March

- The UN's top human rights official, Michelle Bachelet (OHCHR) appealed for business to put rights 'front and centre' when implementing preventative measures to avoid impacting the poorest in society, while the Director-General of the WHO announced that the agency was working with the World Economic Forum to engage private companies globally in meeting the demand for medical products.
- Russia isolated 700 people in St. Petersburg, including many students, due to contact with an Italian student who had been diagnosed the day before.
- Bhutan banned all tourists from arriving in the country for two weeks with immediate effect. This comes after its first confirmed case. Schools will also be closed for two weeks in the Dzongkhags of Thimphu, Paro and Punakha, and international conferences and seminars are postponed.
- After India confirmed its 31st case, India ordered all international passengers to be screened upon entry to the country.
- Samsung Electronics moved all of its phone production from Gumi, South Korea to a factory in Vietnam, as production was constantly being stopped and 6 workers at the Gumi factory had already contracted the virus.

- In Panama, the Health Ministry (Minsa) enabled a hotline (169) to allow people who potentially have coronavirus to consult a doctor. On the same day, it was announced that over 800 people were under medical surveillance, and 30 people had tested negative for the virus. The Minsa also advised against using a surgical mask, as it could cause paranoia within society. Panama has also further enhanced its screening measures at all points of entry.
- In the US, several states introduced measures that order health insurance to not charge people usual fees (co-payment, co-insurance) associated with COVID-19 related healthcare visit or COVID-19 laboratory tests. Several events were cancelled. In Austin, Texas, the major music and media festival SXSW was cancelled for the first time in its 34-year history, a local disaster having been declared despite there being no coronavirus cases in the city itself. In Seattle, Washington, the Emerald City Comic Con was cancelled and postponed until summer. DC Comics cancelled all March convention events, and several Jewish institutions in New York City, most notably Yeshiva University, either closed or took other prophylactic measures. Miku Expo's North American tour dates have also been postponed.
- TwitchCon Europe 2020, scheduled to take place in Amsterdam from 2–3 May 2020, was announced to be cancelled as a precautionary measure.
- The Vis Moot competition, scheduled for April 2020 in Vienna, was cancelled and moved to an online platform.
- The three-day International Indian Film Academy Awards (IIFA) (dubbed Bollywood's Oscars), supposed to be held

from 27 to 29 March, were delayed due to fears of the coronavirus.

- Carnival Cruise Line changed its cancellation policy, making it easier to move guests' cruise dates, and providing onboard credit to those who decide to continue with their March 6-May 31 sailing dates.
- Austria announced 13 new cases, taking its total to 55.
- Belgium confirmed 59 new cases, bringing the total to 109.
- Bhutan announced its first case, an American tourist who had recently also travelled to India after leaving the United States on 18 February.
- Brazil confirmed 5 new cases, bringing the total number to 13.
- Cameroon confirmed its first case, a French citizen.
- Canada confirmed 4 new cases in Ontario, bringing the total to 51 with 26 from Ontario. A husband and wife returned from the cruise ship Grand Princess in California and two men returned from Iran and Las Vegas.
- China confirmed 143 new cases, bringing the total number to 80,552. 30 new deaths were also confirmed, bringing the total to 3,042. Hubei had no cases as a result. In addition, the country detected 4 new cases in Beijing, all visiting Italian nationals.
- Colombia confirmed its first case, a woman who recently travelled from Italy.
- Costa Rica has confirmed its first case involving an American from New York.
- Egypt confirmed 12 additional cases, bringing the total number to 15.

- France confirmed 190 new cases and 2 additional deaths, bringing the total to 613 cases and 9 deaths.
- Germany confirmed 185 new cases, taking it to a total of 534. 105 more cases were later confirmed, bringing the total number to 639.
- The cruise ship Grand Princess announced it had 21 people on board testing positive.
- Greece confirmed 14 additional cases.
- Iceland confirmed 6 additional cases, bringing the total to 43.
- India confirmed 1 more case, bringing the total number to 31.
- Indonesia confirmed 2 more cases, bringing the total number to 4.
- Iran confirmed 1,234 new cases and 16 new deaths, taking its totals up to 4,747 cases and 124 deaths. They also reported 913 people had recovered.
- Italy announced 778 new cases and 49 new deaths.
- Malaysia confirmed 28 new cases, the largest daily increase in the country's number of confirmed cases. This took the country's total to 83.
- The Netherlands reported its first death, and 44 new cases, bringing it to a total of 128 cases.
- New Zealand confirmed its fourth case: a man who is the partner of the second case confirmed on 3 March.
- North Macedonia confirmed 2 additional cases, taking its total to 3.
- Peru confirmed its first case.
- Poland confirmed 4 additional cases (two people that travelled from Italy, 1 person who travelled from United

Kingdom and 1 person who travelled from Germany with the first case confirmed day earlier), taking their total to 5.

- Portugal confirmed 4 additional cases (3 in Porto and 1 in Lisbon), bringing the total to 13. All 3 cases in Porto had a connection with Italy.
- Qatar confirmed 3 new cases, taking it to a total of 11.
- Russia confirmed 6 more cases, bringing the total number to 13.
- Serbia confirmed its first case.
- Singapore confirmed 13 new cases, bringing the total number to 130. This was the largest increase of cases in a single day so far.
- Slovakia confirmed its first case.
- South Korea confirmed 196 more cases, bringing the total number to 6,284. 1 more death was confirmed, bringing the total to 42. Another 309 cases and another death were later confirmed, bringing the total to 6,593 and 43 respectively.
- Spain confirmed 104 additional cases, bringing the total number to 360.
- Sweden confirmed 43 additional cases, bringing the total number to 137.
- Switzerland announced 123 additional cases, raising it to a total of 210 cases and 1 fatality.
- Thailand confirmed 1 new case, bringing the total to 48.
- Togo confirmed its first case.
- In the United Kingdom, the total number of cases were confirmed as 163, a rise of 47 and the highest day-on-day increase.
- The UK Prime Minister announces £46 million in funding for research into a coronavirus vaccine and rapid diagnostic

tests. During a visit to a laboratory in Bedfordshire, he says: "It looks like there will be a substantial period of disruption where we have to deal with this outbreak."

- In the United States, the first 3 cases were confirmed in the state of Maryland. 2 deaths in Florida were confirmed. Officials in the US state of Hawaii have confirmed their first case, a former passenger of the cruise ship Grand Princess. In total, the US confirmed 104 more cases, bringing the total number to 332. 1 more death in Washington State plus 2 in Florida brought the total number of U.S. deaths to 17. In California, a Santa Clara County resident died at home, whose death was attributed later in April to COVID-19. WHO has different data: 19 new cases, 148 in total. 1 new death, 10 in total.
- The Vatican City confirmed its first case.
- Vietnam confirmed 1 more case, bringing the total number to 17. It was the first case in three weeks.

7 March

- Afghanistan confirmed 3 additional cases, taking the total to 4.
- Argentina confirmed its first death, also the first in South America, a 64-year-old man who had travelled to Paris.
- Bahrain confirmed 19 new cases, taking the total number to 79.
- Belgium confirmed 60 additional cases, bringing the total number to 169.
- Brazil confirmed 6 new cases of COVID-19, raising the total number to 19.
- Canada confirmed 6 additional cases, taking the total to 57.

- China confirmed 99 new cases, bringing the total number to 80,651. Deaths increased by 28 to a total of 3,070.
- Egypt confirmed 33 new cases on a Nile cruise ship.
- France's total rose to 949 cases and 16 deaths.
- Germany confirmed 45 new cases, taking it to a total of 684. Another 116 cases were later confirmed, bringing the total number to 800.
- Iran confirmed 1,076 new cases and 21 additional deaths, taking it to a total of 5,823 infected and 145 dead. They also confirmed 16,000 cases were hospitalised as suspect cases and 1,669 cases had recovered. Another MP, Fatemeh Rahbar, died. She had recently been elected to the parliament.
- Iraq confirmed 8 new cases taking the total to 46.
- Italy confirmed 1,247 new cases and 36 new deaths.
- Maldives confirmed its first case, 2 overseas hotel employees.
- Malaysia confirmed 10 more new cases, bringing the total number to 93.
- Malta reported its first 3 cases, an Italian family who were residents in Malta. They had gone on holiday to northern Italy and had been in self-quarantine before being tested for the coronavirus. They were now in isolation at Mater Dei Hospital.
- Moldova confirmed its first case, a person taken to hospital after arriving on a flight from Italy.
- New Zealand confirmed its fifth case of the coronavirus: a woman who was the partner of the third COVID-19 case confirmed in New Zealand.
- Palestine confirms 22 cases.

- Paraguay confirmed its first case.
- Peru confirmed 5 more cases, bringing the total to 6.
- Poland confirmed an additional case, bringing the total to 6.
- Singapore confirmed 8 more cases, bringing the total number to 138.
- South Korea confirmed 174 more cases and 1 more death, bringing the total number to 6,767 and 44 respectively. Another 274 new cases and 4 new deaths were later confirmed, taking the total to 7,041 and 48 respectively.
- Spain confirmed 70 new cases and 2 deaths. The total number of cases was now 516 cases.
- Thailand confirmed 2 new cases, bringing the total to 50.
- The United Arab Emirates confirmed 15 additional cases, taking its total to 45.
- In the United Kingdom, 42 additional cases and 1 additional death were confirmed, taking the total to 206 cases and 2 deaths. 3 additional cases were confirmed in Northern Ireland later in the day, taking the total to 209 cases.
- In the United States, the number of deaths rose to 19 with 16 in Washington, 1 in California, and 2 in Florida. The total for the country increased to 444 confirmed cases. WHO has different data: 65 new confirmed cases, totalling 213. And 1 new death, 11 in total.
- Vietnam confirmed 3 new cases, bringing the total number to 20.
- The Xinjia Express Hotel in Quanzhou City, Fujian Province, China collapsed while containing dozens of close contacts of people with coronavirus. 29 people died as a result.
- The World Health Organization (WHO) stated that the global number of confirmed cases of the new coronavirus disease,

COVID-19, had surpassed 100,000, calling it a 'sombre moment'.

- The International Ice Hockey Federation cancelled the Women's World Championship, scheduled from 31 March to 10 April in Canada, due to concerns about the coronavirus.
- In Singapore, the People's Association suspended activities and classes and activities attended by confirmed cases for 14 days, as well as all singing classes.
- Hong Kong will require all passengers to fill up health declaration forms from 8 March, with residents warned against non-essential travel.

8 March

- Albania confirmed the first 2 cases in the country.
- Austria confirmed 25 additional cases, taking its total to 104.
- Bahrain confirmed 17 new cases, taking the total to 94.
- Bangladesh confirmed its first 3 cases, 2 people who had come from Italy separately, and a contact of 1 of the cases.
- Belgium confirmed 31 additional cases, bringing the total number to 200.
- Brazil confirmed 6 new cases of COVID-19, raising the total number in the country to 25.
- Bulgaria confirmed its first 4 cases.
- Canada confirmed 12 new cases, bringing the total number to 69.
- China confirmed 44 new cases, bringing the total number to 80,695. Deaths increased by 27 to a total of 3,097.
- Egypt confirmed its first death (and the first death in Africa) – a German national who was hospitalised on 1 March and

then suffered respiratory failure caused by acute pneumonia on 7 March.

- France confirmed that the number of cases had risen to 1,126 and 19 deaths. Elisabeth Toutut-Picard became the second Assembly member to be diagnosed with the virus.
- Germany's cases rose to over 1,000 with 1,018 cases confirmed.
- Hong Kong confirmed 4 new cases, taking the total to 114, and a third death.
- India confirmed 5 additional cases, all in Kerala. This took the country's total up to 39.
- Indonesia confirmed 2 additional cases, taking them to 6 cases. One of the new cases was a male crew member from the Diamond Princess.
- Iran confirmed 49 additional deaths, the highest daily toll in the country, taking it to a total of 194 deaths. Total cases had risen to 6,566, an increase of 743.
- Israel confirmed 11 additional cases, taking its total to 29.
- Italy confirmed an additional 1,492 cases and 133 deaths, taking it to a total of 7,375 cases and 366 deaths.
- Kuwait confirmed an additional case, taking its total to 62.
- Latvia confirmed an additional case.
- Lebanon confirmed 4 more cases, bringing the total number to 32.
- Malaysia confirmed 6 new cases, bringing the total to 99.
- Poland confirmed 2 additional cases, taking the total to 8. In the evening, 3 more cases were confirmed, bringing the total number to 11.
- Portugal confirmed 4 additional cases.
- Qatar confirmed 3 additional cases, taking their total to 15.

- Saudi Arabia confirmed 4 additional cases, bringing the total number to 11.
- Singapore confirmed 12 new cases, bringing the total number to 150.
- Spain announced the new total was 616 cases, along with 17 deaths, an increase of 7.
- South Africa confirmed its third case, the wife of the first diagnosed case.
- South Korea confirmed an additional 93 new cases, taking its total to 7,134 and 2 additional deaths, taking the total to 50. Another 179 cases were later confirmed, bringing the total to 7,313.
- Switzerland confirmed there are now 332 confirmed cases, with all those people placed in isolation. There had been 2 deaths.
- The United Kingdom announced an increase of 64 new cases, taking it to a total of 273 cases. The UK also confirmed the third death in the country. 5 new cases were additionally confirmed in Northern Ireland. The third death from coronavirus was reported, at North Manchester General Hospital, as the number of cases in the UK reaches 273, the largest single-day increase so far.
- The United States confirmed 120 more cases, bringing the total number to 564. 2 more deaths were confirmed, bringing the total number to 21. According to WHO, the number of confirmed cases was 213, total deaths 11. No new cases, no new deaths were recorded.
- Vietnam confirmed 10 more cases, bringing the total number to 30.

- Organizers of the Bahrain Grand Prix, the second round of the 2020 Formula One World Championship, decided to hold the 2020 event without any spectators permitted.
- Italy placed more than 16 million people under quarantine in Lombardy and 14 other central and Northern provinces, together with closure of schools, gyms, museums, nightclubs and other venues across the country.
- The President of Portugal cancelled all his public activities and will stay at home in a self-imposed quarantine after receiving a group of students from a school which has since been closed following the detection of a student with COVID-19.
- France banned gatherings of over 1000 people in a bid to curb the spread of the virus.
- All schools and universities in Saudi Arabia have been closed until further notice to control the spread of the virus. In addition, Saudi Arabia bans travel to nine countries (being United Arab Emirates, Kuwait, Bahrain, Egypt, Lebanon, Syria, Iraq, Italy, South Korea), with fines imposed for inaccurate health declarations. Al Qatif was placed under lockdown to contain the outbreak.
- Qatar banned passengers from Pakistan, Bangladesh, Sri Lanka, Philippines, Iran, Iraq, Lebanon, South Korea, Thailand, Nepal, Egypt, China, Syria and India amid fears of spread of the virus.
- Thailand starts requiring travellers from China (including Hong Kong and Macau), Italy and South Korea to present a medical certificate that proves a COVID-free status before entering the country, with those having no certs disallowed.

9 March

- Australia's number of confirmed cases rose to 80, with 6 additional cases.
- Bahrain confirmed an additional 24 cases, taking the total to 118.
- Belgium confirmed 39 additional cases, bringing the total number to 239.
- Brazil confirmed 5 new cases in the state of Rio de Janeiro, raising the total number to 30.
- Brunei's health ministry confirmed a first case of a local man who returned from Kuala Lumpur on 3 March. Symptoms began on 7 March and preliminary tests indicate the person is positive.
- Canada recorded its first COVID-19-related death. The country also confirmed 10 more cases, bringing the total number to 79.
- China confirmed 40 new cases, bringing the total number to 80,735. Deaths increased by 22 to a total of 3,119. There were no locally transmitted cases outside Hubei.
- Colombia confirmed 2 additional cases.
- Cyprus confirmed its first 2 cases.
- Finland confirmed 7 new cases, bringing the total number to 30.
- France saw Guillaume Vuilletet and Sylvie Tolmont confirmed as infected deputies, before Michèle Victory became the fifth deputy of the Assembly to be diagnosed with the virus. The number of cases increased to 1,412. It was also confirmed that the culture minister, Franck Riester, had tested positive.

- Germany reported its first deaths with 2 fatalities. Cases increased to 1,176.
- Guernsey confirmed its first case.
- Hungary confirmed 2 new cases.
- India confirmed 5 additional cases, taking the total to 44.
- Indonesia confirmed 13 additional cases, bringing the total number to 19.
- Iran announced an update to the total cases to 7,161, with a revised number of deaths to 237. New infections are 595 new cases and 43 additional deaths. Those recovered has reached 2,394.
- Ireland confirmed 3 additional cases, taking the country's total to 24.
- Italy saw confirmed cases rise to 9,172 and deaths to 463.
- Kuwait announced 3 additional cases, taking it to a total of 65.
- Lebanon reported 9 new cases, taking the total to 41.
- Malaysia confirmed 18 new cases, taking it to 117.
- Malta confirmed its fourth case.
- The Netherlands announced 56 additional cases.
- Nigeria confirmed its second case, a Nigerian who had contact with the Italian first case.
- Norway declared 11 additional cases. By the end of the day 227 cases had been confirmed.
- Oman reported 2 additional cases, both of whom had travelled to Iran. This took the country's total to 18, 17 of whom had travelled to Iran and 1 to Italy.
- Palestine confirmed 5 new cases in the West Bank.
- Panama announced its first COVID-19 case, a 40-year-old Panamanian woman from Spain.

- The Philippines confirmed 10 additional cases, doubling the current country count to 20. Another 4 cases were later confirmed, bringing the total number to 24.
- Pakistan saw 9 new cases, bringing the total number to 16.
- Poland confirmed 5 more cases, bringing the total number to 16.
- Saudi Arabia confirmed 4 additional cases, increasing the total to 15.
- Scotland confirmed 5 additional case, bringing the total to 11.
- Singapore confirmed 10 more cases, bringing the total number to 160.
- South Africa confirmed another 4 cases, bringing the total number to 7.
- South Korea confirmed 69 new cases and 1 more death, bringing the total to 7,382 and 51 respectively. Another 96 cases were later confirmed, taking it to a total of 7,478.
- Spain's numbers increased to 1,231 cases with 30 deaths, with 32 people having recovered.
- Sweden confirmed 45 additional cases, taking its total to 203. This later rose to 252 cases including the first confirmed local transmission case.
- Switzerland confirmed 42 new cases, rising to a total of 374.
- The United Arab Emirates reported 14 additional cases, taking its total to 59. 4 were Emiratis and the remainder from various other nationalities.
- The United Kingdom's confirmed cases increased by 2, with the confirmation of cases in Wales. Figures released in the afternoon showed the UK had risen to 317 cases. A fourth death was reported, and then a fifth.

- The FTSE 100 plunges by more than 8 percent, its largest intraday fall since 2008, amid concerns over the spread of COVID-19.
- The UK Foreign and Commonwealth Office advises against all but essential travel to Italy due to the COVID-19 outbreak in the country and the nationwide lockdown.
- The first 3 cases are discovered in Dorset
- The United States confirmed 153 additional cases, bringing the total number to 717. 5 more deaths were reported, bringing the total number to 26. According to WHO, the number of confirmed cases is 213, total deaths 11. No new cases, no new deaths were recorded.
- Vietnam confirmed an additional case, taking its total to 31.
- The UN's trade and development agency, UNCTAD, stated that the economic uncertainty caused by the virus would likely cost the global economy $1 trillion in 2020.
- Italy imposes a country-wide quarantine, restricting travel except for necessity, work, and health circumstances. As a result, people flocked to the supermarkets and prison riots erupted.
- Romania bans the flights to and from Italy until 23 March. All schools in Romania are closed from 11 to 22 March.
- Seychelles announced a temporary closing for cruise ships.
- Stock markets crashed worldwide in reaction to the coronavirus outbreak and falling oil prices.
- The BNP Paribas Open tennis tournament, originally scheduled to take place on 11 March in Indian Wells, California, United States, was cancelled after a confirmed case was reported in the local area.

- In Panama, the Panama Metro began to clean its trains more frequently, using different disinfectants. The Minsa announced that 1,073 people are under medical surveillance.
- FIFA and the Asian Football Confederation agree to postpone qualifying matches to be held in March and June due to COVID-19, with matches still allowed to carry on if associations agree with approval from both organisations.
- India starts separating travellers from 12 places (China, South Korea, Japan, Italy, Iran, Singapore, Thailand, Malaysia, Hong Kong, Vietnam, Nepal and Indonesia) in all its airports to deal with the outbreak. Such travellers undergo health screening in separate zones.
- Panama's health ministry began to report daily statistics about COVID-19, with an emphasis on newly infected people.

10 March

- Australia reported 14 new cases, taking the country to a total of 107.
- Austria confirmed 25 additional cases, taking the total to 182.
- Bahrain confirmed 1 additional case, taking the total to 119.
- Belgium confirmed 28 new cases, bringing the total number to 267.
- Bolivia confirmed its first cases, 2 women who had been in Italy, arriving the country without showing any symptoms.
- Brazil confirmed 4 new cases, including the first case in Rio Grande do Sul, raising the total number to 34.
- Brunei confirmed 5 new cases, bringing the total to 6.

- Bulgaria confirmed 2 additional cases, bringing the total to 6.
- Burkina Faso confirmed its first cases with 2 infections, a couple who had returned from France in February.
- China saw only 19 new infections, 17 in Wuhan and 2 imported from overseas. 17 deaths were reported in Hubei. These brought the total number of cases and deaths to 80,754 and 3,136 respectively.
- Democratic Republic of Congo reported its first case, a foreigner who flew into Kinshasa from Belgium who tested positive on arrival and was isolated. It was later confirmed by the Ministry of Health that the information they had originally released was incorrect and that the first case was rather a Congolese citizen returning From France, who had contacted the Health Services two days after his arrival in Congo and had been quarantined in a local neighbourhood.
- Denmark confirmed 174 additional cases, taking it to 264 cases (including 2 in the Faroe Islands).
- France saw cases rise to 1,784 people and 33 people dead, with 86 people in a serious condition.
- Georgia confirmed 8 additional cases, bringing the total to 23.
- Germany's number of case rose to 1,565, with the death roll remaining at 2. 341 new cases were reported in the previous 24 hours.
- Greece confirmed 5 new cases, bringing the total number to 89.
- Hong Kong confirmed an additional 5 cases, taking the total to 120 confirmed and 1 assumed case.
- India saw 18 additional cases, many in Kerala, taking the total to 62.

- Indonesia confirmed 8 more cases, bringing the total number to 27.
- Iran's confirmed cases rose by 881 to 8,042 and deaths rose by 54 to 291.
- Ireland reported 10 additional cases, bringing the total number to 34.
- Israel confirmed 7 more cases, taking the total to 58. The number of cases later shot up to 75.
- Italy confirmed 977 new cases and 168 more deaths, bringing the total to 10,149 and 631 respectively.
- Jamaica confirmed its first case, a Jamaican national who travelled to the country from the United Kingdom.
- Japan confirmed 59 new cases and 3 new deaths.
- Jersey confirmed its first case, a person who returned from Italy.
- Kuwait announced 4 additional cases, increasing the total number to 69.
- Lebanon confirmed its first death from the virus.
- Malaysia confirmed 12 additional cases, taking the total to 129.
- Moldova confirmed 2 additional cases, taking the total to 3. The male and female, have both visited Italy in late February.
- Mongolia announced its first COVID-19 case.
- Morocco confirmed its first death, and 2 additional cases.
- The Netherlands confirmed 61 additional cases and a fourth death.
- Northern Cyprus reported its first case, a 65-year-old German woman who was visiting as a tourist.

- Norway confirmed 147 new cases, with total cases now standing at 374.
- Panama announced its first death and seven new cases, bringing the total number to 8.
- Pakistan confirmed an additional case, bringing the total to 20.
- Palestine recorded an additional case, taking the total to 26.
- The Philippines confirmed 9 more cases, bringing the total number to 33. This comes after the tally was erroneously reported as 35.
- Poland confirmed 8 additional cases, taking the total to 22.
- Qatar confirmed 6 additional cases, taking it to 24 confirmed cases.
- Romania confirmed 8 additional cases, bringing the total number to 25.
- Russia confirmed 4 additional cases, bringing the total to 17.
- San Marino confirmed 11 new cases, taking it to a total of 62 cases and 2 deaths.
- Saudi Arabia confirmed 10 additional cases, taking the total to 20.
- Scotland confirmed 7 new cases, bringing the total to 18.
- Serbia confirmed 3 additional cases, taking the total to 5.
- Singapore confirmed 6 more cases, bringing the total number to 166.
- Slovenia confirmed 15 additional cases.
- South Korea confirmed 35 new cases and 3 more deaths, bringing the total to 7,513 and 54 respectively.
- Spain confirmed 415 new cases and 5 new deaths. The total number of cases rose to 1,674.

- Sweden reported 78 new cases, taking the country's total to 326.
- Thailand confirmed 3 new cases, bringing the total to 53.
- Tunisia announced an additional 3 cases, taking the total to 5.
- Turkey confirmed its first case.
- The United Arab Emirates confirmed 15 additional cases, taking the total to 74.
- The United Kingdom confirmed 54 additional cases, taking it to 373 cases with the sixth confirmed death. Later this increased to 382 cases with the 9 additional cases in Wales.
- Nadine Dorries, Health Minister, becomes the first MP to test positive for coronavirus.
- The United States confirmed 283 additional cases, bringing the total number to 1,000. 5 more deaths were reported, bringing the total number to 31.
- Vietnam confirmed 3 new cases, bringing the total number to 34.
- Australia reported 14 new cases, taking the country to a total of 107.
- Austria confirmed 25 additional cases, taking the total to 182.
- Bahrain confirmed 1 additional case, taking the total to 119.
- Belgium confirmed 28 new cases, bringing the total number to 267.
- Bolivia confirmed its first cases, 2 women who had been in Italy, arriving the country without showing any symptoms.
- Brazil confirmed 4 new cases, including the first case in Rio Grande do Sul, raising the total number to 34.
- Brunei confirmed 5 new cases, bringing the total to 6.

- Bulgaria confirmed 2 additional cases, bringing the total to 6.
- Burkina Faso confirmed its first cases with 2 infections, a couple who had returned from France in February.
- China saw only 19 new infections, 17 in Wuhan and 2 imported from overseas. 17 deaths were reported in Hubei. These brought the total number of cases and deaths to 80,754 and 3,136 respectively.
- Democratic Republic of Congo reported its first case, a foreigner who flew into Kinshasa from Belgium who tested positive on arrival and was isolated. It was later confirmed by the Ministry of Health that the information they had originally released was incorrect and that the first case was rather a Congolese citizen returning From France, who had contacted the Health Services 2 days after his arrival in Congo and had been quarantined in a local neighbourhood.
- Denmark confirmed 174 additional cases, taking it to 264 cases (including 2 in the Faroe Islands).
- France saw cases rise to 1,784 people and 33 people dead, with 86 people in a serious condition.
- Georgia confirmed 8 additional cases, bringing the total to 23.
- Germany's number of case rose to 1,565, with the death roll remaining at 2. 341 new cases were reported in the previous 24 hours.
- Greece confirmed 5 new cases, bringing the total number to 89.
- Hong Kong confirmed an additional 5 cases, taking the total to 120 confirmed and 1 assumed case.
- India saw 18 additional cases, many in Kerala, taking the total to 62.

- Indonesia confirmed 8 more cases, bringing the total number to 27.
- Iran's confirmed cases rose by 881 to 8,042 and deaths rose by 54 to 291.
- Ireland reported 10 additional cases, bringing the total number to 34.
- Israel confirmed 7 more cases, taking the total to 58. The number of cases later shot up to 75.
- Italy confirmed 977 new cases and 168 more deaths, bringing the total to 10,149 and 631 respectively.
- Jamaica confirmed its first case, a Jamaican national who travelled to the country from the United Kingdom.
- Japan confirmed 59 new cases and 3 new deaths.
- Jersey confirmed its first case, a person who returned from Italy.
- Kuwait announced 4 additional cases, increasing the total number to 69.
- Lebanon confirmed its first death from the virus.
- Malaysia confirmed 12 additional cases, taking the total to 129.
- Moldova confirmed 2 additional cases, taking the total to 3. The male and female, have both visited Italy in late February.
- Mongolia announced its first COVID-19 case.
- Morocco confirmed its first death, and 2 additional cases.
- The Netherlands confirmed 61 additional cases and a fourth death.
- Northern Cyprus reported its first case, a 65-year-old German woman who was visiting as a tourist.

- Norway confirmed 147 new cases, with total cases now standing at 374.
- Panama announced its 1st death and 7 new cases, bringing the total number to 8.
- Pakistan confirmed an additional case, bringing the total to 20.
- Palestine recorded an additional case, taking the total to 26.
- The Philippines confirmed 9 more cases, bringing the total number to 33. This comes after the tally was erroneously reported as 35.
- Poland confirmed 8 additional cases, taking the total to 22.
- Qatar confirmed 6 additional cases, taking it to 24 confirmed cases.
- Romania confirmed 8 additional cases, bringing the total number to 25.
- Russia confirmed 4 additional cases, bringing the total to 17.
- San Marino confirmed 11 new cases, taking it to a total of 62 cases and 2 deaths.
- Saudi Arabia confirmed 10 additional cases, taking the total to 20.
- Scotland confirmed 7 new cases, bringing the total to 18.
- Serbia confirmed 3 additional cases, taking the total to 5.
- Singapore confirmed 6 more cases, bringing the total number to 166.
- Slovenia confirmed 15 additional cases.
- South Korea confirmed 35 new cases and 3 more deaths, bringing the total to 7,513 and 54 respectively.
- Spain confirmed 415 new cases and 5 new deaths. The total number of cases rose to 1,674.

- Sweden reported 78 new cases, taking the country's total to 326.
- Thailand confirmed 3 new cases, bringing the total to 53.
- Tunisia announced an additional 3 cases, taking the total to 5.
- Turkey confirmed its first case.
- The United Arab Emirates confirmed 15 additional cases, taking the total to 74.
- The United Kingdom confirmed 54 additional cases, taking it to 373 cases with the sixth confirmed death. Later this increased to 382 cases with the 9 additional cases in Wales.
- The United States confirmed 283 additional cases, bringing the total number to 1,000. 5 more deaths were reported, bringing the total number to 31.
- Vietnam confirmed 3 new cases, bringing the total number to 34.
- The United Nations Educational, Scientific and Cultural Organization (UNESCO) highlighted the unprecedented shuttering of schools globally and restricted access to the UN headquarters in New York.
- Mongolia put multiple cities, including its capital Ulaanbaatar, under quarantine until 16 March after the country's first case was confirmed.
- The Malaysian state of Sabah banned travellers from Iran and Italy from entering. The ban applies to all foreign travellers who have travelled to Iran and Italy within the last 14 days including Malaysians who are non-residents of Sabah.
- All primary and secondary schools in the Czech Republic were closed.

- In Greece, all primary and secondary schools, universities and cram schools (known in Greece as frontistirio) were closed for 2 weeks, starting from 11 March until 24 March. Because 25 March is the national holiday for the Greek War of Independence, schools will reopen on 26 March. These preventive measures were taken in order to limit the spread of coronavirus in Greece. However, according to the Greek minister of education, Niki Kerameus, the school year may be extended if the measures for the closure of all schools get extended. Additionally, the Greek ministry of education prepared a plan to cover up for the lost school days. Among others, this plan includes an extension of the school year, a reduction of the school lessons' duration in 35 minutes in order to increase the teaching hours each day, reduction of Easter holidays, distance learning and cuts on the curriculum. The postponement of university entrance exams from June to July or September was also considered, while the military and student parades across Greece on 25 March were cancelled.
- Panama suspended the school year in Panama City, and activities involving large amounts of people until 7 April. The school year suspension in other parts of the country was set to last until 20 March, but it was later extended to 7 April. The Minsa also announced that 66 people were under medical surveillance.
- RuPaul's DragCon LA 2020, which supposed to take place on 1 to 3 May in Los Angeles has been cancelled. The fate of RuPaul's DragCon in NYC and UK is currently unknown.
- Polish archbishop, the President of the Polish Episcopal Conference said that Polish churches should increase the number of masses, so that fewer people will attend at once.

- The Autonomous Administration of North and East Syria (Also known as Rojava), closed a border crossing underneath its control with neighboring Iraq. The Administration also released a statement asking European journalists following the Syrian Civil War not to visit parts of Syria underneath its control, and that medical checks would be done at all crossings into their territory in response to the Coronavirus.
- Singapore's Ministry of Health announced a suspension of activities for seniors from 11 March for 14 days. This came after many people went out while unwell. Social distancing will be implemented for other activities. Senior care services will continue running with additional precautions.
- Japan unveiled a second package costing $4 billion to cushion the impact of the outbreak, with support mostly for small and medium enterprises.
- Malta stops all flights to Italy immediately after confirming its fourth case, with the ferry now carrying only medicine and cargo.
- New York deploys the National Guard to contain infections in New Rochelle, which is under quarantine.
- The Vatican's Saint Peter's Square and main basilica are closed until 3 April to stop the coronavirus.
- The European Union will propose a law to stop 'ghost flights' in order to help airlines tide through the crisis, ensuring that slots are not given to other operators.
- Several sports events will be played without crowds, including La Liga for the next two rounds, French soccer matches until 15 April, several Bundesliga matches, Barcelona's Champions League, Portugal matches and a

Europa League match between Manchester United and LASK.

- The Spanish Parliament's lower house suspends all sessions for a week after a lawmaker was infected with COVID-19. In addition, schools in several regions are closed, with flights from Italy suspended for two weeks and events with more than 1,000 participants banned in places with viral transmission.
- Thailand approved a stimulus package worth 400 billion baht to cushion the impact of the epidemic. This includes soft loans, funds and tax benefits for those affected, but no handouts.
- Italy will suspend mortgage payments to cushion the economic blow caused by COVID-19.
- Taiwan will allow citizens to buy masks online and collect from convenience stores starting 12 March as part of the mask rationing policy.
- Japan's Cabinet approved draft 'state of emergency' measures for authorities to deal with the outbreak. These include imposing curfews, closing schools, cancelling events and taking over private facilities for medical care.
- Hong Kong will quarantine travellers from Italy, France, Germany, Spain and Japan in designated centres from 14 March in a bid to stop the outbreak.
- Chinese Communist Party general secretary Xi Jinping visits Wuhan and issues a statement claiming that COVID-19 has been eradicated in Wuhan and Hubei province.
- China has developed a robot for throat swabbing to diagnose cases, helping to reduce risks for workers.

11 March

- Hubei's provincial government announces that businesses related to epidemic control, public utilities and daily necessities are allowed to resume work now. Other businesses will be allowed to resume work on 20 March.
- Beijing orders everyone arriving in the city from any country, including those from countries not affected by COVID-19, to undergo home quarantine for 14 days. Those arriving for business trips are to stay in hotels and test for the v
- Albania reported 3 new cases, taking the country's total to 15. The first death in the country was also reported.
- Armenia confirmed 3 new cases, bringing the total number to 4.
- Australia reported 19 new cases, taking the country to a total of 126. American actor Tom Hanks and wife Rita Wilson were diagnosed with the illness during the filming of Baz Luhrmann's upcoming-biographical film Elvis in Australia.
- Austria confirmed 24 additional cases, taking the total to 206.
- Bahrain confirmed 77 additional cases, citizens evacuated from Iran on a flight. This brought the country's total to 189.
- Belgium reported its first death.
- Bosnia and Herzegovina confirmed 7 additional cases.
- Brazil confirmed 34 additional cases, raising the total number to 69.
- Bulgaria reported its first death. It also confirmed 1 additional case, bringing the total to 7.

- China confirmed 24 new cases (including 13 in Hubei) and 22 new deaths, bringing the total number of cases and deaths to 80,778 and 3,158, respectively.
- Colombia confirmed 3 additional cases, bringing the total to 6. Later on the same day, 3 more cases were confirmed, bringing the total to 9.
- Cuba confirmed its first 3 cases.
- Denmark confirmed 180 additional cases, raising the total to 442.
- Egypt confirmed 7 additional cases, 6 of whom were Egyptian. The country now had 67 cases, of which 8 have recovered.
- France reported 487 new cases and 15 fatalities, for a total of 2,281 cases and 48 deaths.
- French Polynesia reported its first case. The person is Maina Sage, a member of the French National Assembly.
- Georgia reported 5 additional cases, increasing the total to 23.
- Germany saw its cases rise to 1,908.
- Greece confirmed 10 additional cases, taking the country's total to 99, 95 of whom were Greek, and 4 were foreign nationals.
- Guyana confirmed its first 2 cases from a 52-year-old woman suffering from underlying health conditions, including diabetes and hypertension. The woman died at the Georgetown Public Hospital.
- Honduras confirmed its first 2 cases, 1 from Spain and 1 from Switzerland.
- Indonesia confirmed 7 more cases, bringing the total number to 34. Its first death was also reported, confirmed by the

United Kingdom's Foreign and Commonwealth Office as a 53-year-old female British national.

- Iran announced that there are now 9,000 infected, with 354 deaths. New infections were 958, with 63 additional deaths. Those recovered total 2,959. Iran's first vice-president, Eshaq Jahangiri, was reported infected.
- Ireland confirmed 9 additional cases, bringing the total number to 43. The first death was also confirmed.
- Israel confirmed 97 cases.
- Italy announced 2,313 new cases and 196 new deaths. Total cases stood at 12,462, with deaths at 827. It was also confirmed that Juventus and Italian footballer Daniele Rugani had tested positive for coronavirus.
- Ivory Coast declared its first case, a local citizen who had recently been in Italy.
- Kuwait reported 3 additional cases, bringing its total to 72.
- Lebanon recorded 8 new cases, taking the total to 59, and a second death.
- Lithuania confirmed 2 additional cases, a married couple that came back from Italy, taking the total to 3 cases.
- Malaysia confirmed 20 additional cases, taking the total to 149.
- The Maldives confirmed 2 additional cases.
- Morocco confirmed 2 additional cases, bringing the total to 5.
- The Netherlands' total increased to 503 cases, and 1 new death was reported.
- Norway confirmed 200 additional cases, taking the total number to 602.
- Paraguay confirmed 3 new cases.

- Panama confirmed several new cases, bringing the total to 14.
- The Philippines confirmed 16 additional cases, bringing the country's total to 49. The second death was also confirmed.
- Portugal announced 18 new cases.
- Qatar reported 6 new cases, increasing the country's total to 24. It later announced 238 new cases in expatriates who came in contact with three infected people and had been quarantined. The revised number of cases is now 262.
- Réunion confirmed its first case.
- Romania confirmed 18 new cases, bringing the total to 47.
- Saudi Arabia reported an additional case, an Egyptian, taking the country's total to 21.
- Scotland confirmed 18 new cases, bringing the total number to 36.
- Singapore confirmed 12 new cases, bringing the total number to 178.
- South Africa confirmed 6 more cases, taking the total to 13.
- South Korea confirmed 242 new cases and 6 new deaths, bringing the total to 7,755 and 60, respectively.
- Spain's cases rose to 2,231, with 54 confirmed deaths.
- Sri Lanka announced 1 additional case, bringing the total number to 2.
- Sweden reported 98 additional cases, taking the total to 500, and announced the first death in the country.
- Taiwan confirmed 1 additional case, raising the country's total to 48.
- Thailand confirmed 6 additional cases, taking the country's cases to 59.

- The United Kingdom confirmed an additional 86 cases, with its overall total now at 456. 2 more deaths were confirmed, bringing the total to 8. The number later increased to 460, with 4 cases declared in Wales, including the first instance of community transmission in Wales.
- The Bank of England cuts its baseline interest rate from 0.75% to 0.25%, back down to the lowest level in history.
- Chancellor of the Exchequer, Rishi Sunak, presents the Johnson Government's first budget, which includes £30 billion in measures to protect the economy from coronavirus.
- The United States confirmed 272 additional cases, bringing the total number to 1,272. 7 more deaths were reported, bringing the total number to 38. The Utah Jazz's Rudy Gobert and Donovan Mitchell were diagnosed with the illness. As a result, the NBA suspended the entire season after the night's games. The Utah Jazz vs Oklahoma City Thunder game was postponed after doctors reported Gobert had the illness. In addition, Michigan confirmed its first 2 cases, raising concerns about the automobile industry's survival.
- Vietnam confirmed 4 additional cases, raising the country's total to 38.
- The World Health Organization declared COVID-19 a pandemic. The declaration followed extensive criticism that the WHO response had been weak and inappropriately favourable toward the government of China.
- Canadian Prime Minister Justin Trudeau announced a CA$1,000,000,000 COVID-19 Response Fund that includes a $50 million contribution to the World Health Organization

and an additional $275 million to fund coronavirus research in Canada.

- All schools and universities in Poland were closed for two weeks.
- The Prime Minister of Denmark announced that all schools, universities and kindergartens would be shut down for two weeks.
- In the United States, the National Collegiate Athletic Association announced that both its Division I Men's Basketball Tournament and Women's Basketball Tournament, scheduled from mid-March to early April, will be held without any spectators in attendance. Boise, Idaho's popular Treefort Music Fest was postponed until 23 to September 27. The 2020 Electronic Entertainment Expo was cancelled.
- California announced a ban on mass gatherings involving 250 or more participants until end-March, with smaller events allowed to go ahead with social distancing of up to 2 metres.
- The U.S. and Canada's National Basketball Association announced that it will suspend the remainder of its 2020 season after players tested positive for the disease.
- U.S. President Donald Trump announced that all travel from Europe (except the UK) into the United States would be suspended for 30 days.
- India suspended visas for travellers, including visa-free travel, from March 13 until April 15, except those on diplomatic, official, employment and project visas. Even travellers allowed to enter will be subject to quarantine orders.

- Israel banned gatherings exceeding 100 people after a spike in cases. Schools will continue to remain open, with universities and other higher learning institutes urged to explore distance learning in case of closure. Companies were asked to let employees work from home.
- The Institut Pasteur de Dakar and DiaTropix teamed up with Mologic, a British biotech firm, to develop "point of need" test kits that can diagnose COVID-19 in 10 minutes.
- Thailand will suspend visa-free arrivals from Hong Kong, South Korea and Italy, as well as visa-on-arrivals from 18 countries, including China and India. In its place will be visa applications and proof of medical certificates.
- Google asks staff in the US and Canada to work from home to reduce the spread of COVID. This comes a week after several other tech firms asked their staff to do so. Twitter follows suit, expanding it to all workers around the world.
- All Premier League and lower matches In England will be played without spectators, with games not shown in pubs to avoid crowding. In addition, a Premier League match between Arsenal and Manchester City is postponed after players interacted with an owner down with the coronavirus, making it the first match to be called off.
- After a confirmed case, one of the Philippines' oldest and exclusive golf clubs, the Wack Wack Golf and Country Club, is closed for disinfection.
- The United States Department of State raised the global travel alert to "Level 3: Reconsider Travel", urging Americans to reconsider travel plans due to the ongoing pandemic.
- March 12

- Stock markets worldwide suffered their greatest single-day fall since the 1987 crash in response to the coronavirus pandemic and the previous day's announcement of the 30-day travel ban between the U.S. and Europe.
- Canadian Prime Minister Trudeau began a self-quarantine for 14 days after his wife Sophie Trudeau tested positive for the virus. Ontario closes schools until at least April 5
- Israel and Sri Lanka closed schools early from March 13, with term holidays lasting until April 20 to stem the spread of the coronavirus. Schools were also asked to refrain from planning excursions during this period.
- Singapore closed mosques for five days starting from March 13 for cleaning as a precaution against the coronavirus, with prayers cancelled for that day. Activities at the mosques will be stopped until March 27. This came after two people were infected from a gathering in Malaysia. Separately, the Catholic Church of Singapore will continue suspending services indefinitely after the World Health Organization declared the coronavirus a pandemic, rescinding an initial plan to resume services on March 14.
- The Osim Sundown Marathon, supposed to be held on May 23 in Singapore, was cancelled due to the coronavirus, with runners having direct entry to next year's event. Several other runs were also postponed.
- The suspension of Cortes Generales, Spain's Parliament, will be extended by 15 days due to the coronavirus.
- Turkey closed all primary, secondary and high schools for a week and universities for three weeks starting from 16 March. All sports matches will be played without spectators until the end of April. Students will continue education from

their homes via the internet and TV channels from 23 March for a week.

- Following the National Basketball Association's suspension of its season one day earlier, other major professional sports leagues in the United States and Canada and sporting organizers do the same. The National Hockey League indefinitely pauses the remainder of its 2020 season, while Major League Soccer imposes a 30-day suspension on its 2020 season. Major League Baseball cancels the remainder of its spring training and delays the start of its 2020 season for at least two weeks. The National Collegiate Athletic Association, which had previously announced that all of its winter championship events, including its Division I Men's Basketball Tournament and Women's Basketball Tournament, would be played with no spectators cancels all championship events until the 2020–21 season. The Professional Golfers' Association of America cancels the Players Championship and other upcoming golf events.
- The World Health Organization says that the COVID-19 pandemic can be controlled as long as countries take the pandemic seriously. This comes after some countries did not take adequate measures to slow transmission, and also after the WHO had stated the outbreak had not reached the status of a pandemic.
- Before midnight, the Government of Estonia declared an emergency situation to last until May 1. Special measures announced for the duration of the emergency situation include a prohibition of all public gatherings, concerts, performances, conferences, sports events, a regular study in all schools and universities (remote forms of study are allowed), closure of museums, cinemas; introduction of

border checks; and visitation limits to hospitals, social service centres and prisons.

- As a result of a McLaren team member testing positive, the entire McLaren team pulled out of the 2020 Australian Grand Prix.
- Euroleague Basketball announces all leagues suspension including the Euroleague and the Eurocup, until an unknown date.
- The 2020 Summer Olympics torch relay began in Olympia, Greece, in a scaled-down ceremony without spectators. It was the first Olympic flame lighting ceremony to be held without public attendance since 1984.
- Several theme parks in the United States have closed due to the coronavirus. In Orlando, Florida, SeaWorld Orlando, Disney World, Disney Cruise Lines, and Universal Orlando Resort closed down (Universal Orlando was originally announced to be closed through March 28.) In California, Disneyland and Universal Studios Hollywood have closed too. Separately, Disneyland also closed its Disneyland Paris park in France.
- Speaking from Blair House during his Saint Patrick's Day official visit to Washington, D.C., Prime Minister of Ireland Leo Varadkar announced that schools, colleges and childcare would close starting March 13 until March 29, recommended cancellation of indoor gatherings of more than 100 people, outdoor gatherings of more than 500 and advised those who could to work from home to do so. As a result, the GAA bans all activities, including training and team gatherings, from 18:00.

- United Kingdom's Prime Minister Boris Johnson advised those with fever or "continuous" cough to self-isolate for seven days, coming after the UK Government moved to the "delay" phase to tackle the pandemic. In addition, schools are advised to cancel overseas trips, and people over 70 and those with pre-existing conditions are advised not to take cruises. Testing will focus on those with symptoms, and people are no longer required to call the National Health Service due to strained capacity, directing them to websites instead. In Northern Ireland, schools and colleges will remain open with the situation under constant review. In Scotland, mass gatherings attracting more than 500 people will be disallowed from next week. In addition, schools will still remain open with an advisory to cancel overseas trips.
- Philippine President Rodrigo Duterte announced a quarantine for Manila. They include stopping all domestic travel into Manila from March 15, closing schools for a month, ban on mass gatherings and entry of foreigners from places where the virus is spreading.
- Several soccer competitions, including La Liga, Eredivisie, Primeira Liga and Major League Soccer, have been suspended due to coronavirus.
- Italy will close all shops except food stores and pharmacies until March 25 to contain the worsening spread there, a day after WHO's declaration of a pandemic.
- The opening event of Tokyo 2020 was announced as a softball game on July 22, despite concerns of COVID-19 spread.

12 March

- Chinese Foreign Ministry spokesperson Zhao Lijian alleges that the US military had brought the virus to Wuhan in a controversial Tweet.
- Hubei will allow industrial production to resume in some areas, as well as lift some travel restrictions.
- Algeria confirmed 5 additional cases and the first death.
- Brazil confirmed 82 new cases, raising the total number to 149.
- Brunei reported 5 new cases, bringing the total number to 11.
- Bulgaria reported 9 new cases from the capital, bringing the total number to 16. They later reported 7 more cases, bringing the total number to 23.
- China reports 8 new cases and 11 deaths, representing a sharp drop in the number of transmissions and fatalities in China. These brought the total number of cases and deaths to 80,786 and 3,169, respectively.
- Colombia confirmed 4 more cases, raising the total to 13.
- Egypt confirmed 13 new cases and 1 new death.
- France's total increased to 2,876 and 61 deaths.
- Germany announced 546 new cases and 2 additional deaths, taking the totals to 2,745 cases and 6 deaths.
- India confirmed its first death, a 76-year-old Indian national with existing health conditions who had recently returned from Saudi Arabia.
- Italy confirmed 189 more deaths, bringing the total number to 1,016, and 2,651 new cases were also confirmed, bringing the total number to 15,113.

- Ireland confirmed 27 new cases, bringing the total to 70. 22 of the new cases were by local transmission.
- Japan reported a total of 624 cases, with 23 dead.
- Kuwait confirmed 8 more cases, taking the total number to 80.
- Malaysia confirmed its first sporadic case after 600 tests. 9 new cases were later confirmed, bringing the total number to 158.
- Norway reported its first death.
- The Philippines confirmed 3 more cases, bringing the total cases to 52.
- Romania confirmed 1 new case, bringing to total number to 48.
- San Marino reported 15 new cases and 3 additional deaths.
- Singapore confirmed 9 more cases, bringing the total number to 187.
- South Korea confirmed 114 new cases and 6 new deaths, bringing the total to 7,869 and 66, respectively.
- Spain confirmed 782 new cases and 31 new deaths, raising the country's total to 3,059 cases and 86 dead.
- Sri Lanka confirmed an additional case, taking the total number to 3.
- St. Vincent & the Grenadines confirmed its first case.
- Switzerland confirmed 212 new cases and 2 additional deaths.
- Thailand confirmed 11 new cases, bringing the total to 70.
- Trinidad & Tobago confirmed its first case, a Swiss national.
- Ukraine reported 2 new cases, bringing the total number to 3.

- The United Kingdom confirmed 136 new cases, bringing the total number to 596. 2 more deaths were also confirmed, bringing the total to 10. It was confirmed that Arsenal head coach Mikel Arteta had tested positive for COVID-19.
- The UK Chief Medical Officers raise the risk to the UK from moderate to high.
- The government advises that anyone with a new continuous cough or a fever should self-isolate for seven days. Schools are asked to cancel trips abroad, and people over 70 and those with pre-existing medical conditions are advised to avoid cruises.
- Following a recent series of major falls, the FTSE100 plunges again, this time by over 10%, its biggest drop since 1987. Other markets around the world are similarly affected by ongoing economic turmoil.
- Public Health England stops performing contact tracing as widespread infections overwhelm capacity.
- The rules published on February 25 for travellers returning from certain countries are withdrawn; they should now follow the same guidelines as other households.
- The United States confirmed 373 additional cases, bringing the total number to 1,645. 3 more deaths were reported, bringing the total number to 41. The Utah Jazz's Donovan Mitchell tested positive for the virus.
- Vietnam confirmed 6 new cases, bringing the total number to 44.
- A team member of McLaren tested positive for the coronavirus, throwing the 2020 Australian Grand Prix into disarray.

- Brazilian President Jair Bolsonaro's communications secretary Fabio Wajngarten tested positive for COVID-19.

13 March

- Antigua and Barbuda confirmed its first case.
- Aruba confirmed its first 2 cases, people who travelled in from New York.
- Bulgaria confirmed 3 new cases, bringing the total number to 26. Bulgaria later confirmed 5 additional cases, bringing the total to 31.
- Brazil confirmed 22 new cases, bringing the total number to 171. President Jair Bolsonaro tested negative for COVID-19.
- Brunei confirmed 14 new cases, bringing the total number to 25.
- The Cayman Islands confirmed its first case.
- Colombia reported 3 more cases, raising the total to 16.
- Costa Rica reported 3 new cases since March 12, bringing the total number of cases to 26.
- Curaçao reported its first case, a Dutch tourist.
- Ethiopia confirmed its first case.
- France's numbers increased to 2,876 cases and 81 deaths.
- Gabon confirmed its first case.
- Germany's case total rose to 3,675.
- Ghana confirmed its first 2 cases, a Norwegian Embassy official and a Turkish citizen.
- Guadeloupe confirmed its first case, a citizen who recently returned from France.
- Guatemala confirmed its first case, a traveller from Italy.

- Guinea reported its first case, an employee of the EU delegation.
- Israel reported a total of 126 cases.
- Italy's cases rose to 17,660, and deaths rose to 1,266, a rise of 250 deaths in 24 hours.
- Kazakhstan confirmed its first 2 cases, which were also the first in Central Asia.
- Kenya confirmed its first case, a Kenyan national who had returned from the United States via London.
- Kosovo confirmed its first 2 cases.
- Lithuania confirmed 3 new cases, bringing the total number to 6. A Spanish citizen from Madrid was confirmed in Vilnius, along with a woman in Klaipėda who arrived from Tenerife, and a man in Kaunas who arrived from Italy on February 29.
- Malaysia confirmed 39 new cases, bringing the total number to 197.
- Palestine confirms 35 coronavirus cases.
- The Philippines confirmed 12 more cases, bringing the total number to 64.
- Panama confirmed several new cases, bringing the total to 27. More new cases were later confirmed, bringing the total to 36.
- Puerto Rico confirmed its first 3 cases, a 71-year-old man and an Italian couple aged 68 and 70.
- Saint Lucia confirmed its first case, a 63-year-old woman who had travelled to the UK.
- Singapore confirmed 13 more cases, bringing the total number to 200. The number of imported cases surpassed that of local cases.

- Slovakia confirmed 11 new cases, bringing the total number to 32.
- South Korea confirmed 110 new cases and 1 new death, bringing the total to 7,979 and 67, respectively.
- Spain's cases rose to 4,231. 35 more deaths were also confirmed, bringing the total to 121.
- Sri Lanka confirmed 3 new cases, bringing the total number to 6.
- Sudan confirmed its first case and the first death, a man in his 50s who travelled to the United Arab Emirates.
- Suriname confirmed its first case.
- Switzerland reported 1,125 cases (of which 116 are undergoing final analysis), a 31% day-on-day increase.
- Thailand confirmed 5 new cases, bringing the total to 75.
- Turkey confirmed its second case. Later in the day, the case count increased to 5. All cases were related to the first case, who contracted the virus from Europe.
- Ukraine reported its first death, a 71-year-old woman from Radomyshl, Zhytomyr Oblast, who recently travelled to Poland.
- The United Kingdom confirmed 202 new cases, bringing the total number to 798.
- Authorities confirm the first death from coronavirus in Scotland, bringing the total deaths across the UK to 11.
- The UK Government restricts the export of three drugs being administered to COVID-19 patients in clinical trials in China: Kaletra, Chloroquine phosphate, and Hydroxychloroquine.
- BBC Radio 1 cancels its Big Weekend music festival, scheduled to take place at the end of May. Organisers subsequently run an alternative event called Big Weekend

UK 2020, with acts appearing on one of five virtual stages and performed from their homes; the event also features past performances from previous Big Weekend events.

- The United States confirmed 559 additional cases, bringing the total number to 2,204. 8 more deaths were reported, bringing the total number to 49.
- U.S. Virgin Islands confirmed the first case in the territory.
- Uruguay confirmed its first 4 cases, all of them having travelled from Milan, Italy.
- Venezuela confirmed its first 2 cases, one a traveller from the United States and the second who had travelled from Spain.
- Vietnam confirmed 3 additional cases, bringing the total number to 47.
- In a video message, UN Secretary-General António Guterres assured the world that the COVID-19 virus would peak and that the global economy would recover, but, until then, "we must act together to slow the spread of the virus and look after each other".
- The World Health Organization issued official advice noting that while the COVID-19 virus outbreak was now designated a pandemic, containment was still possible, and it advised against panic and information while launching a 'COVID-19 Solidarity Response Fund' and stressing the need for everyone to be prepared and follow WHO guidelines.
- With a member of the McLaren team testing positive the day before, and the team withdrawing from the race, F1 and the FIA decided to cancel the opening round of the 2020 Formula One World Championship, the Australian Grand Prix. Later, it was announced that the next two rounds, to be

held in Bahrain and Vietnam, would be postponed. Cricket Australia announced that the three-match series against New Zealand would go ahead but that fans would not be admitted into the venue. The Women's Flat Track Derby Association (WFTDA), the governing body for roller derby in the United States, initiates its response to the pandemic.

- The Auckland Council cancelled the annual Pasifika Festival in Auckland in response to health concerns about the coronavirus.
- The Czech Republic announced a complete travel ban effective midnight on 16 March, banning all foreigners from entering and Czech nationals and long-term resident foreigners from leaving the country. The lockdown will be effective for the duration of the 30-day state of emergency declared on March 12.
- Singapore bans visitors arriving from Italy, France, Spain and Germany from March 15 at 11.59 pm, with Singapore citizens, permanent residents and long-term pass holders returning from these places issued Stay-Home Notices (SHN) lasting 14 days. Port calls for all cruise vessels stopped immediately. Singapore citizens are also advised to defer all non-essential travel to Italy, France, Spain and Germany, review travel plans and exercise caution while travelling. Any traveller showing symptoms at checkpoints will serve SHNs lasting 14 days, even with negative results for COVID-19. All new ticketed cultural, sports and entertainment events with 250 people or more must be deferred or cancelled, with organisers of sold events required to take measures to ensure the safety of participants before being allowed to proceed. Organisers of gatherings are advised to reduce crowds and contact

between people, as well as public venues. Employers are also advised to allow employees to telecommute, stagger work hours and commute at off-peak hours.

- Switzerland issued sweeping restrictions on places of public gatherings, closing schools throughout the country and imposing a ban on public gatherings of more than 100 people until April 30. This is implemented by most cantons as the closure of cinemas, theatres, museums, youth centres, sports centres, fitness centres, swimming pools, wellness centres, discos, pianos-bars, nightclubs, and erotic clubs.
- U.S. President Donald Trump declared a national state of emergency, allocating about US$50 billion of U.S. federal government money for relief efforts. In response, the US stock market Dow Jones Industrial Average posted its largest single-day gain since October 2008.
- In the UK, the Premier League, along with the English Football League and FA Women's Super League, suspended their respective seasons until April after both Arsenal F.C. manager Mikel Arteta and Chelsea F.C. player Callum Hudson-Odoi tested positive for the disease.
- Apple Inc. announced that their annual Worldwide Developers Conference (WWDC) will be held as an online-only conference for the first time as a precaution. They later announced the closure of all Apple Stores outside of Greater China until March 27. Further, a commitment of US$15 million towards the COVID-19 response was announced.
- Australia's chief medical officer advised the government to ban mass gatherings of more than 500 people from stopping the coronavirus.

- In Panama, businesses began to impose and enforce limits on how many food and personal hygiene items a customer may buy at a time.
- Israel bans all mass gatherings, but kindergartens and daycare centres are allowed to stay open.

14 March

- Brazil confirmed 7 more cases, bringing the total number to 178.
- Brunei reported 3 new cases, bringing the total to 40.
- Bulgaria confirmed 6 new cases bringing the total number to 37. One more death was also confirmed, bringing the total number to 2.
- The Central African Republic confirmed its first case.
- China reported 20 new cases, up from 11 cases a day earlier. 16 of the cases were overseas travellers. In response, the Beijing authorities announced that everyone arriving from overseas would be quarantined for 14 days.
- Colombia reported additional 8 more cases, taking the total to 24.
- The Congo Republic confirmed its first case, a person who had travelled from France.
- Denmark confirmed the first death in the country, an 81-year-old man.
- Equatorial Guinea confirmed its first case, a 42-year-old woman who returned from Madrid.
- Eswatini confirmed its first case, a 33-year-old woman who travelled to the United States and then Lesotho before returning home to Eswatini.

- France confirmed 838 new cases, bringing the total number to 4,499. 12 more deaths were confirmed, bringing the total to 91.
- Iran confirmed 1,365 new cases, bringing the total number to 12,729. 97 more deaths were confirmed, bringing the total to 611.
- Ireland confirmed 39 new cases, the largest to date, and one more confirmed death. 129 total confirmed cases and 2 deaths.
- Italy confirmed 3,497 new cases, bringing the total number to 21,157. 175 more deaths were also confirmed, bringing the total to 1,441.
- Malaysia confirmed 41 new cases, bringing the total number to 238.
- Mauritania confirmed its first case.
- Mayotte confirmed its first case.
- Moldova confirmed 4 new cases.
- Namibia confirmed its first cases, two tourists visiting the country.
- New Zealand confirmed its sixth case, a man who had returned from the United States on March 6.
- Palestine confirms 4 new cases, bringing the total to 39 cases.
- The Philippines confirmed 47 more cases, bringing the total number to 111.
- Rwanda confirmed its first case.
- Saudi Arabia confirmed 17 additional cases, with its total rising to 103.
- Seychelles reported its first 2 cases.

- Singapore confirmed 12 more cases, bringing the total number to 212.
- South Korea confirmed 107 new cases and 5 new deaths, bringing the total to 8,086 and 72, respectively.
- Spain confirmed 1,522 new cases, raising its total to 5,753 cases. 62 more deaths were confirmed, bringing the total to 183.
- Sri Lanka confirmed 2 new cases, bringing the total number to 8. Another 3 cases were later confirmed, bringing the total number to 11.
- Panama confirmed several new cases, bringing the total number to 43.
- Thailand confirmed 7 more cases, bringing the total number to 82.
- The United Kingdom confirmed 342 new cases, bringing the total number to 1,140. 10 more deaths were reported, bringing the total to 21.
- A further 10 people are reported to have died from COVID-19, almost doubling the UK death toll from 11 to 21. The government's aim for a "herd immunity" approach generates controversy.
- Vice President of the United States, Mike Pence, announces the US is to extend its European coronavirus travel ban to include the UK from 16 March.
- UK retailers release a joint letter asking customers not to panic-buy products after some supermarkets sell out of items such as pasta, hand gel and toilet paper.
- The United States confirmed 612 new cases, bringing the total number to 2,816. One of the cases was 24-year-old

Christian Wood of the Detroit Pistons. 11 more deaths were reported, bringing the total number to 60.

- Vietnam confirmed 6 additional cases, bringing the total number to 53.
- In response to a rise in imported cases, Beijing authorities announced that everyone arriving from overseas will be quarantined for 14 days.
- The New Zealand Government cancelled the Christchurch mosque shootings memorial service scheduled to be held at Christchurch's Horncastle Arena on March 15 due to COVID-19 concerns. Prime Minister Jacinda Ardern announced that anyone entering New Zealand from midnight on March 15 would have to isolate themselves for 14 days. Cruise ships will be barred from entering New Zealand from midnight March 14 until June 30. In addition, anyone with coronavirus symptoms will not be allowed to enter the Pacific Islands, and those who have been travelling overseas will have to wait for 14 days before travelling to the Pacific.
- Malaysian Prime Minister Muhyiddin Yassin ordered the cancellation or postponement of all public gatherings, including international meetings, sport, social and religious events, until April 30 due to COVID-19 concerns. The Prime Minister also announced that the Government would be evacuating 65 Malaysians in Iran and 323 in Italy in humanitarian missions.
- The US State of Georgia announced they would move their primary election for president from 24 March to 19 May, becoming the second state to do so after Louisiana.
- US President Donald Trump had his physician release a memo that suggested he tested negative for the virus.

- Panama banned all flights from and to Europe and Asia for 30 days. The Panamanian government also began to regulate activities involving over 50 people.
- Cirque du Soleil stops all its shows, including in Las Vegas.

15 March

- The United Nations Secretary-General announced that the UN was putting in places measures to protect staff while affirming that it would continue normal operations.
- All schools in the Banten province of Indonesia are closed until March 28. This comes after the Governor of Banten Wahidin Halim declared the virus an "extraordinary event". Other provinces such as Jakarta, Central Java, West Kalimantan, and West Java also did the same thing.
- Brunei banned all citizens and foreign residents from leaving in response to the coronavirus pandemic. The Ministry of Health has also banned mass gatherings, including weddings and sporting events. In addition, the National Football Association of Brunei Darussalam, the Tutong District Amateur Football Association League, and the Brunei Basketball Association have suspended all matches and games.
- Finland has ceased testing for people returning from trips abroad and all of the people suffering flu symptoms in the country. The tests are now reserved for health professionals only.
- Indian Prime Minister Narendra Modi proposed a SAARC fund called SAARC COVID-19 Emergency Fund to tackle coronavirus via video conference. He proposed setting up a

volunteer basis COVID-19 emergency fund with India committing USD 10 million initially for it.

- South African President Cyril Ramaphosa declared a national state of disaster in terms of the Disaster Management Act and declared measures to be put in place that comprised imposing a travel ban on foreign nationals from high-risk countries, including Italy, Iran, South Korea, Spain, Germany, the United States, the United Kingdom, and China; performing high-intensity screening on travellers from medium-risk countries, such as Portugal, Hong Kong, and Singapore, as well as testing and isolation for South African citizens returning from high-risk countries; closing 35 of the 72 land, sea, and airports of entry; the prohibition of gatherings of more than 100 people; the closing schools from 18 March, 2020, until mid-April 2020; and the suspension of visits to correctional centres (prisons and rehabilitation facilities) for 30 days.
- The Panamanian government began to enforce the temporary closure of all businesses where large (over 50) numbers of people may gather, including pubs, cinemas, grills, casinos, gyms, convention centres and stadiums. Supermarkets may only have up to 50 customers inside at any given time, with ingress being regulated. Activities (like parties and weddings) are banned from having over 50 people present at any given time, and violations are punishable with forceful termination of the activity and a fine. The government also banned people from visiting beaches and other similar places (like large rivers).
- Several fashion companies, including Nike, Lululemon Athletica, Under Armour and Gap Inc., have announced

store closures in the United States and other countries to control COVID-19.

- Akrotiri and Dhekelia bases in Cyprus announced the first 2 cases among British military personnel.
- The Bahamas confirmed their first case, a person with no recent travel history.
- Brunei confirmed 10new cases, bringing the total number to 50.
- Bulgaria confirmed 8 new cases, bringing the total number to 51.
- Cambodia confirmed 4 new cases, bringing the total to 12.
- Finland ceased testing for people returning from trips abroad and all of the people suffering flu symptoms in the country. The tests are reserved for health professionals only.
- Guam confirmed its first 3 cases, 2 people who arrived from Manila and one other person with no recent travel history.
- Indonesia confirmed 21 more cases, bringing the total number to 117. Among the new diagnoses included North Sulawesi and Yogyakarta's first cases.
- Ireland confirmed 40 new cases, the largest to date. 169 total confirmed cases and 2 deaths. The government requested all pubs and bars to close permanently from midnight, in advance of the then-upcoming 17 March Saint Patricks Day public holiday.
- Italy confirmed 3,590 more cases, bringing the total number to 24,747. The country also recorded 368 new deaths, bringing the total number to 1,809. This was the largest death rate in a day for a country since the pandemic started. In addition, Vittorio Gregotti, the Italian architect that

designed the 1992 Barcelona Summer Olympics stadium, died at 92.

- Malaysia confirmed 190 new cases, bringing the total number to 428. Most of these cases were linked to a gathering in Kuala Lumpur.
- Moldova confirmed 11 new cases, bringing the total number to 23.
- New Zealand confirmed 2 new cases, a Wellington man and a Danish woman, bringing the total to 8.
- Saudi Arabia confirmed 15 new cases, bringing the total number to 118
- Singapore confirmed 14 new cases, bringing the total number to 226. This was the highest number of new cases in the country in a single day.
- South Korea confirmed 76 new cases and 3 new deaths, bringing the total to 8,162 and 75, respectively.
- Sri Lanka confirmed 8 more cases, bringing the total to 19. There were 18 active cases with 1 recovered case.
- Panama confirmed several new cases, bringing the total number to 55.
- Thailand confirmed 32 more cases, bringing the total number to 114.
- Turkey confirmed 12 more cases, bringing the total number to 18.
- The United Kingdom confirmed 232 new cases, bringing the total number to 1,372. 14 more deaths were reported, bringing the total to 35.
- The Foreign and Commonwealth Office advises against all but essential travel to Spain.

- The FCO advises against all but essential travel to the United States due to the restrictions imposed in response to the pandemic.
- Health Secretary Matt Hancock says that every UK resident over the age of 70 will be told “within the coming weeks” to self-isolate for “a very long time” to shield them from coronavirus.
- The government announces plans to hold daily televised press conferences to update the public on the fight against the coronavirus pandemic, starting on Monday, 16 March.
- London’s Old Vic becomes the first West End theatre to cancel a performance because of the pandemic when it ends its run of Samuel Beckett’s Endgame two weeks early.
- The Foreign and Commonwealth Office advises against all but essential travel to Spain.

- The FCO advises against all but essential travel to the United States due to the restrictions imposed in response to the pandemic.
- Health Secretary Matt Hancock says that every UK resident over the age of 70 will be told “within the coming weeks” to self-isolate for “a very long time” to shield them from coronavirus.
- The government announces plans to hold daily televised press conferences to update the public on the fight against the coronavirus pandemic, starting on Monday, 16 March.
- London’s Old Vic becomes the first West End theatre to cancel a performance because of the pandemic when it ends its run of Samuel Beckett’s Endgame two weeks early.

- The United States confirmed 669 new cases, bringing the total number to 3,485. 5 more deaths were reported, bringing the total number to 65.
- Uzbekistan confirmed its first case, a citizen who had returned from France.
- Vietnam confirmed 4 additional cases, bringing the total number to 57.

16 March

- Benin confirmed its first case, a 49-year-old man who had travelled to Belgium and Burkina Faso.
- Bulgaria confirmed 2 new cases, bringing the total number to 53. Bulgaria later confirmed 9 more cases, bringing the final total to 62.
- Costa Rica confirmed 40 cases.
- Cyprus confirmed 13 new cases, taking the total to 46.
- Egypt confirmed 40 new cases, taking the total to 166. It also confirmed 2 additional deaths.
- France confirmed that cases had risen to 6,633 with 148 deaths.
- Germany's cases rose to 7,272 with 17 deaths.
- Greece confirmed 21 new cases for a total of 352.
- Greenland confirmed its first case.
- Guatemala confirmed 5 more cases, bringing the total to 6 and the first death in the country from the virus.
- Indonesia confirmed 17 more cases, 134 in total.
- Iran's cases rose to 13,938, with its death toll rising by 129 to 853. The deaths included Hashem Bathaie Golpayenagi, Grand Ayatollah and a representative of the Tehran Province in Iran's Assembly of Experts.

- Ireland confirmed 54 new cases, the largest to date. 223 total confirmed cases and 2 deaths.
- Italy's confirmed cases rose to 27,980 and deaths to 2,158. This total included 3,233 new cases and 349 new deaths.
- Jordan confirmed 4 new cases, taking its total to 15.
- Kuwait confirmed 11 new cases, taking the total to 123.
- Liberia confirmed its first case.
- Malaysia announced another 125 cases, taking it to a total of 553, with many of the new cases linked to a recent religious festival in the country.
- Moldova announced another 6 cases, taking its total to 29.
- Oman confirmed 2 additional cases, raising the total to 24.
- Qatar reported 64 new cases taking it to 401.
- Singapore confirmed 17 more cases, bringing the total number to 243. This was the biggest spike of new cases in a single day.
- Somalia confirmed its first case.
- South Korea confirmed 74 new cases, bringing the total to 8,236.
- Spain reported 9,942 cases and 342 deaths.
- Sri Lanka confirmed 11 more cases, bringing the total to 29.
- Tanzania confirmed its first case.
- Thailand confirms 33 new cases, bringing the total to 147.
- Turkey announced that the number of cases had risen to 47, with 29 new cases confirmed.
- The United Kingdom confirmed a total of 1,543 positive tests, up from 1,372.
- The UK death toll from the pandemic reaches 55, with the number of cases of the illness passing 1,500.

- Prime Minister Boris Johnson advises everyone in the UK against "non-essential" travel and contact with others to curb coronavirus, as well as to work from home if possible and avoid visiting social venues such as pubs, clubs or theatres. Pregnant women, people over the age of 70 and those with certain health conditions are urged to consider the advice "particularly important", and will be asked to self-isolate within days. The Department for Digital, Culture, Media & Sport states, "it is advised that large gatherings should not take place".
- The UK government issues a call for businesses to support the supply of ventilators and ventilator components; the NHS has access to 8,175 ventilators, but it is thought that up to 30,000 may be needed.
- The BBC delays its planned changes to TV licences for the over-75s from June to August because of the pandemic.
- Theatres in London, as well as elsewhere around the UK, close following Boris Johnson's advice that people should avoid such venues.
- The United States confirmed 974 new cases, bringing the total number to 4,459. 22 more deaths were reported, bringing the total number to 87.
- Ukraine confirmed 2 new cases: two women, one of whom recently returned from Italy. Later in the day, 2 more cases were confirmed, bringing the total to 7.
- Vietnam confirmed 4 additional cases, bringing the total number to 61.
- Actor Idris Elba tests positive for COVID-19. This comes after Tom Hanks and Rita Wilson both announced positive results last week.

- The Chinese National Bureau of Statistics releases figures showing that industrial output fell 13.5%, fixed asset investment fell 24.5%, private sector investment fell 26.4%, and retail sales shrank 20.5% in January–February 2020 as a result of the coronavirus pandemic.
- The United Nations World Health Organization issued advice on 'Five Things You Should Know Now about the COVID-19 Pandemic' and on safeguarding mental health during the pandemic, while WHO Director-General Tedros Adhanom Ghebreyesus "blasted" the slow virus testing response and stressed, "Once again, our message is: test, test, test."
- The Australian Border Force suspends the removal operations of New Zealand citizens to New Zealand up to March 30, effective midnight 16 March.
- Canadian Prime Minister Justin Trudeau announces restrictions to entry into Canada, allowing only Canadian and American citizens, permanent residents, the closest family of citizens, diplomats, and aircrew. Any Canada-bound passengers showing symptoms of COVID-19 would be refused to board. Saskatchewan Premier Scott Moe announces the closure of all primary and secondary schools in the province effective 20 March.
- Costa Rican Health Minister Daniel Salas confirmed 41 cases of coronavirus. The government also decreed a state of national emergency. Classes were suspended in all public and private schools and colleges until April 4. Borders would be closed starting Wednesday, 18 March and last until April 12. Costa Ricans and permanent residents have no entry restrictions. Those entering must remain in quarantine for at least 14 days.

- Guatemalan President Alejandro Giammattei announced that Guatemala will close its borders for two weeks as part of measures to contain the virus.
- Slovakian prime minister Peter Pellegrini said the government was preparing cash worth 1.2 million euros ($1.3 million) to purchase masks from a contracted Chinese supplier. He then said, "However, a dealer from Germany came there first, paid more for the shipment, and bought it."
- Malaysian Prime Minister Muhyiddin Yassin bans Malaysian citizens from going overseas and foreigners from entering Malaysia from 18 to March 31. Malaysians returning from overseas will have to go through health checks and a 14-day self-quarantine.
- Pink Dot SG, an event in support of the LGBT community in Singapore supposed to be held on June 27, is cancelled due to the pandemic the first time it did so. In its place will be a live streaming session where people can tune in.
- US President Donald J. Trump refers to COVID-19 as the "Chinese virus," drawing allegations of racism from Chinese and WHO officials.
- Also, in the United States, the annual Kentucky Derby has been rescheduled from May 2 to September 5, 2020, and this was the first time since the 1945 event took place outside of the regular May schedule.
- The UK government advises the British public to minimise all unnecessary social contact, suggesting that people should work from home if possible and avoid visiting social venues such as pubs, clubs or theatres.
- Trials by Moderna to test a potential vaccine start with 45 volunteers roped in.

- Hong Kong will impose a daily fee from 17 March for people under quarantine staying in temporary facilities to deter abuse of such areas.
- The Philippines starts imposing home quarantine measures, and starts a stay-at-home order in Luzon, with all work and transportation suspended except for essential services. These measures will last until April 13 at the minimum.
- The Malaysian state of Sawarak will issue all visitors and residents with a 14-day stay-home notice to fight the pandemic from 18 March. All official government events with more than 50 people will be cancelled until further notice. Sawarak will close all educational institutions for two weeks from 17 March, with school holidays extended for a week until March 29. All public sports facilities are also closed.
- Spain will extend its state of emergency beyond the initial 15 days, with border closures considered too.
- The Tokyo 2020 torch relay will go ahead with some ceremonies cancelled due to COVID-19.
- The Czech Republic locks down several towns in the eastern side of the country and bans the movement of people except for work and other essential activities until 24 March. This comes a day after a rule to close all restaurants and most shops for at least 10 days.
- Thailand proposed measures to tackle the virus, including the postponement of Songkran from 13 to April 15, suspending activities in universities, schools and tuition centres and closing crowded venues temporarily like boxing stadiums, cinemas and entertainment facilities. At the same time, extra compensation for healthcare staff was approved, and distribution of confiscated masks will be done.

17 March

- Barbados reported its first 2 cases, people who recently returned from the US.
- Bulgaria confirmed 5 new cases, bringing the number to 67, and then an additional 14 new cases, bringing the total number to 81.
- Brazil confirmed the first death in the country, a 62-year-old man in the state of São Paulo.
- France confirmed that 7,730 people had now tested positive with 175 deaths.
- The Gambia reported its first case.
- Hungary reported 11 new cases, bringing the total number to 50.
- Indonesia reported 38 new cases, bringing the total number to 172.
- Ireland confirmed 69 new cases, the largest to date. 292 total confirmed cases and 2 deaths.
- Italy confirmed an increase to 31,506 cases and 2,503 deaths.
- Kuwait confirmed 7 new cases, taking the total to 130.
- Malaysia reported its first 2 deaths, a 60-year-old pastor in Sarawak and a 34-year-old man from Johor who had attended a Muslim religious gathering. 120 new cases were also confirmed, bringing the total number to 673.
- Montenegro reported its first 2 cases. 1 infected was from Podgorica, and the other from Ulcinj. Montenegro was the last country in Europe without any confirmed cases.
- The Netherlands confirmed 1,705 cases and 43 deaths.

- New Zealand confirmed 4 new cases, bringing the total to 12.
- Pakistan confirmed its first death.
- Panama confirmed several new cases, bringing the total number to 86.
- The Philippines reported 45 new cases, taking the total to 187.
- Singapore confirmed 23 new cases, bringing the total number to 266. This was the highest number of new cases in the country in a single day so far.
- Sint Maarten confirmed its first case, a 26-year-old local resident who travelled to UK and Miami.
- Slovakia confirmed 25 new cases, bringing the total number to 97.
- South Korea confirmed 84 new cases and 6 new deaths, bringing the total to 8,320 and 81, respectively.
- Thailand confirmed 30 new cases, bringing the total to 177.
- Ukraine reported 7 new cases and its 2nd death, bringing the total number of cases to 14.
- The United Kingdom reported 407 new cases, with the total rising from 1,543 to 1,950.
- The Chancellor, Rishi Sunak, announces that £330bn will be made available in loan guarantees for businesses affected by the virus.
- The Foreign and Commonwealth Office advises against all non-essential international travel due to the pandemic and the border restrictions put in place by many countries in response.
- The UK government provides a £3.2million emergency support package to help rough sleepers into

accommodation. With complex physical and mental health needs, in general, homeless people are at significant risk of catching the virus.

- The BBC announces major changes to the schedule across the network. While programmes such as Politics Live, Victoria Derbyshire, The Andrew Neil Show, Newswatch, The Travel Show and HARDTalk have been suspended, others such as Newsnight and The Andrew Marr Show will continue with a smaller number of production staff. Question Time is moved to an earlier 8 pm Thursday timeslot and will be broadcast without an audience from a fixed location. Podcasts programmes Americast, Beyond Today and The Next Episode, are also suspended.
- Cinema chains Odeon, Cineworld, Vue and Picturehouse announce they will be closing all their UK outlets in response to the advice to avoid visiting such venues.
- The United States confirmed 1,676 new cases, bringing the total number to 6,135. 25 more deaths were reported, bringing the total number to 112. The Brooklyn Nets announced that four of their players had tested positive, including forward Kevin Durant.
- Vietnam confirmed 5 more cases, bringing the total number to 66.
- As Southeast Asian countries reported over 480 cases of COVID-19 and eight deaths, the World Health Organization called for countries to “act now” and urgently scale-up “aggressive” measures to address the disease.
- UN agencies, the International Organization for Migration and the UN refugee agency, UNHCR, announced they had temporarily halted resettlement travel for refugees.

- The United Nations' agency for children, UNICEF, offered advice on how parents and carers could talk to children about the coronavirus.
- New Zealand Health Minister David Clark announced that New Zealand Government will deport foreign tourists who flout government requirements to self-quarantine for two weeks. Later, Immigration New Zealand detained two foreign tourists for refusing to comply with self-quarantine requirements. That same day, Finance Minister Grant Robertson announced a NZ$12.1 billion COVID-19 coronavirus business package to aid businesses, beneficiaries, and health services affected by the COVID-19 outbreak.
- Jon Landau, the co-producer of the Avatar film sequels, announced that film production at New Zealand–based Stone Street Studios had been suspended in response to the coronavirus outbreak. However, filming will continue in Los Angeles.
- Panama banned all non-resident foreigners from entering the country. Panamanian authorities also began to use the #QUEDATEENCASA (#STAYATHOME) hashtag on social media in an attempt to convince people to stay at home in self-quarantine.
- The UEFA announced the upcoming Euro 2020 will be postponed to June 11 to July 11, 2021, marking the first time in the 60-year history of the UEFA championship that has ever been postponed.
- The upcoming 2020 French Open, the second Grand Slam tennis event of the year, announced that it will be postponed

from September 20 to October 4, 2020, in response to the coronavirus outbreak in France.

- In the US, several tourism spots, including the Statue of Liberty and Ellis Island, White House, Broadway, and Smithsonian museums, have shut down.

18 March

- Bermuda confirmed its first 2 cases.
- Bangladesh confirmed its first death.
- Costa Rica confirmed its first death.
- Djibouti confirmed its first case.
- El Salvador confirmed its first case.
- Guatemala confirmed 2 additional cases, bringing the total to 8.
- Ireland confirmed 74 new cases, the largest to date. 366 total confirmed cases and 2 deaths.
- Italy reported 4,207 new cases and 475 new deaths. The total number of cases reached 35,713, and the total death toll rose to 2,978.
- Kyrgyzstan reported its first cases, three people who had recently returned from a pilgrimage to Saudi Arabia.
- Malaysia confirmed 117 new cases, bringing the total number to 790.
- Mauritius announced its first 3 cases.
- Moldova confirmed its first death and 6 new cases, bringing the total to 36.
- Montserrat confirmed its first case, a person who visited the United Kingdom.
- New Caledonia confirmed its first 2 cases.

- New Zealand confirmed 8 new cases, bringing the total to 20.
- Nicaragua confirmed its first case, imported from Panama.
- Palestine confirms 44 cases.
- Panama confirmed several new cases, bringing the total to 109.
- Singapore confirmed 47 new cases, bringing the total number to 313. This was the highest number of new cases in the country in a single day so far.
- Slovakia confirmed its first death.
- South Korea confirmed 93 new cases and 3 new deaths, bringing the total to 8,413 and 84, respectively.
- Thailand confirmed 35 new cases, bringing the total to 212.
- The United Kingdom confirmed 676 new cases, taking it to a total of 2,626. 32 additional deaths were announced, taking the total to 104.
- Pound sterling falls below $1.18, its lowest level since 1985. Bank of England governor Andrew Bailey, commenting on the UK and wider economic situation, says: "It's obviously an emergency. I think we're living in completely unparalleled times... It's going to be a very big downturn – we know that."
- The UK death toll from coronavirus exceeds 100, with 32 new cases taking the total to 104.
- The government announces that all schools in the country will shut from the afternoon of Friday, 20 March, except for those looking after the children of key workers and vulnerable children. No exams will take place this academic year, Education Secretary Gavin Williamson confirms.
- Princess Beatrice cancels her wedding reception at Buckingham Palace and will take further advice on whether

to carry on with a private wedding ceremony, scheduled to take place on May 29.

- The 50th anniversary Glastonbury Festival is cancelled as a result of the pandemic.
- The government announces emergency legislation to bring in a ban on new evictions for three months as part of measures to help protect renters in social and private rented accommodation.
- The BBC announces that due to the coronavirus pandemic, filming on Casualty, Doctors, EastEnders, Holby City, Pobol y Cwm and River City is suspended until further notice. Weekly episodes of EastEnders will also be reduced from four to two to keep it on the air for as long as possible.
- MP Lloyd Russell-Moyle announces that he has tested positive for the virus.
- The United States confirmed 2,601 more cases, bringing the total number to 8,736. 37 more deaths were reported, bringing the total number to 149.
- Vietnam confirmed 10more cases, bringing the total number to 76.
- Zambia reported its first 2 cases.
- The Director-General of the United Nations World Health Organization United Nations announced the beginning of the first vaccine 'solidarity trial' had begun, calling it "an incredible achievement" and urging the world to maintain "the same spirit of solidarity" that had helped fight Ebola.
- The United Nations International Labour Organization released projections showing that millions of people would fall out of employment due to the pandemic and called for an internationally coordinated policy response, as had

happened in the 2008 financial crisis, to lower the impact on global unemployment significantly.

- The Eurovision Song Contest, planned to be held in Rotterdam, The Netherlands, was cancelled.
- The New Zealand Ministry of Foreign Affairs and Trade (MFAT) urged all New Zealanders travelling overseas to return home in response to the spread of the coronavirus.
- New Zealand and Australian Governments cancelled Anzac Day services scheduled to be held at Gallipoli in Turkey in response to travel restrictions and the coronavirus outbreak.
- After cases increased quickly, Singapore announced that Stay-Home Notices will apply to all travellers arriving in Singapore from 20 March. Travellers are also advised to delay travel plans, with more social distancing measures soon.
- Panama imposed a nationwide curfew, effective every day from 9 pm to 5 pm the next day. The curfew can be enforced with everyone, regardless of age, race, etc. It was imposed to prevent the spread of the virus. Panamanian president Nito Cortizo ordered the construction of a modular hospital, similar to China's purpose-built hospitals, to be completed within a month. Panama also closed its land border with Costa Rica and began to operate a Whatsapp number to allow people to consult a doctor. Panamanian authorities later began to explore the possibility of a mandatory nationwide quarantine and allowing only one person per household to buy groceries and pharmaceuticals.
- The United Kingdom announced that all schools, colleges and nurseries would be closed from 21 March until further notice - with the exception for children of "key workers" and

vulnerable children - and that A-Level and GCSE examinations in May and June would be cancelled in England and Wales.

- Several automakers, including BMW, Kia, Toyota and Honda, temporarily suspended production for several weeks in the US and Europe.
- After an indefinite postponement due to the coronavirus, the 2020 ASEAN Para Games will now be scheduled from 3 to October 9.
- South Korea will pump in more money to relieve economic pressures caused by the coronavirus to the tune of about $5 billion to $10 billion. In addition, a cap on foreign currency forward positions for local banks will be raised to 50% from the current 40% from 19 March, as well as raise the ceiling for foreign banks to 250% from the current 200%. In addition, there will be tightened border checks for all overseas travellers to stamp out potential cases.

19 March

- The UN World Health Organization Director-General reported that China had reported no new domestic cases and stated that the WHO was working to ensure the supply chain for protective equipment and tests.
- UN Secretary-General António Guterres held his first virtual press conference, stating, "more than ever before, we need solidarity, hope and the political will to see this crisis through together".
- Australian Prime Minister Scott Morrison announced that Australia would be closing its borders to all non-residents and non-Australian citizens from 9 pm on 20 March. After the

advisory, Qantas and Jetstar announced a suspension of flights from late March, with two-thirds of its employees standing down until the end-May. In Tasmania, Premier Peter Gutwein announced that all non-essential travellers arriving into the state will be required to undergo quarantine for two weeks, with spot checks to ensure compliance. The rule takes effect on 20 March at midnight.

- Royal New Zealand Returned and Services' Association cancelled all Anzac Day services scheduled for April 25. New Zealand Health Minister David Clark advised the cancellation of mass indoor events with more than 100 people with the exception of workplaces, schools, supermarkets and public transport. Prime Minister Jacinda Ardern closed New Zealand's border to non-citizens and non-residents with the exception of Samoan and Tongan citizens travelling to New Zealand for essential reasons, "essential health workers", and those seeking to enter the country for humanitarian reasons.
- Argentine President Alberto Fernández announced a mandatory quarantine, in effect from midnight on 20 March until March 31.
- Playboy magazine ceases print production in part to disruptions in its supply chain. The mayor of Boise, Idaho, Lauren McLean, orders the closure of all restaurants and bars (with the exception of those with take-out, delivery, or drive-thru options) for 30 days, effective as of 12:01 am. Friday.
- In the United States, Californian Governor Gavin Newsom issued a stay at home order for all residents of the state, with residents only allowed to leave their homes for essential purposes, coming after modelling showed a surge risk.

Earlier on, the Governor asked President Donald Trump to send a hospital ship to Los Angeles to prepare for a surge of patients. In Los Angeles, Mayor Eric Garcetti also ordered a similar stay at home order for residents there.

- The United States Department of State raised the global travel alert to "Level 4: Do Not Travel", the highest possible alert it can issue, urging Americans abroad to return immediately as well as not to travel abroad due to the pandemic. The State Department will also suspend normal visa services in most countries, with the exception being urgent travel for emergency or within 72 hours from the following day.
- Angola confirmed its first case, a Chinese businessman.
- Chad confirmed its first case, a Moroccan national who had travelled to the country from Cameroon.
- China reported no new cases of local infections but confirmed 34 new cases from overseas arrivals.
- Fiji confirmed its first case.
- Guatemala confirmed 1 additional case, raising the total to 9.

- Haiti reported its first 2 cases.
- Ireland confirmed 191 new cases, the largest to date with more than two and a half times the confirmed cases of 18 March and a third death, bringing the total number of cases to 557. Approximately 7,000 tests have been administered to date and the Minister for Health, Simon Harris, believes there will be 15,000 tests given a day starting within the next few days.
- The Isle of Man confirmed its first case, a person who recently returned from Spain.

- Italy's number of cases rose to 41,035 from a previous 35,713, up by 5,322, a faster rate of growth than the past three days. They also overtook China as the country with the most deaths, registering 3,405 dead, a rise of 427 from the day before.
- Malaysia confirmed 110 new cases, bringing the total number to 900.
- New Zealand confirmed 8 new cases, bringing the total to 28.
- Niger confirmed its first case, a local 36-year-old man who travelled a lot to Togo, Ghana, Ivory Coast and Burkina Faso due to work.
- Ibrahim Milhem confirmed 3 new cases bringing the total to 47. He said in the daily briefing that 2 cases were students returning home from France and quarantined before being in contact with anyone. The third is for a person from Nablus previously suspected of having the disease and was kept in the home, quarantine.
- Palestine confirms 3 new cases, bringing the total to 47.
- Panama reported several new cases, bringing the total number to 137.
- Pakistan confirmed 70 additional cases.
- Russia confirmed its first death.
- Singapore confirmed 32 new cases, bringing the total number to 345.
- South Korea confirmed 152 new cases and 7 new deaths, bringing the total to 8,565 and 91, respectively.
- Spain reported a large increase in cases, with 17,147 cases and 767 deaths.
- Thailand confirmed 60 new cases, bringing the total to 272.

- The United Kingdom's total of diagnosed cases rose to 3,229, an increase of 603, with the death toll rising to 144.
- The first COVID-19 death is confirmed in Northern Ireland.
- The Ministry of Defence announces the formation of the COVID Support Force, enabling the military to support public services and civilian authorities in tackling the outbreak. Two military operations are also announced: Operation Rescript, which focuses on the outbreak in the United Kingdom, and Operation Broadshare, which focuses on British military activities overseas.
- In an emergency move, the Bank of England cuts interest rates again, from 0.25% to just 0.1%. This is the lowest rate in the Bank's 325-year history.
- The government announces £1.6bn for local authorities to help with the cost of adult social care and support for the homeless, and £1.3 billion to the NHS and social care to allow up to 15,000 people to be discharged from hospital.
- The UK government no longer deems COVID-19 to be a "high consequence infectious disease" (HCID) following opinions from the UK HCID group and the Advisory Committee on Dangerous Pathogens.
- The United States confirmed 4,397 more cases, bringing the total number to 13,133. 46 more deaths were reported, bringing the total number to 195. The Denver Nuggets, Los Angeles Lakers, Philadelphia 76ers, and the Boston Celtics all reported that some of their players had tested positive for the virus. The players had not been named.
- Vietnam confirmed 9 more cases, bringing the total number to 85.

20 March

- Cape Verde confirmed its first case, a 62-year-old English tourist.
- East Timor confirmed its first case.
- Guatemala confirmed 3 additional cases, bringing the total to 12.
- Ireland confirmed 126 new cases, less than that of 19 March. 683 total confirmed cases and 3 deaths.
- Madagascar reported its first 3 cases.
- Malaysia confirmed its third death. In addition, 130 new cases were confirmed, bringing the total number to 1,030.
- New Zealand confirmed 11 new cases, bringing the total to 39.
- Palestine confirms a new case, bringing the total to 48. Authorities also report that 17 have recovered.
- Panama reported over 60 new cases, bringing the total number to 200.
- Papua New Guinea confirmed its first case.
- Singapore confirmed 40 new cases, bringing the total number to 385.
- South Korea confirmed 87 new cases and 3 new deaths, bringing the total to 8,652 and 94, respectively.
- Thailand confirmed 50 new cases, bringing the total to 322.
- Uganda confirmed its first case.
- Ukraine confirmed 15 new cases, bringing the total number to 41.
- The United Kingdom confirmed that positive test results had risen to 3,983, and there had been 177 deaths.

- Chancellor Rishi Sunak announces that the government will pay 80% of wages for employees not working, up to £2,500 a month, as part of "unprecedented" measures to protect people's jobs.
- Prime Minister Boris Johnson orders all cafes, pubs and restaurants to close from the evening of 20 March, except for take-away food, to tackle coronavirus. All the UK's nightclubs, theatres, cinemas, gyms and leisure centres are told to close "as soon as they reasonably can".
- The United States confirmed 5,630 more cases, bringing the total number to 18,763. 63 more deaths were reported, bringing the total number to 258.
- Vietnam confirmed 6 more cases, bringing the total number to 91.
- Zimbabwe confirmed its first case.

21 March

- New Zealand Prime Minister Jacinda Ardern introduces a four-level COVID-19 alert system. New Zealand is currently on Level 2, where people over the age of 70 or with compromised immune systems are encouraged to stay at home, and all non-essential domestic travel to be curtailed. Several local body councils around New Zealand in Auckland, Wellington, Christchurch, Dunedin, Lower Hutt and Porirua closed public facilities, including swimming pools, libraries, recreation centres, community centres, art galleries, and museums.
- In Australia, a human biosecurity emergency was declared by the federal government under the Biosecurity Act 2015, after a National Security Committee meeting the previous

day with state and territory governments. The Department of Health had earlier devoted a web page to the pandemic, as had the states.

- Global streaming services Netflix and YouTube reduce their video quality in the European Union to help prevent Internet gridlock as tens of millions of Europeans work at home or self-isolate.
- Disney will close the Aulani resort in Hawaii from 24 March until the end of the month to protect against the coronavirus.
- South Korea's Prime Minister Chung Sye-kyun advised the closure of religious, sports and entertainment facilities and avoiding socialising and travel for the next 15 days in a bid to control the outbreak, with penalties should rules be flouted. In addition, up to 3.8 trillion won will be provided for small businesses and the disadvantaged to tide through the crisis.
- Åland Islands confirmed their first 2 cases.
- China reports no new cases of local infections but confirms 41 new cases from overseas travellers, bringing the total number of overseas infected to 269.
- Eritrea confirmed its first case, a 39-year-old Eritrean national with permanent residence in Norway.
- Guatemala confirmed 5 new cases, bringing the total to 17.
- Indonesia confirmed 81 new cases, bringing the total to 450. The number of deaths rose by 6 to 38.
- Ireland confirmed 102 new cases, less than that of 20 March, with a total of 785 total confirmed cases and 3 deaths.
- Malaysia confirmed 5 more deaths, bringing the total to 8. Separately, 153 new cases were confirmed, bringing the total number to 1,183.

- New Zealand reported 13 new cases, bringing the total to 52.
- Palestine confirms 4 new cases, bringing the total to 52.
- The Philippines recorded 77 new cases, bringing the total number to 307.
- Singapore confirmed its first 2 deaths, a 64-year-old Indonesian man and a 75-year-old Singaporean woman. 47 new cases were later confirmed, bringing the total number to 432.
- South Korea confirmed 147 new cases and 8 new deaths, bringing the total to 8,799 and 102, respectively.
- Transnistria confirmed its first 2 cases.
- The United Kingdom confirmed that positive test results had risen to 5,018, and there had been 233 deaths.
- The UK Environment Secretary George Eustice urges shoppers to stop panic buying, as supermarkets around the UK struggle to keep up with demand. Tesco, Asda, Aldi, and Lidl are reported to have begun a recruitment drive for up to 30,000 new staff.
- The Driver and Vehicle Standards Agency announces that all pending practical and driving theory tests are to be postponed for at least three months in the case of practical tests and up to and including April 20 for theory tests. All candidates are to receive notification of when their tests are rescheduled.
- The United States confirmed 4,886 more cases, bringing the total number to 23,649. 44 more deaths were reported, bringing the total number to 302.
- Vietnam confirmed 3 more cases, bringing the total number to 94.

22 March

- China reported 39 new cases, down from 46 a day earlier. All of these cases were overseas travellers.
- Dominica confirmed its first case, a 54-year-old man who recently arrived from the United Kingdom.
- Grenada confirmed its first case, a woman who recently travelled to the UK.
- Indonesia confirmed 64 new cases, bringing the total number to 514.
- Ireland confirmed 121 new cases, more than that of 21 March, and a fourth death, with a total of 906 total confirmed cases and 4 deaths.
- Malaysia confirmed 2 more deaths, bringing the total to 10. There were also 123 new cases confirmed, bringing the total number to 1,306.
- Mozambique confirmed its first case.
- New Zealand reported 14 new cases, bringing the total to 66.
- Palestine updates the number of cases to 59.
- Romania confirmed its first death, a 67-year-old man suffering from cancer. A total of 367 cases had since been recorded.
- Singapore confirmed 23 new cases, bringing the total number to 455.
- South Korea confirmed 98 new cases and 2 new deaths, bringing the total to 8,897 and 104, respectively.
- Syria recorded its first case.
- The United Kingdom confirmed that positive test results had risen to 5,683, and there had been 281 deaths.

- The Nursing and Midwifery Council announces that more than 5,600 former nurses have registered to offer their services in the fight against coronavirus.
- Boris Johnson warns that “tougher measures” may be introduced if people do not follow government advice on social distancing.
- Downing Street confirms Foreign Secretary Dominic Raab will act in place of Prime Minister Boris Johnson if he becomes “incapacitated”.
- The press reports the UK’s virus’s youngest victim so far, an eighteen-year-old with underlying health problems.
- The British television channel ITV suspends the production of several television programmes, including Coronation Street, Emmerdale.
- ITV also announce Its daytime programmes Lorraine and Loose Women will temporarily cease live broadcasting.
- The United States confirmed 10,351 more cases, bringing the total number to 34,000. 111 more deaths were reported, bringing the total number to 413.
- Ukraine confirmed 26 more cases, bringing the total number to 73.
- Vietnam confirmed 19 more cases, bringing the total number to 113.
- In response to a rise in imported cases, the Civil Aviation Administration of China decided to divert international flights bound for Beijing to 12 designated airports for quarantine.
- The Canadian Olympic Committee and the Canadian Paralympic Committee have called for the postponement of the 2020 Tokyo Olympic Games, warning that they will not send athletes if the Games go ahead on July 24.

- India observed a 14-hour long curfew both to try and combat the coronavirus pandemic and assess the country's ability to fight the virus.
- Singapore bans all travellers starting from 23 March, 11:59 pm. This comes after a spike in imported cases of COVID-19. Only people working in essential services like healthcare services and transport will be allowed into Singapore during this time. In addition, the Singapore-Malaysia Special Working Committee has agreed to have Malaysians with work permits to continue working in Singapore. Discussions are ongoing.
- Italy said that the 680,000 face masks and ventilators it ordered from China were confiscated by Czech Republic police, who said they did so in an anti-trafficking operation. Despite acknowledging the mistake, the Czech kept 380,000 of the seized equipment in the country while sending 110,000 items to Italy as compensation.
- A stimulus vote in the United States to lessen the coronavirus impact fails to pass after falling short of the required votes. This comes after several Democrats voted against the bill due to insufficient worker protections.
- McDonald's will close their restaurants in UK and Ireland from 23 March, with Nando's following suit. Other retailers in the UK have since announced closures. In addition, Waterstones will close all stores from 23 March after staff expressed concerns over their safety.

23 March

- Belize confirmed its first case, a local resident who recently returned from Los Angeles.
- Indonesia confirmed 65 new cases, bringing the total number to 579.
- Ireland confirmed 219 new cases, the largest increase to date, and 2 deaths, with a total of 1,125 total confirmed cases and 6 deaths.
- Malaysia confirmed 4 more deaths, bringing the total to 14. There were also 212 new cases confirmed, bringing the total number to 1,518.
- Myanmar confirmed its first 2 cases.
- New Zealand confirmed 36 new cases, bringing the total number to 102.
- Panama confirmed several new cases, bringing the total number to 345. Panama also confirmed several new deaths, bringing the total number to 6.
- Singapore confirmed 54 new cases, bringing the total number to 509.
- South Korea confirmed 64 new cases and 7 new deaths, bringing the total to 8,961 and 111, respectively.
- The Turks and Caicos Islands confirmed their first case.
- The United Kingdom confirmed that positive test results had risen to 6,650, and there had been 335 deaths.
- British Prime Minister Boris Johnson announces in a televised speech that the government has implemented a stay-at-home instruction. The British public must stay at home, except for one form of exercise a day (such as jogging, walking or cycling), shopping for essential items,

meeting any medical need, providing care for a vulnerable person, or travelling to work if it cannot be done from home. All non-essential businesses are required to close. The stay-at-home instruction is to be kept under constant review, with a formal review due after three weeks.

- The government announces emergency measures to safeguard the nation's rail network, with season ticket holders given refunds if working from home and rail franchise agreements nationalised for at least six months to prevent rail companies from collapsing.
- In a televised address, Boris Johnson announces new strict rules apply to the entire United Kingdom with the aim to slow the spread of the disease by reducing transmission of the disease between different households. The British public is instructed that they must stay at home, except for certain "very limited purposes" – shopping for essential items (such as food and medicine); one form of outdoor exercise each day (such as running, walking or cycling), either alone or with others who live in the same household; for any medical need, or to provide care to a vulnerable person, and to travel to and from work where this is "absolutely necessary" and the work in question cannot be done from home. However, when these restrictions came into force on March 26, the statutory instrument for England omitted any limit on the number of exercise sessions. All non-essential shops, libraries, places of worship, playgrounds and outdoor gyms are closed, and police are given powers to enforce the measures, including the use of fines.
- Vietnam confirmed 10 more cases, bringing the total number to 123.

- The United Nations Secretary-General called for the world's first global ceasefire to support the bigger battle against COVID-19, a "common enemy that is now threatening all of humankind".
- The UN health agency, the WHO, and international football's governing body, FIFA, launched a joint campaign, 'Pass the Message to Kick Out Coronavirus', including a WhatsApp helpline.
- The International Telecommunication Union launched a new platform to assist global networks under increasing strain and facing rising demand during the pandemic to remain "safer, stronger and more connected".
- Former American film producer and convicted sex offender Harvey Weinstein tests positive for the coronavirus.
- UN-Habitat announced the impacts of the pandemic could be considerably higher on urban poor living in slums, where overcrowding could prevent handwashing and recommended measures like social distancing and self-isolation.
- The UN Children's Fund (UNICEF) and its relief partners in Syria warned that disruptions to water in the country's war-battered northeast could worsen the risks posed by the pandemic.
- In response to a spike in cases, the New Zealand Government has raised the national COVID-19 alert level to three in preparation for a nationwide lockdown that will come into effect midnight March 26. As part of the nationwide lockdown that will come into effect on March 26, the COVID-19 alert level will be raised to four. Schools, all indoor and outdoor events, most businesses, and cafes will be required

to shut down. However, essential services such as supermarkets, petrol stations, and health services will remain open. The Government also released a list of "essential services" that will be allowed to operate during the four-week lockdown.

- Former American film producer and convicted sex offender Harvey Weinstein tests positive for the coronavirus.
- Singapore announced that all arriving travellers would be required to fill up online health declaration forms before undergoing immigration clearance from March 27 as a protection measure against the coronavirus.
- Wuhan eases its two-month lockdown on residents, including allowing those from compounds deemed virus-free to leave their homes and return to work if they did not have a temperature and could provide a green code of health. Non-residents were allowed to apply to leave the city. Resumption of train services.
- The United Nations Secretary-General called for the world's first global ceasefire to support the bigger battle against COVID-19, a "common enemy that is now threatening all of humankind".
- The UN health agency, the WHO, and international football's governing body, FIFA, launched a joint campaign, 'Pass the Message to Kick Out Coronavirus', including a WhatsApp helpline.
- The International Telecommunication Union launched a new platform to assist global networks under increasing strain and facing rising demand during the pandemic to remain "safer, stronger and more connected".

- UN-Habitat announced the impacts of the pandemic could be considerably higher on urban poor living in slums, where overcrowding could prevent handwashing and recommended measures like social distancing and self-isolation.
- The UN Children's Fund (UNICEF) and its relief partners in Syria warned that disruptions to water in the country's war-battered northeast could worsen the risks posed by the pandemic.
- In response to a spike in cases, the New Zealand Government has raised the national COVID-19 alert level to three in preparation for a nationwide lockdown that will come into effect midnight March 26. As part of the nationwide lockdown that will come into effect on March 26, the COVID-19 alert level will be raised to four. Schools, all indoor and outdoor events, most businesses, and cafes will be required to shut down. However, essential services such as supermarkets, petrol stations, and health services will remain open. The Government also released a list of "essential services" that will be allowed to operate during the four-week lockdown.
- Singapore announced that all arriving travellers would be required to fill up online health declaration forms before undergoing immigration clearance from March 27 as a protection measure against the coronavirus.
- The International Olympic Committee, International Paralympic Committee and the Tokyo 2020 Organising Committee announce that the 2020 Tokyo Olympic Games and the 2020 Tokyo Paralympic Games will be postponed to a date beyond 2020 but no later than summer 2021. Marking

the first time in the 124-year history of the Olympic Games that has ever been postponed rather than cancelled.

- United Nations Secretary-General António Guterres welcomed the Group of 20 industrialized powers (G20) decision to convene a virtual emergency summit on the pandemic and recommended three areas for discussion.
- The United Nations High Commissioner for Human Rights called for an easing of sanctions against countries under sanctions, like Iran, to “allow their medical systems to fight the disease and limit its global spread”.
- United Nations Special Envoy to Syria Geir Pedersen called for a country-wide truce to fight the pandemic.
- The New Zealand Government has extended all temporary visas until late September 2020, allowing travellers whose visas expire before April 1 to remain if they are unable to leave the country. Foreign Minister Winston Peters has urged New Zealanders stranded overseas to consider sheltering “in place” due to travel restrictions. Peters has estimated there were 80,000 New Zealanders stranded overseas, 17,000 of whom have registered with the Ministry of Foreign Affairs and Trade’s “Safe Travel” programme.
- Poland’s government announced further restrictions on people leaving their homes and on public gatherings to further limit the spread of SARS-CoV-2 infections. The new limits constrained gatherings by default to a maximum of two people (with an exception for families); an exception for religious gatherings, such as mass in the Catholic Church, funerals and marriages in which five participants and the person conducting the ceremony were allowed to gather; and an exception for workplaces. Non-essential travel was prohibited, with the exception of travelling to work or home,

SARS-CoV-2 control related activities, or "necessary everyday activities". Everyday activities qualifying as "necessary" included shopping, buying medicines, visiting doctors, walking dogs, jogging, cycling and walking, provided that no more than two people participate and contact with others was avoided. The restrictions were initially defined for the period from March 25 to April 11 inclusive.

- India's prime minister Narendra Modi announced a total lockdown, effective from midnight on March 25.
- Panama extended its curfew to 12 hours in length, starting at 5 pm and ending at 5 am of the next day. The Panamanian government also announced fines of up to US$100,000 for those who refuse to stay in self-quarantine after being diagnosed. Several businesses began to cover their glass windows with plywood panels and/or bricks to prevent looting. The first of several Lufthansa 747-400s landed in the Tocumen International Airport to repatriate 700 German tourists. Later in the day, the Panamanian government established a nationwide lockdown until further notice, with citizens only allowed to go outside for 3 hours a day, with the allowed exit time depending on their last ID or passport number digit. So, for example, if one's ID number ends in 7, that person will be allowed to go outside at 6:30 am and will have to return home at 9:30 am. Citizens over 60 will only be allowed to be outside from 11:00 am to 1:00 pm.
- The 2020 Rock & Roll Hall of Fame induction ceremony was postponed to November 2020.
- Chinese Premier Li Keqiang reports that the spread of domestically transmitted cases has been basically blocked, and the outbreak has been controlled in China.

24 March

- China reports 78 newly confirmed cases, including 74 imported cases, bringing the total number of imported cases to 427. In addition, the NHC reported 7 deaths in Wuhan.
- Easter Island reports its first case.
- Indonesia confirmed 107 new cases, the largest increase it has had to date, bringing the total number of cases to 686.
- Ireland confirmed 204 new cases, fewer than that of 23 March, and 1 death, giving a total of 1,329 total confirmed cases and 7 deaths.
- Italy confirmed 5,249 new cases and 743 new deaths, taking the country to a total of 69,176 cases and 6,820 deaths.
- Laos reported its first 2 cases.
- Libya confirmed its first case.
- Malaysia reported 106 new cases, bringing the total number to 1,624. Malaysia also reported 1 death, bringing the total number of deaths to 15.
- New Caledonia reported 2 new cases, bringing the total to 9.
- New Zealand confirmed 40 new cases and started including probable cases in its count. The inclusion brings New Zealand's total to 155.
- Palestine reports a new case, bringing the total number to 60.
- Panama confirmed 98 new cases, bringing the total number to 443, and 2 deaths, bringing the total number to 8.
- Singapore confirmed 49 new cases, bringing the total number to 558.
- South Korea confirmed 76 new cases and 9 new deaths, bringing the total to 9,037 and 120, respectively.

- The United Kingdom confirmed that positive test results had risen to 8,077, and there had been 422 deaths. The 8,077 cases included 6,843 in England, 584 in Scotland, 478 in Wales and 172 in Northern Ireland.
- The UK records its highest number of coronavirus deaths in one day, after a further 87 people die across the country, bringing the total to 422.
- For the first time, all of the UK's mobile networks send out a government text alert. The message reads: "GOV.UK CORONAVIRUS ALERT. New rules are in force now: you must stay at home. More info and exemptions at gov.uk/coronavirus Stay at home. Protect the NHS. Save lives."
- Health Secretary Matt Hancock announces the government will open a temporary hospital, the NHS Nightingale Hospital at the ExCeL London, to add extra critical care capacity in response to coronavirus pandemic.
- The Church of England closes all its buildings.
- BBC News announces that it is delaying plans to cut 450 news jobs due to the pressure of covering the coronavirus pandemic.
- The International Olympic Committee, International Paralympic Committee and the Tokyo 2020 Organising Committee announce that the 2020 Tokyo Olympic Games and the 2020 Tokyo Paralympic Games will be postponed to a date beyond 2020 but no later than summer 2021. Marking the first time in the 124-year history of the Olympic Games that has ever been postponed rather than cancelled.
- United Nations Secretary-General António Guterres welcomed the Group of 20 industrialised powers (G20)

decision to convene a virtual emergency summit on the pandemic and recommended three areas for discussion.

- The United Nations High Commissioner for Human Rights called for an easing of sanctions against countries under sanctions, like Iran, to "allow their medical systems to fight the disease and limit its global spread".
- United Nations Special Envoy to Syria Geir Pedersen called for a country-wide truce to fight the pandemic.
- The New Zealand Government has extended all temporary visas until late September 2020, allowing travellers whose visas expire before 1 April to remain if they are unable to leave the country. Foreign Minister Winston Peters has urged New Zealanders stranded overseas to consider sheltering "in place" due to travel restrictions. Peters has estimated there were 80,000 New Zealanders stranded overseas, 17,000 of whom have registered with the Ministry of Foreign Affairs and Trade's "Safe Travel" programme.
- On 24 March, Poland's government announced further restrictions on people leaving their homes and on public gatherings to further limit the spread of SARS-CoV-2 infections. The new limits constrained gatherings by default to a maximum of two people (with an exception for families); an exception for religious gatherings, such as mass in the Catholic Church, funerals and marriages in which five participants and the person conducting the ceremony were allowed to gather; and an exception for workplaces. Non-essential travel was prohibited, with the exception of travelling to work or home, SARS-CoV-2 control related activities, or "necessary everyday activities". Everyday activities qualifying as "necessary" included shopping, buying medicines, visiting doctors, walking dogs, jogging,

cycling and walking, provided that no more than two people participate and contact with others was avoided. The restrictions were initially defined for the period from 25 March to 11 April inclusive.

- India's prime minister Narendra Modi announced a total lockdown, effective from midnight on 25 March.
- Panama extended its curfew to 12 hours in length, starting at 5 pm and ending at 5 am of the next day. The Panamanian government also announced fines of up to US$100,000 for those who refuse to stay in self-quarantine after being diagnosed. Several businesses began to cover their glass windows with plywood panels and/or bricks to prevent looting. The first of several Lufthansa 747-400s landed in the Tocumen International Airport to repatriate 700 German tourists. Later in the day, the Panamanian government established a nationwide lockdown until further notice, with citizens only allowed to go outside for 3 hours a day, with the allowed exit time depending on their last ID or passport number digit. So, for example, if one's ID number ends in 7, that person will be allowed to go outside at 6:30 am and will have to return home at 9:30 am. Citizens over 60 will only be allowed to be outside from 11:00 am to 1:00 pm.
- The 2020 Rock & Roll Hall of Fame induction ceremony was postponed to November 2020.

25 March

- The British Virgin Islands reported their first 2 cases.
- Guinea-Bissau reported its first 2 cases.

- Ireland confirmed 235 new cases, the largest increase to date, and 2 deaths, giving a total of 1,564 total confirmed cases and 9 deaths.
- Latvia reported 24 new cases, among them the first 5 untraceable cases, raising the total number to 221.
- Malaysia confirmed 4 more deaths, bringing the total to 19. There were also 172 new cases confirmed, bringing the total number to 1,796.
- Mali reported its first 2 cases.
- New Zealand reported 50 new cases, including probable cases, bringing the total number of confirmed and probable cases to 205.
- Palestine confirms its first death. Authorities also confirm 2 news cases, bringing the total to 62.
- Peru confirmed 2 deaths, bringing the death toll to 9.
- Saint Kitts and Nevis reported its first 2 cases.
- Singapore confirmed 73 new cases, bringing the total number to 631.
- South Korea confirmed 100 new cases and 6 new deaths, bringing the total to 9,137 and 126, respectively.
- The United Kingdom confirmed that positive test results had risen to 9,529, and there had been 463 deaths.
- HRH Charles, Prince of Wales, heir apparent to the British throne, tests positive for the COVID-19 virus.
- Parliament shuts down for a month.
- British Transport Police deploys 500 officers to patrol the UK's rail network in an effort to discourage non-essential journeys. New measures are also introduced on the London Underground to reduce passenger numbers.

- British diplomat Steven Dick, deputy ambassador to Hungary, dies in Budapest after contracting the virus.
- The police will be given the power to use "reasonable force" to enforce the lockdown regulations.
- The first two working NHS doctors die from COVID-19 on the same day, one a GP, the other a surgeon.
- The Contingencies Fund Act 2020 receives royal assent.
- Hubei's Health Commission eliminates all travel restrictions in and out of the province, with the exception of Wuhan.
- The United Nations launched a major humanitarian appeal and $2 billion coordinated global humanitarian response plan to aid the most affected and most vulnerable countries and prevent COVID-19 from "circling back around the globe".
- Echoing the 23 March appeal to warring parties across the globe for an immediate global ceasefire, United Nations Secretary-General António Guterres called on those fighting in Yemen to cease hostilities and increase efforts to counter a potential COVID-19 outbreak.
- The United Nations High Commissioner for Human Rights, Michelle Bachelet, urged quick action by governments to prevent COVID-19 from devastating prisons and other places of detention.
- The World Bank and IMF called for a global debt payment suspension in light of the COVID-19 pandemic.
- In response to a sharp spike in coronavirus cases to 205, New Zealand's Civil Defence Minister Peeni Henare declared a national state of emergency lasting seven days, which may be extended. This supplements the Coronavirus alert level 4 rating that comes into action at 11:59 pm.

- Diamond Comics Distributors, a major distributor for most major US publishers, including Marvel Comics and DC Comics, announces that it would stop shipping new comics to stores commencing 1 April.
- Diamond's sister company Alliance Game Distributors also adopted a similar policy, shutting down both its distribution systems the previous day.
- Egypt begins disinfection on the Giza pyramid complex.

26 March

- Anguilla reported its first 2 cases.
- Iran reported 2,389 new cases and 175 deaths within the last 24 hours, bringing Iran's total death toll to 2,234.
- Ireland confirmed 255 new cases, the largest increase to date, and 10 deaths, the largest jump in deaths to date (previously 2 deaths in one day), giving a total of 1,819 total confirmed cases and 19 deaths.
- Malaysia confirmed 4 more deaths, bringing the total to 23. There were also 235 new cases confirmed, bringing the total number to 2,031.
- New Zealand reported 78 confirmed and probable cases, bringing the total to 283. A total of 27 people have recovered from the virus.
- Palestine confirmed 13 new cases, bringing the total to 86.
- Panama confirmed 116 new cases, bringing the total to 674, and confirmed a new death, bringing the total to 9.
- Russia confirmed 182 cases, bringing the total to 842.
- Singapore confirmed 52 new cases, bringing the total number to 683.

- South Korea confirmed 104 new cases and 5 new deaths, bringing the total to 9,241 and 131, respectively.
- Spain confirmed a further 655 deaths, taking the country's death toll to 4,000.
- The UK Government announces that some self-employed will be paid 80% of profits, up to £2,500 a month, to help them cope during the economic crisis triggered by COVID-19.
- At 8 pm, millions of people around the country take part in a "Clap for Carers" tribute, applauding the NHS and other care workers.
- The Health Protection (Coronavirus, Restrictions) (England) Regulations 2020 (SI 350) (the 'Lockdown Regulations') come into effect, significantly extending the range of businesses that are required by law to close with immediate effect, including all retail businesses not on an approved list. These regulations also include significant restrictions on freedom of movement: "no person may leave the place where they are living without reasonable excuse".
- The number of UK coronavirus deaths increases by more than 100 in a day for the first time, rising to 578, while a total of 11,568 have tested positive for the virus.
- The National Theatre launches National Theatre at Home, a two-month programme whereby a different production from its archives will be streamed for free each week. The project begins with Richard Bean's comedy One Man, Two Guvnors, featuring James Corden.
- The United Nations Secretary-General emphasised to world leaders at the G20 virtual summit that a sustainable global economy must arise once the COVID-19 pandemic is

reversed, as the G20 committed to injecting over $5 trillion into the global economy to counteract the effects of the COVID-19 pandemic.

- The United Nations Conference on Trade and Development (UNCTAD) reported via its latest Investment Trends Monitor report that foreign direct investment flows were likely to drop by 30 to 40 per cent during 2020 and into 2021, reflecting a far more serious economic situation than initially projected.
- A group of 42 experts representing nearly every independent rights specialist working within the United Nations Human Rights Council-mandated system stressed that in addition to public health and emergency measures to counter the COVID-19 pandemic, countries had to respect the fundamental individual human rights.
- The head of the United Nations Children's Fund, UNICEF, highlighted that life-saving vaccinations must not "fall victim" to the COVID-19 pandemic.
- Jeanine Hennis-Plasschaert, the United Nations Secretary-General's Special Representative for Iraq, issued a message urging citizens to support government efforts to halt further spread of COVID-19.
- A European Commission summit is held, during which the heads of government of Spain, Italy and other European Union countries argue for the issuance of joint debt to help their economies recover from the crisis (dubbed "corona bonds"), which is opposed by Germany and the Netherlands.
- India announces a 1.7 trillion INR economic stimulus plan to help millions of people affected by a nationwide lockdown. The Minister of Finance Nirmala Sitharaman also confirmed that the Indian Government plans to distribute five kilograms

of staple food grains like wheat or rice for each person free of charge in order to feed about 800 million poor people over the next three months.

- Russia halts all international air traffic with the exception of flights repatriating Russian citizens back to the country. Moscow closes all restaurants, bars, parks, and shops but allows grocery stores and pharmacies to remain open.
- Panama began to limit the number of people that may attend a funeral. Now only five attendees will be allowed per funeral. The Panama Metro closed some of its stations due to a reduction in ridership.
- The United States Senate passes a US$2.2 trillion emergency relief package, which is to date the biggest rescue deal in US history. US President Trump pledges that the United States would cooperate with China in combating the COVID-19 pandemic, signalling a fresh détente between Washington and Beijing after weeks of rising tensions. That same day, following a video call summit with other G20 leaders, Trump stated that the US was cooperating with international allies to stop the spread of the coronavirus and to increase information sharing.
- The United Arab Emirates imposes a night curfew and begins disinfection across streets.
- South Korea will require all long-term visitors arriving from the United States to self-isolate for two weeks, taking effect from 27 March. A rule that requires long-term visitors from Europe to undergo compulsory tests and a two-week quarantine took effect the same day.

27 March

- China reported 67 new imported cases, bringing the total number of infected cases to 81,285.
- Ireland confirmed 302 new cases, the largest increase to date, and 3 deaths. This gave a total of 2,121 confirmed cases and 22 deaths. The government issued strict guidelines beginning at midnight where people must stay at home with specific exceptions such as essential employees for essential businesses. Notably, residents would be allowed to leave solely for going to the grocery store, pharmacy, for a medical appointment, or for exercise with a maximum 2 km radius from their house where social distancing must be practised and exercise time must be kept short.
- Italy confirmed a new highest single-day death toll with 919 deaths (surpassing Spain's total released earlier in the day), increasing the country's total to 9,134. Overall confirmed cases of infection rose by 5,959 to 86,498.
- Malaysia confirmed its 24th death, a 35-year-old man who travelled to Indonesia earlier in the month. Another 2 deaths were later confirmed, bringing the total to 26. There were also 130 new cases confirmed, bringing the total number to 2,161.
- New Zealand confirmed 85 new confirmed and probable cases, bringing the total to 368.
- Palestine confirms 7 new cases, bringing the total to 91.
- Panama confirmed 112 new cases, bringing the total to 786, and confirmed 5 new deaths, bringing the total to 14.
- Singapore confirmed 49 new cases, bringing the total number to 732.

- South Africa confirmed its first death at the same time as when the lockdown in the country began.
- South Korea confirmed 91 new cases and 8 new deaths, bringing the total to 9,332 and 139, respectively.
- Spain recorded the highest single-day death toll worldwide to date, with 769 deaths. There were now 64,059 confirmed cases, up from 56,188.
- The United States confirmed at least 101,242 cases based on figures collated by Johns Hopkins University, overtaking China (81,782) and Italy (80,589). The US death toll surpassed 1,500.
- The UK Prime Minister Boris Johnson and Health Secretary Matt Hancock both test positive for COVID-19. Johnson will self-isolate in 10 Downing Street, and Hancock is self-isolating at home whilst working.
- Chief Medical Adviser Chris Whitty and Labour Party MP Angela Rayner, the Shadow Secretary of State for Education, also confirm they have been suffering symptoms and are self-isolating.
- Leon Restaurants sets up the "Feed NHS" initiative to deliver 5,600 free meals a day to NHS critical care staff at London hospitals.
- The 2020 Cambridge Folk Festival is cancelled.
- Dominic Cummings, Johnson's lead adviser, drives 250 miles to Durham with his wife and child. When this came to public notice in May, he explained that "there was nobody in London that he could reasonably ask to look after his child".
- News reports citing a government document reported that a 57-year-old woman, who tested positive for the coronavirus disease on 10 December 2019 and was described in The

Wall Street Journal on 6 20 March20, may have been patient zero in the coronavirus pandemic.

- The first oil refinery shutdowns in India and Europe were announced while global refinery runs drop in response to plunging demand as countries worldwide implement lockdowns.
- Baskut Tuncak, United Nations Special Rapporteur on the implications for human rights of the environmentally sound management and disposal of hazardous substances and wastes, called on states and business leaders to ensure that 'health care heroes' working on the frontlines receives adequate protective equipment.
- Executive Director of the United Nations Population Fund, Natalia Kanem, pledged support for those suffering from invisible impacts of the pandemic, including women and girls with disrupted access to life-saving sexual and reproductive health care.
- In Colombia, President Iván Duque announced the extension of the national quarantine in April.
- Malaysian Prime Minister Muhyiddin Yassin announces the RM 250 billion Prihatin stimulus package to help people, businesses and the economy to weather the effects of the COVID-19 pandemic. The Prihatin stimulus package consists of RM128 billion for welfare assistance, RM100 billion to support small and medium businesses, RM2 billion to strengthen the country's economy, and an RM20 billion stimulus package that was announced previously.
- Japan's professional basketball league B.League cancels the remainder of the season in response to the coronavirus pandemic.

- British Prime Minister Boris Johnson and Health Secretary Matt Hancock test positive for COVID-19.
- Shenzhen Bioeasy Biotechnology began to replace the defective test kits it had sent to Spain.
- The United States House of Representatives pass the Coronavirus Aid, Relief, and Economic Security Act via voice vote, and was signed by Donald Trump afterwards. The USNS Mercy arrives in Los Angeles for assistance. Fanatics, Nike, Under Armour and others began to produce face masks.
- The government of the Republic of Ireland announced restrictions on movement to be in place until 12 April.
- South Korea requires all airlines to check the temperatures of passengers arriving into the country from 30 March, with anyone having a temperature at 37.5 degrees Celsius not allowed into the country.
- In response to a rise in imported cases, the Chinese Government announces that it will close China's borders to foreigners starting on 28 March in an effort to stop imported cases of the coronavirus from entering China. The ban also includes foreigners with visas and residency permits. Other measures include restricting both Chinese and foreign airlines to a single route and destination a week.

28 March

- Ireland confirmed 294 new cases and 14 deaths, the largest death toll to date. This gave a total of 2,415 confirmed cases and 36 deaths.
- Italy surpassed 10,000 deaths attributed to the virus.

- Malaysia confirmed a new death, bringing the total to 27. There were also 159 new cases confirmed, bringing the total number to 2,320.
- New Zealand reported 83 new cases, including 78 confirmed and 5 probable cases, bringing the total to 451.
- Palestine confirmed 6 new cases, bringing the total to 97.
- Panama confirmed 115 new cases, bringing the total to 901, and confirmed 3 new deaths, bringing the total to 17.
- Singapore confirmed 70 new cases, bringing the total number to 802.
- South Korea confirmed 146 new cases and 5 new deaths, bringing the total to 9,478 and 144, respectively.
- The United Kingdom confirmed that positive test results had risen to 17,089, and there had been 260 new deaths, increasing the total to 1,019.
- Alister Jack, the Secretary of State for Scotland, announces that he is self-isolating after experiencing coronavirus symptoms.
- A further 260 deaths take the number of fatalities past 1,000, with a total of 1,019 deaths having occurred so far; 17,089 people have tested positive.
- At 11 pm, new regulations come into force in Northern Ireland, giving authorities the power to force businesses to close, and impose fines on them if they refuse, as well as on people leaving their homes without a “reasonable excuse”. The measures introduced by the Northern Ireland Executive bring Northern Ireland into line with the rest of the UK.
- Nickolay Mladenov, the United Nations Special Coordinator for the Middle East Peace Process, praised the coordination

between the Israeli and Palestine authorities for their reaction to the pandemic.

- After 63 new cases are confirmed in the United Arab Emirates, the country announced that disinfection and curfew will be extended to 5 April.
- In Nicaragua, many citizens began to express anger and disappointment at their government for not doing enough to control the virus.
- In the United States, the FDA authorised the emergency use of a quick COVID-19 testing kit developed by Abbott laboratories.
- Clashes break out on a bridge connecting Hubei and the neighbouring Jiangxi province when Hubei travellers attempt to storm a Jiangxi checkpoint. This clash was the result of a disagreement between police from both provinces over how to verify people from Hubei allowed to enter Jiangxi. In response, provincial authorities have announced that checkpoints will be removed, and no special documentation would be needed to cross.

29 March

- Ireland confirmed 200 new cases and 10 deaths. This gives a total of 2,615 confirmed cases and 46 deaths.
- Israel reported 628 new cases, bringing the total to 4,247. The country also reported three new deaths, bringing the total number to 15.
- Malaysia reported 7 new deaths, bringing the total to 34. The country also confirmed 150 new cases, bringing the total number to 2,470.

- New Zealand reported 60 new confirmed and 3 new probable cases, bringing the total number of confirmed and probable cases to 514. The country also recorded its first death.
- Palestine confirms 9 new cases, bringing the total to 108.
- Panama confirmed 88 new cases, bringing the total to 989, and confirmed 7 new deaths, bringing the total to 24.
- Singapore confirmed its third death. At the same time, 42 new cases were confirmed, bringing the total to 844.
- South Korea confirmed 105 new cases and 8 new deaths, bringing the total to 9,583 and 152, respectively.
- The government will send a letter to 30 million households warning that things will "get worse before they get better" and that tighter restrictions could be implemented if necessary. The letter will also be accompanied by a leaflet setting out the government's lockdown rules along with health information.
- Dr Jenny Harries, England's deputy chief medical officer, suggests it could be six months before life can return to "normal" because social distancing measures will have to be reduced "gradually".
- The first NHS nurse dies of COVID-19.
- The United Nations donated 250,000 face masks to New York City health workers.
- Malaysian Minister of Defence Ismail Sabri Yaakob confirmed that 649 people had been detained as of yesterday, while 73 people had pleaded guilty to various offences, including illegal public gatherings, obstructing public officials, and breaking through police blockades.

- The New Zealand Police launch a new online form on their website for people to report COVID-19 Alert Level 4 restriction breaches, including isolation breaches and businesses operating illegally.
- Panama began to make its own reagents for COVID-19 test kits.
- The Argentine government announced the extension of the mandatory nationwide quarantine, originally intended to end on 31 March, until mid-April.
- South Korea makes a two-week quarantine mandatory for all travellers, including those arriving for short-term visits, which will take effect from 1 April. Foreigners will also be required to pay for costs incurred during quarantine.
- According to a Guardian report, Western and African expatriates have encountered increased racial hostility and discrimination in response to a shift in recent cases reported in China from local to "imported" ones. Hostility towards foreigners has taken the form of being denied entry to restaurants, shops, gyms, and hotels, being subjected to further screening, and verbal abuse and ostracism.

30 March

- Botswana recorded its first 3 cases.
- France reported 418 deaths in the past 24 hours, bringing the total number of fatalities to 3,024. France has 44,550 confirmed cases.
- Iran confirmed 2,757 official deaths, with more than 40,000 confirmed cases.
- Ireland confirmed 295 new cases and 8 deaths. This gave a total of 2,910 confirmed cases and 54 deaths.

- Malaysia reported 3 new deaths, bringing the total to 37. The country also confirmed 156 new cases, bringing the total number to 2,626.
- New Zealand reported 76 new cases, bringing the total number of confirmed and probable cases to 589.
- Palestine confirmed 7 new cases, bringing the total number of cases to 115.
- Panama confirmed 86 new cases, bringing the total to 1,075, and reported 27 deaths so far.
- Singapore confirmed 35 new cases, bringing the total number to 879.
- South Korea confirmed 78 new cases and 6 new deaths, bringing the total to 9,661 and 158, respectively.
- Spain reported that 812 people have died from the coronavirus in the period between Sunday and Monday.
- In the United States, New York's official death toll exceeded 1,000.
- In Hungary, the National Assembly passes a law allowing Prime Minister Viktor Orbán to rule by decree. Other measures include imprisonment for spreading misinformation and maintaining a national state of emergency.
- The International Olympic Committee and the International Paralympic Committee move the 2020 Summer Olympics and 2020 Summer Paralympics 364 days from their original schedules, to be held between 23 July and 8 August 2021 and 24 August and 5 September 2021, respectively.
- In Israel, Prime Minister Benjamin Netanyahu goes into self-isolation after coming into contact with infected people.

- Japan bans entry by foreign citizens travelling from the United States, China, South Korea and most of Europe. Returning Japanese citizens will be required to self-quarantine for 14 days.
- In Nigeria, authorities in Lagos place the city under a two-week lockdown commencing on Monday night.
- As the number of reported deaths rises to 1,408, Patrick Vallance, the UK's chief scientific adviser, says there are early signs that social distancing measures are "making a difference". Transmission of the virus within the community is thought to be decreasing, and hospital admission data suggests cases are not rising as fast as anticipated.
- Foreign Secretary Dominic Raab announces an arrangement between the government and major UK airlines to fly home tens of thousands of British nationals who are stranded abroad by the coronavirus outbreak.
- Dominic Cummings, the Prime Minister's Chief Adviser, is reported to be self-isolating after experiencing coronavirus symptoms.
- Vehicle owners are granted a six-month exemption from MOT tests, enabling them to continue using their vehicles for essential travel.
- All Gatwick Express services are suspended until further notice on the grounds of significantly reduced demand for travel to Gatwick Airport.
- The United States Department of State advised Americans to return to the US while the Government is able to help, citing the risk of being stuck overseas for long periods of time. In Russia, Moscow authorities have placed the capital into lockdown after many residents ignored official requests

to stay at home. Under strict isolation measures, residents are not allowed to leave their homes unless for a medical emergency, to travel to essential jobs, obtain groceries and medicine, and to walk their dogs.

- South Korea requires all travellers returning from overseas to undergo two weeks of quarantine from 1 April.
- President of Uganda Yoweri Museveni imposes a lockdown to contain the spread of the coronavirus, including banning private cars from the roads for 14 days.
- The United Nations calls for a US$2.5 trillion emergency package to help developing countries cope with the economic impact of the COVID-19 pandemic.
- The United Nations World Health Organization Director-General called for a global increase in the production of protective equipment and medical supplies.
- Fernand de Varennes, the United Nations Special Rapporteur on minority issues, issued a statement noting that COVID-19 was stoking xenophobia, hate and exclusion, including against Chinese and other Asians.
- The United Nations Group of Eminent International and Regional Experts on Yemen urged for a general release of inmates in Yemen to avert a nationwide coronavirus outbreak.
- The United Nations Special Envoy for Syria reiterated calls for a "complete, immediate nationwide ceasefire" as a response to the coronavirus.
- In the United States, President Trump extends the country's national shutdown and social distancing rules until 30 April. Ford and General Electric unveiled plans to manufacture 50,000 ventilators in 100 days. The FDA authorised the

emergency use of anti-malarial drugs hydroxychloroquine and chloroquine for the treatment of seriously ill COVID-19 patients. Some Instacart and Amazon workers protested, demanding more stringent hygiene and safety standards.

- The US government and Johnson & Johnson plan to manufacture at least 1 billion doses of a potential vaccine. Testing would start in September with potential emergency approval by early 2021.
- Chinese Communist Party general secretary Xi Jinping announces that the Government will introduce measures to help small and medium-sized enterprises affected by the COVID-19 pandemic.

31 March

- Burundi confirmed its first 2 cases.
- China reported 48 new confirmed "imported cases" of the coronavirus but no new domestically transmitted cases on 30 March.
- Guam confirmed 2 new cases, bringing the total number to 58.
- Ireland confirmed 325 new cases, the most to date, and 17 deaths, the most to date. This gave a total of 3,235 confirmed cases and 71 deaths.
- Malaysia reported 6 new deaths, bringing the total death toll to 43. In addition, 140 new cases were confirmed, bringing the total number to 2,766.
- New Zealand confirmed 58 new confirmed and probable cases, bringing the total number to 647. 74 people have recovered.

- Palestine confirmed 2 new cases, bringing the total to 117, including 10 in Gaza.
- Panama confirmed 106 new cases, bringing the total to 1,181, and reported 3 new deaths, bringing the total to 30.
- Sierra Leone confirmed its first case.
- Singapore confirmed 47 new cases, bringing the total number to 926.
- Sint Eustatius confirmed its first 2 cases.
- Somaliland confirmed its first 2 cases.
- South Korea confirmed 125 new cases and 4 new deaths, bringing the total to 9,786 and 162, respectively.
- The largest UK daily death toll of the outbreak so far is reported, with 381 deaths taking the total to 1,789.
- The number of people in hospital with COVID-19 passes 10,000.
- A significant rise in anxiety and depression among the UK population is reported following the lockdown. The study, by researchers from the University of Sheffield and Ulster University, finds that people reporting anxiety increased from 17% to 36%, while those reporting depression increased from 16% to 38%.
- The captain of a U.S. Navy aircraft carrier USS Theodore Roosevelt that has more than 100 cases of coronavirus, wrote a stunning plea for help to senior military officials.
- The United Nations Secretary-General launched a comprehensive socioeconomic plan, Shared Responsibility, Global Solidarity: Responding to the Socioeconomic Impacts of COVID-19, to “defeat the virus and build a better world”.
- The United Nations children’s fund (UNICEF) warned that COVID-19 would seriously impact the health care system in

the Democratic Republic of the Congo (DRC), already battling deadly measles and cholera epidemics that had resulted in the deaths of thousands of children.

- The United Nations in Somalia, echoing the Secretary-General's call for "an immediate global ceasefire to put aside violence, mistrust, hostilities and animosity, and to focus on battling the virus, not each other", appealed to Somalis to "come together in this fight against the pandemic".
- Hilal Elver, the United Nations Special Rapporteur on the Right to Food, issued a statement noting that the continued imposition of sanctions, especially on Syria, Venezuela, Iran, Cuba and Zimbabwe, were seriously impacting the fundamental right to sufficient and adequate food.
- The UN Deputy Special Representative for Afghanistan told Security Council members that, in the light of the COVID-19 pandemic, political parties in Afghanistan were being urged to prioritise national interests and join peace talks with the Taliban.
- The Malaysian Defence Minister Datuk Seri Ismail Sabri Yaakob announced that all Malaysians returning from overseas would have to undergo two weeks of quarantine at designated sites across the country.
- The New Zealand Government extends the country's state of national emergency by seven days.
- The Panamanian government began to enforce limits on profit margins for critical cleaning and hygiene supplies. The government also announced the implementation of an absolute quarantine: now, citizens will only be allowed to be outside on alternating days depending on the gender

specified on their ID card, with everyone staying at home during Sundays.

- The Solomon Islands closes all schools in the country as a precautionary measure against COVID-19.
- General Electric laid off 2,600 employees in an attempt to save money on operating costs.
- South Korea will start the new school year with online classes from 9 April after multiple delays caused by the virus.
- By 31 20 March20, the virus had spread to much of the globe, and there were at least 730,000 cases confirmed, with more than 36,000 deaths. Only the following countries and territories had not reported any cases of SARS-CoV-2 infections:
- Strict surveillance measures are being enforced at airports, seaports and border crossings to prevent the disease wide-spreading into countries/territories which either share a border with or are located in the neighbourhood of Mainland China. Accordingly, some countries are thermally monitoring passengers arriving at their major international airports, while flights to and from infected countries have ceased operating. More seriously, countries such as North Korea and Papua New Guinea have banned travellers from all Asian countries.
- Land and sea borders are being closed over the fears of the virus. For example, Hong Kong, Mongolia, North Korea, and Russia have closed their borders with Mainland China, while Papua New Guinea closed its land border with Indonesia. Singapore has closed its borders to all recent travellers of China.

- Visas have also been suspended in some countries. Vietnam ceased issuing visas to Chinese citizens, excepting diplomatic work. Kazakhstan, Malaysia, Sri Lanka and the Philippines also suspended visa issuances: on arrival with Chinese citizens, toward the entire infected area of China and toward Hubei-related visitors who previously had travel history or currently hold a passport issued by Hubei and its neighbourhood's authorities.
- Evacuations of each country's citizens have been done, and most of them are repatriated and quarantined for at least 14 days. Travel restrictions and advisories have been issued, mainly to East Asian and European countries.
- The pandemic has caused lockdowns in some places, such as Wuhan of China, Daegu of South Korea, Luzon of the Philippines, Italy, Denmark, France, Malaysia, Czech Republic, Spain, and India. Public or mass gatherings are prohibited or restricted, including schools and workplaces. A lot of concerts and sports events are cancelled.

Pandemic Chronology April 2020

1 April

- Albania reported 16 new cases, bringing the total number to 259.
- France reported 509 new deaths in the past 24 hours, bringing the total number to 4,023.
- Germany reported 5,435 new cases, bringing the total number to 67,366. The country also reported 149 deaths, bringing the total to 732.
- Hong Kong reported that a cat has tested positive for the coronavirus, bringing the total number of infected pets in the territory to three.
- Indonesia reported 149 new cases and 21 deaths, bringing the total number of cases to 1,677 and deaths to 157, while 103 had recovered.
- Iran confirmed 2,987 new cases, bringing the total to 47,593. Iran also reported 138 deaths, bringing the total to 3,036. The country also reported that 15,473 had recovered from COVID-19.
- Ireland confirmed 212 new cases, significantly fewer new cases than 31 March, and 14 deaths. This gave a total of 3,447 confirmed cases and 85 deaths. About 1,500 people were being tested per day at this stage.
- Italy reported 4,782 new cases, bringing the total number to 110,574. The country also reported 727 deaths, bringing the total to 13,155.
- Libya reported 2 new cases, bringing the total to 10.

- Malaysia confirmed 142 new cases, bringing the total to 2,908. The country's health authorities also confirmed that 108 patients had recovered.
- New Zealand confirmed that 61 new cases (47 confirmed and 14 probable) were reported, bringing the total to 708 (647 confirmed and 61 probable).
- Palestine confirmed 17 new cases (15 in the West Bank and two in Gaza), bringing the total to 134.
- Panama confirmed 136 new cases, bringing the total number to 1,317. Several new deaths were reported, bringing the total number to 32.
- The Philippines reported 227 new cases and 8 more deaths, bringing the total number of cases to 2,311 and deaths to 96.
- Qatar reported 54 new cases, bringing the total to 835.
- Singapore confirmed 74 new cases, bringing the total number to 1,000.
- South Korea confirmed 101 new cases and 3 new deaths, bringing the total to 9,887 and 165, respectively. 5,560 people had recovered.
- Spain reported 864 deaths and 102,136 infections.
- Turkey reported 2,348 new cases and 63 new deaths, bringing the total number of deaths to 277.
- Ukraine confirmed 149 new cases and 3 new deaths, bringing the total number to 794 and the number of deaths to 20.
- The United Kingdom reported 563 deaths within the past 24 hours, bringing the total number to 2,352. The country's youngest reported person to die of the virus was a 13-year-old boy named Ismail Mohamed Abdulwahab.

- The UK government confirms that a total of 2,000 NHS staff have been tested for coronavirus since the outbreak began, but Cabinet Office Minister Michael Gove says a shortage of chemical reagents needed for COVID-19 testing means it is not possible to screen the NHS's 1.2 million workforces. Gove's statement is contradicted by the Chemical Industries Association, which says there is not a shortage of the relevant chemicals and that at a meeting with a business minister the week before, the government had not tried to find out about potential supply problems.
- The contactless payment limit for in-store spending is raised from £30 to £45.
- Multinational pharmaceutical company Roche denies the existence of a deal to supply Wales with COVID-19 tests after First Minister Mark Drakeford and Health Minister Vaughan Gething blame the collapse of a deal for a shortage of testing kits.
- The United States confirmed a total of over 200,000 cases and 4,076 deaths. The United States Department of State reported the deaths of two local employees at US diplomatic missions in Indonesia and the Democratic Republic of Congo.
- The World Health Organization reported that deaths from COVID-19 had more than doubled in the previous week and would soon reach 50,000 globally, with the global caseload heading towards one million.
- The UN Department of Economic and Social Affairs reported in a new analysis that the global economy could shrink by up to one per cent in 2020 due to the COVID-19 pandemic, or

even further if restrictions on economic activities were continued without sufficient fiscal responses.

- The UN High Commissioner for Refugees (UNHCR) outlined a series of measures the UNHCR was taking to respond to the coronavirus public health emergency and prevent further spread, especially those to reinforce health and the 'WASH' systems (water, sanitation and hygiene), including distributing soap and increasing water access.
- The Executive Director of the UN Children's Fund warned that an outbreak of COVID-19 in the world's refugee camps was "looking imminent".
- The UNHCR and International Organization for Migration emphasised that the worldwide COVID-19 emergency was compounding the already desperate situation for many refugees and migrants from Venezuela. The United Nations Economic and Social Commission for Western Asia issued a new policy brief noting that COVID-19 would be responsible for pushing a further 8.3 million people in the Arab region into poverty. The UN system in Nigeria announced that it was working with its partners to reduce the spread of the coronavirus, especially in the northeast, where communities and camps house millions of internally displaced people uprooted by the Boko Haram insurgency.
- World Meteorological Organization (WMO) Secretary-General Petteri Taalas urged governments to support national early warning and weather observing capacities despite the "severe challenges" caused by COVID-19, as the WMO's Global Observing System came under strain due to the lack of data from commercial airliners.
- Eritrea Africa announced a three-week lockdown, commencing 2 April to combat the spread of COVID-19.

- Sierra Leone Africa declared that a three-day lockdown would come into effect on Saturday (4 April).
- President of the United States Donald Trump posted his "Coronavirus Guidelines for America" on Twitter after warning that the United States faced a "very painful" two weeks as it confronted the virus. That same day, the White House projected that the United States could face between 100,000 and 240,000 deaths as a result of the COVID-19 pandemic.
- The US Food and Drug Administration reported that it was facing a shortage of malaria drugs, including hydroxychloroquine and related chloroquine, due to a surge in demand caused by the coronavirus pandemic.
- The United States Department of Homeland Security and Department of Justice suspended hearings for asylum seekers in Mexico until 1 May.
- Panama began to enforce an absolute quarantine measure, during which male and female citizens would only be allowed to be outside their homes on alternating days of the week.
- President of Brazil Jair Bolsonaro made remarks minimising the impact of the coronavirus and highlighting that confinement and quarantine measures could hurt the Brazilian economy.
- South American airliner LATAM Airlines Group announced that it would cut 95% of flight operations. The airline would maintain 39 domestic routes in Brazil, 13 in Chile and 4 international routes.
- The United States reported that 6.7 million people had filed for unemployment benefits in the past week.

- Following intervention by President Trump, Fort Lauderdale authorities allowed two coronavirus-stricken cruise liners, MS Zaandam and MS Rotterdam, to dock at Port Everglades.
- Governor of New York Andrew Cuomo announced that New York state only had enough ventilators for the next six days. In response, President Trump invoked the Defense Production Act to ramp up the production of both ventilators and protective face masks by US companies. In addition, the President extended an offer to Iran to help with the coronavirus pandemic.
- Boeing CEO Dave Calhoun announced a voluntary layoff plan in response to the economic setbacks experienced by the aviation industry.
- The World Bank approved a plan to invest US$160 billion in emergency aid over the next 15 months to help countries deal with the coronavirus.

2 April

- Belgium reported a total of 1,001 deaths and 15,348 cases.
- Canada reported 1,115 new cases, bringing the total to 10,132. Canada also reported 22 new deaths, bringing the total to 127.
- Germany reported 6,156 new cases, bringing the total number to 73,522. The country also reported 140 deaths, bringing the total to 872.
- India has confirmed a total of 50 deaths and 1,965 cases nationwide.
- Iran reports 124 deaths, reaching a total of 3,160. Health authorities confirmed 50,468 infected cases.

- Ireland confirmed 402 new cases and 13 deaths. This gave a total of 3,894 confirmed cases and 98 deaths.
- Israel confirmed 31 deaths and 6,211 infected cases, with 107 in serious condition.
- Italy reports 760 deaths, bringing the total to 13,915.
- Malawi confirmed its 3 first cases.
- Malaysia confirmed 208 new cases, taking the total number of cases to 3,116. 5 deaths were also reported, taking the death toll to 50.
- New Zealand confirmed 89 new cases (76 confirmed and 13 probable), bringing the total to 797. Of the cases, 92 had recovered, and 13 were hospitalised.
- The Netherlands reports 166 deaths, bringing the death toll to 1,339. The country also reports 14,697 cases.
- Palestine confirmed 21 new cases bringing the total to 155.
- Panama reported 158 new cases and 5 new deaths, bringing the total numbers to 1,475 and 37, respectively.
- The Philippines reports 11 new deaths and 332 new cases, bringing the total number of deaths to 107 and infected cases to 2,633.
- Russia reports 771 new cases, bringing the total to 3,548. A total of 30 people have died.
- Singapore confirmed its fourth death. At the same time, 49 new cases were confirmed, bringing the total number to 1,049.
- South Korea confirmed 89 new cases and 4 new deaths, bringing the total to 9,976 and 169, respectively.
- Spain reports a total of 10,003 deaths and 110,238 cases.
- Switzerland's death toll rises to 432 and reports 18,267 positive tests.

- Ukraine confirmed 103 new cases and 2 new deaths, bringing the total number of cases to 897 and the total number of deaths to 22.
- The United Kingdom reports 569 deaths, bringing the total to 2,921. Health authorities report that 163,194 people have been tested, with 33,718 testing positive.
- Matt Hancock, MP, who returns to give the daily government briefing after completing his self-isolation, sets a target of carrying out 100,000 tests a day by the end of the month (encompassing both swab tests and blood tests).
- The UK government writes off historical debts totalling £13.4bn of over 100 hospital trusts, an action which had been under consideration since before the onset of the pandemic.
- At 8 pm, the UK gives another national round of applause for NHS staff and other key workers.
- UK Health Secretary Matt Hancock announced that the British Government would intend to build a diagnostics industry to test 100,000 people a day for the coronavirus. First Minister of Scotland Nicola Sturgeon admitted that the number of deaths in Scotland had been under-reported due to mistakes in notifying the Government about new fatalities. In response to a call by British Prime Minister Boris Johnson, several British engineers, aerospace and Formula One companies, including BAE Systems, Rolls Royce, Ford and Airbus, announced that they would join forces to produce 1,500 ventilators.
- The United States confirmed a total of over 225,000 cases and 5,345 deaths.

- Zambia reports 3 new cases, bringing the total to 39. Zambia also reports its first death.
- There are over 1,000,000 confirmed cases and 50,000 confirmed deaths in the world.
- The United Nations General Assembly passed resolution A/RES/74/270: Global solidarity to fight the coronavirus disease 2019 (COVID-19). The United Nations postponed the COP26 climate summit postponed to 'safeguard lives'.The International Organization for Migration sounded the alarm over conditions in crowded reception centres in Greece as the first migrants tested positive for COVID-19.UN High Commissioner for Human Rights, Michelle Bachelet, warned of the plight of hundreds of thousands of now unemployed migrant workers in India, calling for 'domestic solidarity' in the coronavirus battle.
- The World Food Programme (WFP) warned that food insecurity levels for five million people in the Sahel region of Africa were "spiralling out of control", with the COVID-19 pandemic potentially impacting humanitarian supply chains.
- On World Autism Awareness Day, the UN Secretary-General appealed for the rights of persons with autism to be taken into account in efforts to address the COVID-19 pandemic.
- Albania extended lockdown, closing schools, eateries, and other public venues, which has been in force since mid-March and due to end on 3 April.
- President of Russia Vladimir Putin sent a military plane to the United States carrying medical supplies and masks to help the United States fight the coronavirus as a goodwill gesture to US President Trump. That same day, Putin approved legislation allowing the Russian government to

declare a state of national emergency to combat the COVID-19 outbreak.

- UK Housing Secretary Robert Jenrick announced that the British Government would aim to test 25,000 people a day by mid-April from its present capacity of 12,750 a day. The All England Lawn Tennis Club also announced that the Wimbledon tennis championship, scheduled to have been held between 29 June and 12 July, had been cancelled in response to the coronavirus pandemic.
- The Union of European Football Associations suspended all Champions League and Europa League matches due to the coronavirus pandemic.
- The Championships, Wimbledon was cancelled for the first time since 1945.
- Reporters without Borders launched its "Tracker 19" tool to document state censorship, disinformation and their effect on people's access to news and information during the COVID-19 global pandemic.
- The Qatari Ministry of Administrative Development, Labour and Social Affairs (MADLSA) announced that workers in quarantine and treatment across the country would be paid in full, ordering employers and companies to follow government policy and creating a hotline for workers to voice their grievances.
- Turkey sent a military aeroplane carrying masks, face gears, eye gears, overalls and anti-bacterial fluids to Spain and Italy.
- Iranian authorities closed streets and shops in the capital Tehran to help contain the spread of the coronavirus.

- In Lebanon, the Human Rights Watch NGO criticised Lebanese municipal authorities for imposing discriminatory measures against Syrian refugees, including curfews.
- The Saudi Ministry of Interior imposed a 24-hour curfew on Mecca and Medina. Besides essential workers, residents would be allowed to buy groceries and access medical care.
- The United Arab Emirates government allowed national carrier Emirates to launch a number of flights from 6 April to repatriate visitors and expatriates to their home countries.
- Cyprus extended a ban on commercial flights with 28 countries for two weeks in order to contain the spread of the coronavirus.
- German authorities reported that 1.1 million self-employed and small businesses had applied for financial assistance. The German government already paid €1 billion in financial assistance, with another €1.8 billion being approved.
- Greek authorities quarantined a migrant camp after 23 asylum seekers tested positive for the coronavirus.
- In Ireland, Tánaiste Simon Coveney extended movement restrictions limiting travel to buying groceries, exercising, and essential family visits beyond 12 April. Israeli Minister of Health Yaakov Litzman and his wife tested positive for COVID-19. The Portuguese Assembly of the Republic extended the state of emergency by another 15 days in response to a sharp rise in the death toll to 200. Portuguese Prime Minister Antonio Costa also announced that airports would close between 9 and 13 April, allowing only flights repatriating citizens or transporting goods.
- President of Romania Klaus Iohannis announced that Romanian doctors, nurses, and personnel dealing with the

coronavirus pandemic would receive a monthly bonus of €500.

- In Russia, the Mayor of Moscow Sergei Sobyanin extended a partial lockdown and movement restrictions on residents until 1 May. Residents of Moscow, which has been experiencing a heavy caseload, have since Monday been allowed to leave their homes only to buy food or medicine nearby, get urgent medical treatment, walk the dog or take out the rubbish.
- Spanish authorities released figures showing that 898,922 workers had lost their jobs since 12 March. Catalonian President Quim Torra appealed for help from the Spanish Army.
- Mayor of Istanbul Ekrem Imamoglu called for a lockdown in response to a spike in cases to 15,000, with 60% occurring in Istanbul.
- The Ukrainian government accepted Tesla CEO and philanthropist Elon Musk's offer to deliver ventilators to Ukraine.
- The 2020 United Nations Climate Change Conference, scheduled to be held in Glasgow in November 2020, was postponed to 2021. Israeli Prime Minister Benjamin Netanyahu ordered all Israeli citizens to wear face masks in public as part of national efforts to combat COVID-19.

3 April

- Albania reports 27 new cases with a total death toll of 17.
- Canada confirms that it has 10,132 cases and 127 deaths. Ontario alone has reported 3,255 confirmed cases and 67 deaths.

- China confirms 4 new deaths, bringing the death toll to 3,322. China also reports 40 asymptomatic cases of coronavirus.
- Egypt confirms 120 new cases, bringing the total to 985. Egypt also reports 8 new deaths, bringing the total to 66.
- The Falkland Islands reports its first case.
- France reports 588 new deaths, bringing the total number of hospital deaths to 5,091. This figure excludes the 1,416 deaths in rest homes, bringing the total death toll to 6,507.
- Greece reports a total of 1,425 cases and 53 deaths.
- India reports 1,965 total cases, with many cases being traced to a tablighi jamaat in New Delhi held in March.
- Indonesia's death toll rises to 170, with a total of 1,790 confirmed infections.
- Iran reports 134 new deaths, bringing the death toll to 3,294. Official figures claim that 53,183 are infected and that 17,935 have recovered.
- Ireland confirmed 424 new cases and 22 deaths. This gave a total of 4,273 confirmed cases and 120 deaths.
- Iraq officially reports 772 cases and 54 confirmed deaths. This figure has been disputed by three doctors, a health ministry official, and a senior political official, who claimed that thousands have been infected.
- Italy confirms 766 new deaths, bringing the total death toll to 14,681. The country also confirmed 2,339 new cases, bringing the total number to 85,388.
- Kyrgyzstan reports its first death from the coronavirus.
- Latvia confirms its first coronavirus-related death, a 99-year-old woman with various underlying chronic conditions.

- Malaysia confirms 217 new cases, bringing the country's total to 3,333. The country also reports 3 more deaths, bringing the total death toll to 53.
- The Netherlands reports 1,026 new cases, bringing the total number to 15,723. The country also confirms 148 more deaths, bringing the total to 1,487.
- Panama reported 198 new cases and 4 new deaths, bringing the total numbers to 1,673 and 41, respectively.
- New Zealand confirms 71 new confirmed and probable cases, bringing the total to 868.
- Palestine confirms 32 cases, bringing the total to 193.
- Singapore confirms its fifth death. At the same time, 65 new cases were confirmed, bringing the total number to 1,114.
- South Korea reports 86 new cases and 5 new deaths, bringing the total to 10,062 and 174, respectively. 27,000 people are under self-quarantine.
- Spain reports 950 deaths, bringing the total to 10,000.
- Sweden reports 612 new cases, bringing the total to around 6,000. The country's death toll reaches nearly 333.
- Ukraine reports 175 new cases, bringing the total number to 1,072, as well as 5 new deaths, bringing the total number to 27.
- The United Kingdom reports 684 deaths, bringing the total to 3,605. UK health authorities confirm that 173,784 have been tested, with 38,168 being positive.
- NHS Nightingale Hospital London, the first temporary hospital to treat coronavirus patients, opens at the ExCel Centre in East London, employing NHS staff and military personnel, with 500 beds and a potential capacity for 4,000. It is the first of several such facilities planned across the UK.

- Figures published by the Cabinet Office indicate UK road traffic levels have fallen by 73% since the lockdown measures were introduced and are at their lowest since 1955.
- With warm weather forecast for some areas during the upcoming weekend, Matt Hancock warns people to stay at home, telling them this is an instruction "not a request".
- The Queen holds the first virtual meeting with the Privy Council.
- The United States reports 26,000 new cases, bringing the total to 228,000. The US death toll reaches 950, bringing the total to 5,374. New York State reports 562 deaths, bringing the death toll to 2,935.
- According to figures released by Johns Hopkins University, 58,773 people have died as a result of COVID-19, and there are at least 1,094,068 confirmed cases.
- In a joint statement, the UN refugee agency (UNHCR), the International Organization for Migration, the UN human rights office (OHCHR) and the World Health Organization stressed that "refugees, migrants and displaced persons are at heightened risk of contracting the new coronavirus disease" as health systems threatened to be overwhelmed.
- The United Nations Human Rights Commissioner Michelle Bachelet welcomed the decision by many governments to release hundreds of thousands of prisoners to slow the transmission of the new coronavirus within prison systems.
- The UN Secretary-General warned of a surge in domestic violence due to lockdowns.
- The World Food Programme (WFP) released a major report, "COVID-19: Potential impact on the world's poorest people:

A WFP analysis of the economic and food security implications of the pandemic", noting that the global food chain was holding, while pointing out that food exports by major producers could be impacted if the exporting countries panicked.

- The UN Secretary-General reiterated his call for a global ceasefire and urged unity in mobilising "every ounce of energy" to defeat the coronavirus pandemic.
- At a press briefing, the Director-General of the Ghana Health Service announced the commencement of local production of nose masks as part of efforts to arrest the spread of the pandemic in Ghana.
- Josep Borrell, the High Representative of the European Union, issued a statement stating that sanctions should not get in the way of the delivery of medical equipment and supplies to countries trying to contain COVID-19.
- German State Minister of the Interior for Berlin Andreas Geisel accused the United States of committing "modern piracy" by allegedly diverting a shipment of 200,000 masks from an American 3M's Chinese factory in Thailand intended for Germany. In response, the US Embassy spokeswoman Jillian Bonnardeaux issued a statement on 6 April denying that the US had any "knowledge" of the diversion of the mask shipment from Thailand. 3M also said they had no knowledge of the shipment, stating, "We know nothing of an order from the Berlin police for 3M masks that come from China." Berlin police later confirmed that the shipment was not seized by U.S. authorities but was said to have simply been bought at a better price, widely believed to be from a German dealer or China. This revelation outraged the Berlin opposition, whose CDU parliamentary group leader Burkard

Dregger accused Geisel of "deliberately misleading Berliners" in order "to cover up its own inability to obtain protective equipment".

- The Hungarian Government announces the creation of a US$4 billion fund to rejuvenate the economy, using rerouted government resources and the national employment fund.
- Spanish Prime Minister Pedro Sánchez announces the extension of Spain's lockdown until 25 April to curb the spread of the coronavirus.
- Ukraine sends a team of 20 medical personnel to assist Italian medical authorities in the central Marche region.
- Saudi Arabia extended the starting date of a 24-hour curfew to 3 pm on Friday in Dammam, Ta'if and al-Qatif in order to combat the coronavirus. King Salman invests 9 billion riyals (US$2.3 billion) in financial support for 1.2 million Saudi citizens working in the private sector.
- President of Guatemala Alejandro Giammattei banned internal travel and gathering at beaches before and during the Easter holidays in order to combat the spread of the coronavirus.
- The Chinese Government donated 1,000 ventilators to New York state with the help of Chinese billionaires Jack Ma and Joseph Tsai. New York Governor Andrew Cuomo signed an executive order allowing state authorities to requisition unused ventilators and personal protective equipment from hospitals.
- The United States Centers for Disease Control and Prevention (CDC) initiated antibody tests to help determine how many people had been infected with the coronavirus, including those who have never developed symptoms.

- Jared Moskowitz, head of Florida Division of Emergency Management, blasted the American company 3M for selling N95 masks directly to foreign countries for cash instead of the United States. Moskowitz stated that 3M agreed to authorise distributors and brokers to represent they were selling the masks to Florida, but instead, his team for the last several weeks "get to warehouses that are completely empty." He then said the 3M authorised U.S. distributors later told him the masks Florida contracted for never showed up because the company instead prioritised orders that come in later, for higher prices, from foreign countries (including Germany, Russia, and France). As a result, Moskowitz highlighted the issue on Twitter, saying he decided to "troll" 3M.
- The United States Department of Labor reported that the US economy lost 701,100 jobs in March, ending 113 months of job growth. The US unemployment rate rose to 4.4 per cent.
- US President Trump also invoked the Defense Production Act to force 3M to prioritise US orders over international orders and to stop exporting American-made respirators to Canada and Latin America. In response, Canadian Prime Minister Justin Trudeau warned that it would be a mistake for the US to block the flow of medical supplies into Canada.
- Washington State Governor Jay Inslee extended stay-at-home orders until 23 May. These orders would keep non-essential businesses closed and most of the state's residents at home.

4 April

- Albania reports 29 new cases, bringing the total to 333 with a total of 18 deaths.
- China reports 19 new cases (18 imported and one in Wuhan), bringing the total number of confirmed cases to 81,639. China also reports 4 new deaths, bringing the death toll to 3,326.
- France records nearly 5,400 deaths, including 884 previously unreported cases in rest homes.
- Georgia confirms its first death, with the country reporting a total of 157 cases.
- Germany reports 6,082 new cases, bringing the total to 85,778. The country also reports 1,158 deaths.
- Indonesia confirms 106 new cases, bringing the total to 2,092. The country reports 10 new deaths, bringing the death toll to 191.
- Iran confirms 55,743 cases, of whom 4,103 are in critical condition. The country also reports 158 deaths, bringing the death toll to 3,542.
- Ireland confirmed 331 new cases and 17 deaths. This gave a total of 4,604 confirmed cases and 137 deaths.
- Israeli authorities report a total number of 7,428 cases and 41 deaths.
- Italy confirms 766 new deaths, bringing the death toll to 14,681. Italy reports 4,585 new cases, bringing the total to 119,827.
- Japan reports 118 new cases in Tokyo, raising the total to about 3,000. The country also has reported a total of 73 deaths.

- Kuwait reports its first death. The country also reports 62 new cases, increasing the total to 479 cases.
- Malaysia reports 150 new cases, bringing the total to 3,486. Malaysia also records 4 new deaths, bringing the total to 57.
- The Netherlands confirms 164 deaths, bringing the death toll to 1,651.
- Panama reported 128 new cases and 5 new deaths, bringing the total numbers to 1,801 and 46, respectively.
- New Zealand confirms 82 new cases (50 confirmed and 32 probable), bringing the total number to 950. It is reported that 127 people have recovered and that over 3,600 people have been tested on Friday.
- The Philippines reports 76 new cases, bringing the total to 3,094. The country also reports 8 new deaths, bringing the total to 144.
- Portugal confirms a total of 266 deaths and 10,524 cases.
- Qatar reports 250 new cases, bringing the total to 1,213. 16 people have recovered, bringing the total number of recoveries to 109.
- Singapore confirms its sixth death. At the same time, 75 new cases were confirmed, bringing the total number to 1,189.
- South Korea confirms 94 new cases and 3 new deaths, bringing the total to 10,156 and 177, respectively.
- Spain reports 809 new deaths, bringing the total death toll to 11,744. The number of confirmed cases rises to 124,736.
- Switzerland's number of infected cases rises to 20,278 and the death toll to 540.
- Turkey confirms 76 new deaths, bringing the death toll to 501. The country also reports a total of 23,934 cases. 786

patients have recovered, while 1,311 remain in intensive care.

- Ukraine reports 153 new cases and 5 new deaths, bringing the total numbers to 1,225 and 32, respectively.
- The United Kingdom reports a total death toll of 4,313. 183,190 people have also been tested, with 41,903 positive cases being confirmed.
- The United States reports a total of 300,915 cases and 8,162 deaths, based on figures by Johns Hopkins University. New York state reports 113,704 cases and a total of 3,565 deaths.
- The first 4 cases are confirmed in the disputed territory of Western Sahara.
- According to Johns Hopkins University, the number of coronavirus cases worldwide exceeds 1.1 million.
- The UN chief of peacekeeping operations Jean-Pierre Lacroix stressed that UN peacekeepers were continuing in their mission to help fragile countries navigate conflict and COVID-19, as he echoed the Secretary-General's call for an immediate global ceasefire.
- The United Nations reported it was forced to significantly scale back its activities on Mine Awareness Day, which usually involves football games on cleared minefields.
- Albania imposed a 40-hour lockdown over the weekend in response to a spike in cases.
- Airbus delivered 4 million masks from China to Europe.
- The Bulgarian National Assembly extends a national state of emergency until 13 April.

- French authorities converted a large refrigerated warehouse at the Rungis fresh food market into a temporary morgue to hold 1,000 bodies.
- The Swedish health care company Mölnlycke announced that France had seized millions of face masks and gloves that the company imported from China to Spain and Italy. The company's general manager, Richard Twomey, denounced France for "confiscating masks and gloves even though it was not its own. This is an extremely disturbing, unbecoming act."
- Greece quarantined a second migrant camp near Athens after a 53-year-old Afghan man tested positive for COVID-19. The Israeli government declared Bnei Brak a restricted zone due to the town's high rate of infections and placed the town under lockdown, limiting travel to and from the town. Israeli authorities also required that ritual washing for deceased Jewish and Muslim victims of COVID-19 be done by personnel wearing full protective gear to contain the spread of the disease. Swiss police surrounded Geneva's main prison after 40 prisoners refused to return to their cells, complaining about insufficient measures to combat the spread of the coronavirus.
- Turkey imposed a partial curfew on Turkish citizens under the age of 20 years, which came into effect at midnight. Turkish authorities also shut down the borders of 31 cities to most vehicles, excluding those transporting essential supplies.
- In the United Kingdom, the ExCel exhibition centre in London was opened as a temporary 4,000-bed hospital, branded 'NHS Nightingale' having been constructed over the previous nine days. It was opened by Prince Charles over a

video link. British biomedical scientists and National Health Service staff also reported that a shortage of equipment was preventing them from carrying out more coronavirus tests.

- In the UK t is announced that a five-year-old has died from the virus, believed to be the youngest victim to date.
- The results of the 2020 Labour Party leadership election and the 2020 Labour Party deputy leadership election are announced, in which Keir Starmer is elected as the leader of the Labour Party, succeeding Jeremy Corbyn, and Angela Rayner is elected as deputy leader of the party. The results are released by email after a public event to announce the results was cancelled due to the pandemic.
- Médecins Sans Frontières (Doctors Without Borders) President Christos Christou urged European countries not to hoard medical supplies and equipment and to allow their export to vulnerable countries in Southeast Asia, the Middle East and Africa. He also called on developed countries to increase their production of medical supplies.
- Bahrain reopens Bahrain International Airport to transit by international travellers but limits entry to citizens and residents.
- President of Egypt Abdel Fattah el-Sisi postpones several megaprojects, including the Grand Egyptian Museum and moving the capital from Cairo to a new planned city.
- Prime Minister of Pakistan Imran Khan issued a statement on Twitter that the Indian subcontinent faced a difficult choice of having to balance between imposing a lockdown to contain the spread of the coronavirus and ensuring that people would not die of hunger and the economy would not collapse.

- Saudi Arabia imposes a lockdown and partial curfew in seven neighbourhoods in Jeddah. Residents in the affected neighbourhoods can only obtain groceries, and medical services between 6 am and 3 pm local time.
- The Tunisian Assembly of the Representatives of the People ceded power to Prime Minister Elyes Fakhfakh's government for two months, allowing them to issue decrees, sign purchase agreements and seek finance without consulting parliament.
- The United Arab Emirates extends an overnight curfew indefinitely, requiring people to stay at home between 8 pm and 6 am local time. During the curfew, UAE authorities will disinfect streets, parks, and public transport facilities.
- President of Malawi Peter Mutharika announces several measures to support small and medium businesses, including tax breaks, reducing fuel allowances and increasing risk allowances for health workers. The President also announces that he and his Cabinet will take a 10 per cent salary cut.
- 198 markets in the Eastern Region of Ghana were disinfected as part of the drive to control the pandemic. The Ministry of Local Government and Rural Development teamed up with Moderpest Company and Zoomlion Ghana for the exercise.
- The Nigerian Government announces the creation of a 500 billion naira (US$1.39 billion) coronavirus crisis intervention fund to upgrade its healthcare infrastructure.
- Al Jazeera reports that thousands of people have been detained across Central America for violating lockdown measures and curfews: Honduras (2,250 people),

Guatemala (5,705), Panama (over 5,000 including 424 for violating rules that limit men and women to leave homes on alternate days).

- United States Attorney General William Barr issues an executive order allowing the Bureau of Prisons to release vulnerable prisoners from federal correctional facilities into home detention. Priority will be given to facilities affected by COVID-19, including Oakdale in Louisiana, Elkton in Ohio, and Danbury in Connecticut.
- Josep Borrell, the High Representative of the European Union, issued a statement stating that sanctions should not get in the way of the delivery of medical equipment and supplies to countries trying to contain COVID-19.
- German State Minister of the Interior for Berlin Andreas Geisel accused the United States of committing “modern piracy” by allegedly diverting a shipment of 200,000 masks from an American 3M’s Chinese factory in Thailand intended for Germany. In response, US Embassy spokeswoman Jillian Bonnardeaux issued a statement on 6 April denying that the US had any “knowledge” of the diversion of the mask shipment from Thailand. 3M also said they had no knowledge of the shipment, stating, “We know nothing of an order from the Berlin police for 3M masks that come from China.” Berlin police later confirmed that the shipment was not seized by U.S. authorities but was said to have simply been bought at a better price, widely believed to be from a German dealer or China. This revelation outraged the Berlin opposition, whose CDU parliamentary group leader Burkard Dregger accused Geisel of “deliberately misleading Berliners” in order “to cover up its own inability to obtain protective equipment”.

- The Hungarian Government announces the creation of a US$4 billion fund to rejuvenate the economy, using rerouted government resources and the national employment fund.
- Spanish Prime Minister Pedro Sánchez announces the extension of Spain's lockdown until 25 April to curb the spread of the coronavirus.
- Ukraine sends a team of 20 medical personnel to assist Italian medical authorities in the central Marche region.

5 April

- Albania reports 28 new cases, bringing the total to 361. The country reports a total of 20 deaths and 104 recoveries.
- Canada reports a total of 258 deaths and 14,426 cases.
- China reports 39 new cases (all but one imported) and 78 new asymptomatic cases. China reports 1 death.
- Ethiopia reports its first 2 deaths, a 60-year-old woman and a 56-year-old man.
- France reports a total of 90,848 cases. France also reports 357 deaths, bringing the total to 8,078. There are over 28,891 hospitalised patients.
- Germany reports a total of 96,092 cases.
- Haiti reports its first death.
- Iran reports 150 deaths, bringing the total to 3,603. Iran has recorded a total of 58,226 cases, 22,011 recoveries, and 4,057 critical cases.
- Ireland confirmed 390 new cases and 21 deaths. This gave a total of 4,994 confirmed cases and 158 deaths.
- Italy reports a total of 124,632 cases and new 525 deaths.
- Japan reports more than 130 cases in Tokyo, bringing the number of cases in the capital above 1,000.

- Malaysia reports 179 new cases, bringing the number of cases to 3,662.
- New Zealand reports 89 new cases (48 confirmed and 41 probable), bringing the total to 1,039 (870 confirmed and 169 probable). In addition, 29 more recoveries were reported, bringing the total to 156.
- Panama reported 187 new cases and 8 new deaths, bringing the total numbers to 1,988 and 54, respectively.
- Qatar reports 279 new cases, bringing the total to 1,604.
- Russia reports 658 new cases, bringing the total to 5,389. The country also reports a total of 45 deaths.
- Saint Pierre and Miquelon confirm its first case.
- Singapore confirms 120 new cases, bringing the total number to 1,309. This is the highest number of new cases in a day.
- South Korea confirms 81 new cases and 6 new deaths, bringing the total to 10,237 and 183, respectively.
- South Sudan confirms its first case.
- Spain reports 674 new deaths, bringing the total to 12,418 deaths. The country reports a total of 130,759 cases.
- Turkey reports 73 new deaths and 3,135 new cases, bringing the total number of deaths to 574 and the number of cases to 27,069.
- Ukraine reports 83 new cases and 5 new deaths, bringing the total numbers to 1,308 and 37, respectively.
- The United Kingdom reports 621 deaths, bringing the total to 4,934. A total of 47,806 people have tested positive for the coronavirus.
- Queen Elizabeth II makes a rare broadcast to the UK and the wider Commonwealth, something she has done on only

four previous occasions. In the address, she thanks people for following the government's social distancing rules, pays tribute to key workers, and says the UK "will succeed" in its fight against coronavirus but may have "more still to endure".

- Prime Minister Boris Johnson is admitted to the hospital for tests after testing positive for coronavirus ten days earlier.
- Matt Hancock says the goal for the number of ventilators has been reduced to 18,000 and that the NHS has between 9,000 and 10,000 available.
- The results of the 2020 Labour Party leadership election and the 2020 Labour Party deputy leadership election are announced, in which Keir Starmer is elected as the leader of the Labour Party, succeeding Jeremy Corbyn, and Angela Rayner is elected as deputy leader of the party. The results are released by email after a public event to announce the results was cancelled due to the pandemic.
- The United States reports a total of 311,544 cases. New York state also reports 594 deaths, bringing the total to 4,159.
- Johns Hopkins University reports that the number of global confirmed cases has passed 1.2 million with 64,753 confirmed deaths.
- The United Arab Emirates' Cabinet announces that it will strengthen the country's "strategic stockpile." The country's Vice President and Prime Minister, Mohammed bin Rashid Al Maktoum announces that factories will be redirected to support the country's health sector.
- US President Trump urges Americans worried about the coronavirus to take a drug known as hydroxychloroquine,

which is used to treat malaria, arthritis and lupus, contradicting advice from US federal public health advisers.

- In the Czech Republic, 300 pilots launch a “Pilots to the People” project to use their private planes to distribute medical supplies across the country.
- In Jerusalem, the annual Palm Sunday parade is cancelled due to health concerns. An online service is instead held at the Co-Cathedral of the Most Holy Name of Jesus. UK Health Secretary Matt Hancock warns that the UK Government may restrict outdoor exercise if people flout lockdown rules. UK Prime Minister Boris Johnson, who tested positive for COVID-19 ten days ago, is admitted to hospital. Queen Elizabeth II gives a special address to the nation, calling for unity and global cooperation in response to the COVID-19 pandemic.
- Catherine Calderwood resigns as the Chief Medical Officer for Scotland for breaking her own department’s advice on self-isolation by visiting her second home twice.

6 April

- The Czech Republic reports a total of 4,591 cases, 72 deaths, and 96 recoveries.
- Egypt reports 149 new cases, bringing the total to 1,322. The country reports 7 new deaths, bringing the total to 85 and 259 recoveries.
- France reports a total of 8,078 deaths, including 6,494 hospital deaths.
- Germany reports 3,677 new cases, bringing the total to 95,391.

- Indonesia reports 218 new cases, bringing the total to 2,491. The country also reports 11 deaths, bringing the total to 209 and 192 recoveries.
- Iran reports a total of 3,739 deaths and 60,500 cases.
- Ireland confirmed 370 new cases and 16 deaths. This gave a total of 5,364 confirmed cases and 174 deaths.
- Italy's death toll rises by 636. The country also reports 3,599 new cases, bringing the total to 132,547.
- Kenya has reported a total of 158 cases and 6 deaths.
- Kosovo reports 2 new deaths, bringing the total death toll to 3.
- Malaysia reports 131 new cases, bringing the total to 3,793. Malaysian authorities also report 236 new recovered cases. Malaysia also reports a new death, bringing the death toll to 62.
- New Zealand reports 39 newly confirmed and 28 probable cases, bringing the total to 1,106 confirmed and probable cases.
- Panama reports 112 new cases and 1 new death, bringing the total numbers to 2,100 and 55, respectively.
- The Philippines reports 414 new cases, bringing the total to 3,660. The country also reports 11 deaths, bringing the total to 163 and 73 recoveries.
- Romania has reported a total of 4,057 cases and 157 deaths.
- Russia reports 954 new cases, bringing the total to 6,343. The country reports a total of 47 deaths.
- São Tomé and Príncipe reports its first 4 cases.

- Singapore confirms 66 new cases, bringing the total number to 1,375. Of the new cases, 35 were linked to clusters at foreign dormitories.
- South Korea confirms 47 new cases and 3 new deaths, bringing the total to 10,284 and 186, respectively.
- Switzerland reports a total of 584 deaths and 21,652 cases.
- Thailand reports 51 new cases, bringing the total to 2,220. The country also reports 3 new deaths, bringing the total to 26.
- Turkey reports 3,148 new cases, bringing the total to 30,217. The country also reports 75 deaths, bringing the total to 649.
- Ukraine reports a total of 1,319 cases and 38 deaths.
- The United Arab Emirates reports a total of 1,799 cases and 10 deaths.
- The United Kingdom reports 439 new deaths, bringing the total to 5,373. The UK also reports a total of 51,608 cases.
- The death toll from COVID-19 in the UK exceeds 5,000. The total number of reported cases is nearly 52,000.
- Prime Minister Boris Johnson is taken into intensive care at St Thomas' Hospital. It is announced that First Secretary of State Dominic Raab will deputise for him.
- National Express suspends all its long-distance coach services.
- In the United States, Johns Hopkins University reports a total of 10,000 deaths and 347,000 confirmed cases. A Malayan tiger named Nadia became the first known non-human animal in the country to test positive for the coronavirus.
- The UN Working Group of Experts on People of African Descent warned that structural discrimination could be worsening inequalities surrounding access to healthcare and

treatment, potentially leading to a rise in disease and death rates among people of African descent.

- UNESCO invited young innovators, data scientists and designers, especially those now out of school, to join a month-long hackathon, CodeTheCurve, to provide digital solutions to the global pandemic.
- On the International Day of Sport for Development and Peace, as millions of people were stuck indoors, the World Health Organization urged people to continue to practice sport and exercise through its #BeActive campaign.
- Alibaba Group CEO Jack Ma donates 500 ventilators, 200,000 suits and face shields, 2,000 thermometers, one million swabs and extraction kits and 500,000 gloves to all 54 African countries.
- Kenyan President Uhuru Kenyatta announces a halt to all movement in parts of the country affected by COVID-19, including the capital Nairobi, coming into effect on 7 pm on 6 April for a period of 21 days.
- The Nigerian Government requests a US$6.9 billion fund from international lenders to alleviate the economic impact of the coronavirus.
- The Independent Communications Authority of South Africa introduces an emergency release of broadband spectrum to meet a spike in internet usage caused by the coronavirus pandemic.
- Chancellor of Austria Sebastian Kurz announces plans to reopen small non-essential businesses and DIY shops on 14 April, followed by all shops and malls on 1 May, in order to loosen the nationwide lockdown.

- Danish Prime Minister Mette Frederiksen announces that Denmark will reopen daycare centres and schools for children in the first and fifth grade, commencing 15 April, if the number of coronavirus cases remains stable.
- Israeli Prime Minister Benjamin Netanyahu implements a national lockdown for the Passover period, beginning 7 April and ending 10 April, including banning Israelis from leaving their homes on Wednesday evenings, when families travel for Passover seder meals. In Italy, Poste Italiane makes an agreement for the Carabinieri to deliver mail to Italian pensioners who are 75 years old and above.
- Polish Prime Minister Mateusz Morawiecki announces plans to increase testing from 6,000-7,000 to 8,000-9,000 a month in response to predictions that infections will peak in May and June.
- Romanian President Klaus Iohannis extends the national state of emergency by 30 days.
- Spain mobilises 60,000 retired medical personnel in order to facilitate the "contagion slowdown."
- Sweden's central bank, Sveriges Riksbank, extends its 500 billion Swedish crowns loan scheme (US$49 billion) to individual companies affected by the coronavirus pandemic.
- A spokesman for UK Prime Minister Boris Johnson announces that the country now has 10,000 ventilators in its health system. The 2020 Open Championship was originally scheduled to be held between 16 and 19 July at Royal St George's Golf Club in Sandwich, England. The British media company, Daily Mail and General Trust, which publishes the Daily Mail, asks staff to take a pay cut with the difference made up in shares, to help the company cope with the loss

of advertising revenue and lower circulation caused by the coronavirus pandemic.

- World Health Organization (WHO) Director-General Tedros Adhanom advises that public demand for face masks could create a shortage for medical personnel.
- The 2020 Masters Tournament, originally scheduled to be held on 12–15 November at Augusta National Golf Club in Augusta, Georgia, is postponed.
- Apple Inc. CEO Tim Cook announces that his company will produce and ship 1 million face shields for use by medical workers at its factories in the US and China, focusing on the US for initial distribution.
- In Canada, Premier of Ontario Doug Ford criticises the United States for blocking the supply of three million masks over the weekend.
- In the United States, New York State Governor Andrew Cuomo extends an order closing non-essential businesses and schools until 29 April. Governor of South Carolina Henry McMaster orders all residents to stay at home except for purchasing groceries and exercising.
- Iranian Foreign Ministry spokesperson Abbas Mousavi announces that Iran will not seek American help and demands that Washington lifts its sanctions against Iran. The Supreme Leader of Iran, Ali Khamenei, announces the withdrawal of €1 billion from the country's sovereign wealth fund to invest in Iran's health services and the unemployment insurance fund.
- Saudi Arabia imposes 24-hour lockdowns on the governorates of Jeddah, Taif, Qatif and Khobar, and the cities of Riyadh, Tabuk, Dammam, Dhahran and Hofuf.

- The World Health Organization teamed up with Global Citizen to launch 'One World Together At Home", a global television and streaming event curated by Lady Gaga, to celebrate frontline health care workers in their battle against the pandemic.

7 April

- Abkhazia confirms its first case.
- Artsakh confirms its first case.
- Brazil reports a total of 13,717 cases and 667 deaths.
- Canada reports 1,241 new cases, bringing the total to 17,063. The country also reported a total of 345 deaths.
- China reports no new coronavirus deaths for the first time since it started publishing figures on COVID-19 last year. Chinese authorities also report 32 new imported cases and 30 new asymptomatic cases, bringing the total to 1,033.
- France reports more than 10,000 total deaths, including 7,091 hospital deaths and 3,237 deaths in retirement homes.
- Germany reports 3,834 cases, bringing the total to 99,225. The country's death toll also rose by 173 to 1,607.
- Indonesia reports 247 new cases, bringing the total to 2,738. The country also reports 12 new deaths, bringing the total to 221. In addition, 204 people have recovered.
- Iran reports 2,089 new cases, bringing the total to 62,589. The country also reports 133 deaths, bringing the total to 3,872.
- Ireland confirmed 345 new cases and 36 deaths, the largest to date. This gave a total of 5,709 confirmed cases and 210 deaths.

- Malaysia reports 170 new cases, bringing the total to 3,963. Health authorities also report 1 death, bringing the death toll to 63. In addition, 80 patients have recovered, bringing the total number of recoveries to 1,321.
- New Zealand reports 54 new cases, bringing the total to 1,160. 241 people have also recovered.
- The Philippines report 104 new cases, bringing the total to 3,764. The country also reports 14 new deaths, bringing the total to 177.
- Qatar reports 225 new cases, bringing the total to 2,057. The country reports 6 deaths.
- Russia reports 1,154 new cases, bringing the total to 7,497. The country also reports 11 new deaths, bringing the death toll to 58.
- Singapore confirms 106 new cases, bringing the total number to 1,481.
- South Sudan reports its second case.
- Switzerland reports a total of 641 deaths and 22,242 cases.
- Turkey reports 3,892 new cases, bringing the total to 34,109. The death toll rose by 76 to 725 while the country reported a total of 150 recoveries.
- Ukraine reports 143 new cases and 7 new deaths, bringing the total numbers to 1,462 and 45, respectively.
- In the United States, New York state reports 731 new deaths, bringing the death toll in that state to 5,489.
- According to Johns Hopkins University, over 1.3 million people globally have been affected by the coronavirus. More than 74,500 people have died, while nearly 285,000 have recovered.

- Radio New Zealand and Reuters report that over 20,000 Pakistani migrant workers are stranded in the United Arab Emirates. ACF Animal Rescue rescue pet cats, dogs, and rabbits from an abandoned pet market in Karachi's Empress Market.
- The Tunisian Interior Ministry warns that people infected with the coronavirus can be prosecuted for manslaughter if they do not abide by governmental directives to self-isolate and cross-contaminate others.
- Benin's government ordered residents in several cities and towns to wear face masks. The Benin government also placed a "cordon sanitaire" on 12 areas, including the capital Porto-Novo and largest city Cotonou, banning travel, public gatherings and shutting down public transportation. This came into effect the following day.
- The Czech Republic extends the state of emergency until late April. Czech Prime Minister, Andrej Babiš' government had initially sought to extend the state of emergency until 11 May but lacked sufficient parliamentary support.
- Finland extends tightened border controls until 13 May in order to contain the spread of COVID-19.
- Slovenian Prime Minister Janez Janša announces that the Slovenian government could ease lockdown measures on factories and service providers if current trends towards the decline of the coronavirus continue.
- UK Prime Minister Boris Johnson remains in intensive care while Foreign Secretary Dominic Raab serves as acting-Prime Minister. British Chief Scientific Adviser Patrick Vallance states that while the UK has not seen a rise in the

number of coronavirus cases, it remains too early to tell whether the outbreak has peaked.

- Radio New Zealand and Reuters report that over 20,000 Pakistani migrant workers are stranded in the United Arab Emirates. ACF Animal Rescue rescue pet cats, dogs, and rabbits from an abandoned pet market in Karachi's Empress Market.
- The Tunisian Interior Ministry warns that people infected with the coronavirus can be prosecuted for manslaughter if they do not abide by governmental directives to self-isolate and cross-contaminate others.
- Brazilian Health Minister Luiz Henrique Mandetta warns that the country faces a shortage of respirators.
- Canadian Prime Minister Justin Trudeau confirms that the Canadian Government is working with the United States Government to allow the movement of medical supplies to Canada following complaints that Washington had blocked the shipment of face masks. United States Secretary of State Mike Pompeo has announced that the Trump Administration will focus on keeping key medical supplies, including personal protection equipment, in the United States. Secretary of the Treasury Steven Mnuchin calls upon Congress to approve an additional US$250 billion subsidy for a small business relief programme by Saturday. This would supplement a US$350 billion relief programme for small businesses that was launched earlier on Friday.

8 April

- Bangladesh reports a total of 218 cases and 20 deaths.
- Belarus reports 205 new cases, bringing the total to 1,066. The country has reported a total of 13 deaths.
- China reports 62 new cases (nearly all imported), bringing the total number of imported cases to 1,042. China has reported a total of 81,802 cases since the beginning of the outbreak.
- The Czech Republic reports a total of 5,000 cases and 195 deaths.
- Egypt reports 9 new deaths, bringing the death toll to 94. The country also reports a total of 1,450 cases.
- Ethiopia reports a total of 52 cases and 2 deaths.
- France reports 541 new hospital deaths, bringing the death toll to 10,869. French authorities also report 7,148 people in intensive care.
- Germany reports 254 new deaths, bringing the total to 1,864. The country reports a total number of 103,228 cases.
- Indonesia reports 218 new cases, bringing the total to 2,956. Indonesia also reports 19 new deaths, taking the total to 240. 222 have recovered.
- Iran reports 121 new deaths, bringing the death toll to 3,993. The country also reports 1,997 new cases, bringing the total to 64,586. Iran also reports 3,956 infected people.
- Ireland confirmed 365 new cases and 25 deaths. This gave a total of 6,074 confirmed cases and 235 deaths.
- Israel reports 156 new cases, bringing the total to 9,400. The country also reports 6 new deaths, bringing the total to 71. 147 are in critical condition, while 801 have recovered.

- Japan reports 144 new cases in Tokyo, bringing the total number of cases to 4,768. The country has reported a total of 98 deaths.
- Malaysia reports 156 new cases, bringing the total number to 4,119. The country also reports 2 more deaths, bringing a total of 65 deaths.
- Myanmar reports a total of 22 cases and 3 deaths.
- New Zealand reports 50 new cases (26 confirmed and 24 probable), bringing the total to 1,210. 41 new recoveries were reported, bringing the total to 282.
- Pakistan reports a total of 3,546 cases, 57 deaths, and 458 recoveries.
- Peru reports a total of 107 deaths and 2,954 confirmed cases.
- The Philippines reports 106 new cases, bringing the total to 3,870. The country also reports 5 deaths, bringing the death toll to 182. The Philippines reports 12 new recoveries, bringing the total to 96.
- Poland confirms a total of more than 5,000 cases. The country also reports 22 new deaths, bringing the total to 435. Poland has so far tested 100,000 people.
- Russia reports 1,175 new cases, bringing the total to 8,672. 5 new deaths reported, bringing the total to 63.
- Singapore confirms 142 new cases, bringing the total number to 1,623. In addition, a person was later confirmed to have COVID-19 after he died, which was caused by a heart condition.
- Somalia reports its first death. Authorities also reported 4 new cases, bringing the total to 12.
- Switzerland reports a total of 705 deaths and 22,789 cases.

- Thailand reports 3 new deaths, bringing the death toll to 30. The country has a total of 2,369 cases.
- Turkey reports a total of 38,226 confirmed cases, 812 related deaths, and 1,846 recovered cases. Turkish health authorities have also conducted 24,9900 cases.
- Ukraine reports 206 new cases and 7 new deaths, bringing the total numbers to 1,668 and 52, respectively.
- The Emirate of Dubai, which is part of the United Arab Emirates, reports a total of 2,659 cases and 12 deaths.
- The United Kingdom reports 938 new deaths, bringing the death toll to 7,097.
- The United States reports 400,000 confirmed cases and a total of 12,900 deaths.
- The Resolution Foundation, using figures from the British Chambers of Commerce, reports that more than nine million workers are expected to be furloughed under the government's job retention scheme, with an estimated cost to the taxpayer of between £30 and 40bn.
- Egyptian Prime Minister Mostafa Madbouly extends a nighttime curfew that will start at 8 pm until 23 April to combat the spread of coronavirus. The country's airports will remain closed.
- The Iranian President Hassan Rouhani appeals to the International Monetary Fund to give the country the US$5 billion emergency loan that Tehran had requested to fight the coronavirus pandemic.
- The Jordanian Finance Minister Mohammed Al Ississ states that Jordan will be able to repay its foreign debt obligations despite the loss of economic revenue caused by the coronavirus pandemic.

- The Lebanese Ministry of Social Affairs launches a 75 billion Lebanese pound aid relief programme. This includes one-time cash assistance of 400,000 Lebanese pounds (US$140) to about 187,500 families.
- The Pakistani Government announces that it plans to increase its daily COVID-19 testing capacity to at least 25,000 tests a day by late April and to increase the supply of personal equipment to doctors from 9 April.
- In the United Arab Emirates, the Emirate of Dubai's justice department suspends marriages and divorces as a result of the COVID-19 pandemic.
- Negotiations between European Union finance ministers over an economic rescue package break down due to disagreements between the Netherlands and Italy over what conditions should be attached to Eurozone credit for governments fighting the pandemic. Mauro Ferrari, the head of the European Research Council, resigns in protest at his dissatisfaction with the European Union's response to the COVID-19 pandemic.
- The French Government extends the nation's lockdown until 15 April.
- The President of Turkey's Directorate of Communications announces that the Turkish Government will be tracking the mobile phones of citizens to enforce the quarantine through an app called the "Pandemic Isolation Tracking Project."
- The World Health Organization's Europe director Hans Kluge issues a statement advising governments not to relax measures aimed at containing the coronavirus.
- Brazilian President Jair Bolsonaro announces that Brazil will purchase the anti-malaria drug hydroxychloroquine despite

scientists warning that there is insufficient evidence that the drug treats COVID-19.

- President of Peru Martin Vizcarra extends the national state of emergency until 26 April.
- The United States President Trump criticises the World Health Organization (WHO)'s handling of the coronavirus pandemic and alleged that the international organisation had pursued a "very China-centric" approach. In response, the WHO's Director-General Tedros Adhanom has defended his agency's handling of the COVID-19 pandemic in response to President Trump's criticism, urging world leaders not to politicise the pandemic. Uruguay approves a humanitarian flight to evacuate Australian and New Zealand passengers from the Aurora Expeditions cruise ship Greg Mortimer, where 60% of the passengers have tested positive for COVID-19. The New York Times reports that genomic analysis of New York infections indicate the immediate origin of its cases were travellers from Europe instead of Asia and that weeks before its first confirmed infection, the virus has likely present in New York during mid-February.
- The U.S. Customs and Border Protection (CBP) and the Federal Emergency Management Agency (FEMA) issue a joint announcement that they will seize exports of medical supplies, including respirators, surgical masks and surgical gloves, until they can determine whether it should be returned for use in the US, purchased by the US Government, or exported. This followed an earlier memorandum on 1 April by President Trump empowering federal agencies to keep medical supplies within US borders.

- Governor of New York Andrew Cuomo issues a directive for flags to be flown at half-mast in New York state to honour victims of the coronavirus.
- Google announces that it will give gamers two months of free access to Stadia Pro to cope with COVID-19 lockdowns. This offer is available in 14 countries and will be rolled out over 48 hours.
- Twitter CEO Jack Dorsey contributes 28% of his fortune to create a US$1 billion fund known as StartSmall, focusing initially on global relief efforts for the coronavirus pandemic.
- Egyptian Prime Minister Mostafa Madbouly extends a nighttime curfew that will start at 8 pm until 23 April to combat the spread of coronavirus. The country's airports will remain closed.
- The Iranian President Hassan Rouhani appeals to the International Monetary Fund to give the country the US$5 billion emergency loan that Tehran had requested to fight the coronavirus pandemic.
- The Jordanian Finance Minister Mohammed Al Ississ states that Jordan will be able to repay its foreign debt obligations despite the loss of economic revenue caused by the coronavirus pandemic.
- The Lebanese Ministry of Social Affairs launches a 75 billion Lebanese pound aid relief programme. This includes one-time cash assistance of 400,000 Lebanese pounds (US$140) to about 187,500 families.
- The Pakistani Government announces that it plans to increase its daily COVID-19 testing capacity to at least 25,000 tests a day by late April and to increase the supply of personal equipment to doctors from 9 April.

- In the United Arab Emirates, the Emirate of Dubai's justice department suspends marriages and divorces as a result of the COVID-19 pandemic.
- Ethiopian Prime Minister Abiy Ahmed declares a state of emergency to combat the spread of COVID-19. Ethiopian authorities have already banned public gatherings, closed schools, and required employees to work from home.
- South African President Cyril Ramaphosa orders that the Minister of Communications, Telecommunications and Postal Services Stella Ndabeni-Abrahams be placed on "special leave" for two months for breaching lockdown requirements by having lunch with a former official in her home.

9 April

- Brazil reports its first case among the Yanomami people in the Amazon: a 15-year-old boy.
- Canada reports a total of 19,774 cases. Canadian authorities report a total of 461 deaths.
- Chinese authorities in the northeastern city of Suifenhe report 40 new cases, all returning Chinese nationals who had come from nearby Russia.
- Egypt reports 139 new cases, bringing the total to 1,699. Egyptian authorities also report 15 new deaths, bringing the total to 115.
- Hungary reports a total of 980 confirmed cases and 66 deaths.
- Ireland confirmed 500 new cases, the largest to date, and 28 deaths. This brings the total to 6,574 cases and 265 deaths.

- Malaysia reports 109 new cases and 2 new deaths, bringing the total number of cases and deaths to 4,228 and 67, respectively. The country also reports that 72 people are in intensive care but that 121 people have been discharged.
- The Netherlands reports 1,213 new cases, bringing the total to 21,762. Dutch authorities have reported a total of 2,396 deaths.
- New Zealand reports 29 new cases (23 confirmed and 6 probable), bringing the total to 1,239 (992 confirmed and 247 probable). The country also reports 35 new recoveries, bringing the total to 317.
- Pakistan has a total of 3,713 confirmed cases and 62 deaths.
- Russia reports 1,459 new cases, bringing the total to more than 10,000. The country also reports 13 deaths, bringing the total to 76.
- Singapore confirms 287 new cases, bringing the total number to 1,910.
- South Korea reports 39 new cases, bringing the total to 10,423. The country also reports 4 deaths, bringing the total to 204.
- Spain reports 683 new deaths, bringing the death toll to 15,238. The country reports a total of 152,446 cases.
- Turkey reports 96 new deaths, bringing the total to 908. Turkey also confirms 4,056 new cases, bringing the total to 42,282.
- Ukraine reports 224 new cases and 5 new deaths, bringing the total numbers to 1,892 and 57, respectively.

- The United Kingdom reports 881 new deaths, bringing the total to 7,987. British authorities have also tested a total of 243,321 people, with 65,077 testing positive.
- The United States reports over 15,000 deaths linked to the coronavirus.
- Vietnam announces that 15,461 people, including 1,000 healthcare workers linked to a coronavirus outbreak at a Hanoi hospital, have all tested negative for the disease.
- 2 new cases are confirmed in the disputed territory of Western Sahara, bringing the total to 6.
- According to figures released by Johns Hopkins University, there has been a total of 1,502,618 cases, 89,915 deaths, and 339,775 recoveries.
- Dominic Raab says the UK is "starting to see the impact" of the restrictions, but it is "too early" to lift them and urges people to stay indoors over the upcoming Easter weekend. With warm weather forecast again for Easter, this message is echoed by police and tourist destinations. Johnson was moved out of intensive care but remained in hospital.
- At 8 pm, the nation stages a third round of applause for NHS staff and other key workers.
- Dr John Nkengasong, the Director of the Africa Centres for Disease Control and Prevention (Africa CDC), condemns remarks made on 1 April by two French scientists, Professors Jean-Paul Mira and Camille Locht, that a potential tuberculosis vaccine for the coronavirus be tested on Africa as "disgusting and racist." Mira had issued an apology for his statements via his employer, the Paris network of hospitals, on 3 April, while Locht could not be reached by that date for comment.

- The entire Parliament of Botswana, including President of Botswana Mokgweetsi Masisi, will be quarantined for 14 days and tested for the coronavirus after a health worker screening lawmakers for the virus herself tested positive overnight.
- South African President Cyril Ramaphosa defends the World Health Organization (WHO) in response to criticism by US President Trump. President Ramaphosa also extended the country's lockdown, which had been started on 27 March and was due to last 21 days, by a further two weeks.
- Ugandan President Yoweri Museveni issues a Twitter post discouraging people from jogging in groups and instead encouraging them to exercise indoors.
- German Chancellor Angela Merkel has called for "patience" during the coronavirus crisis, stating that society will have to "live with the virus" until a vaccine becomes available.
- Hungarian Prime Minister Viktor Orbán extends the nation's lockdown indefinitely.
- Russian retailers report a surge in the sales of alcoholic beverages over the past few weeks during the lockdown. According to market research firm Nielsen, the sale of vodka, whisky and beer rose 31%, 47% and 25%, respectively.
- UK Prime Minister Boris Johnson is released from intensive care but remains in hospital.
- Iranian Supreme Leader Ali Khamenei urges Iranians to spend Ramadan at home during the lockdown. Public gatherings are banned while schools and universities have been closed.

- The Pakistani Government distributes a one-time Rs12,000 (US$70) grant to 12 million low-income families.
- Canada reports a record 1 million job losses in March, with the national unemployment rate soaring to 7.8%. Canadian health authorities also estimate that between 11,000 and 22,000 could die from COVID-19 in Canada.
- The US Centers for Disease Control issues new guidelines advising people working in essential services like healthcare and food supply to check their temperatures before going to work, wear face masks, and practise social distancing. According to figures, 6.6 million Americans have filed for unemployment as a result of the coronavirus pandemic.
- The Japanese company Fujifilm enters the second phase of its Avigan anti-flu clinical trial on 50 patients at three hospitals in Massachusetts.
- The Nicaraguan Government releases 1,700 prisoners in response to the coronavirus pandemic but excludes political prisoners.
- The United Nations delivers 90 tons of medical supplies, sanitation equipment, and water to Venezuela, including 28,000 PPE kits for health workers, oxygen concentrators, pediatric beds, water quality control products and hygiene kits. The Bangkok-based United Nations Human Rights Office for Southeast Asia calls upon governments to protect the health of migrants from COVID-19 by releasing them from detention centres and suspending deportations.
- Uber's Vice President of safety and insurance, Gus Fuldner, announces that the company will be shipping millions of masks to active drivers and food delivery people around the world to help combat the spread of COVID-19.

- Iranian Supreme Leader Ali Khamenei urges Iranians to spend Ramadan at home during the lockdown. Public gatherings are banned while schools and universities have been closed.
- The Pakistani government distributes a one-time Rs12,000 (US$70) grant to 12 million low-income families.
- Hundreds have protested against lockdown restrictions imposed by state governors in the Brazilian cities of Rio de Janeiro, Sao Paulo and the capital Brasilia. Brazilian President Jair Bolsonaro has criticized the lockdown measures, claiming that the "fear was excessive" and that people want a return to normality.
- Honduran security minister Jair Meza has extended the country's curfew until 26 April in an attempt to curb the spread of the coronavirus.
- Panama has detained about 1,700 undocumented migrants heading to the United States in a jungle camp in La Penita near the Colombian border after 17 coronavirus cases were detected among them. These infected individuals have been removed from the camp, whose facilities are designed to host 200 people.
- US President Donald Trump and Turkish President Recep Tayyip Erdoğan agreed to continue their close bilateral cooperation to combat the coronavirus during a phone interview. Governor of New York Andrew Cuomo issued a statement stating that the outbreak in New York state is "on the descent." President Trump has also reiterated a US offer to help Iran deal with the coronavirus pandemic if Tehran requested it.

- The World Health Organization and non-profit NGO Global Citizen have sponsored a two-hour One World: Together at Home television broadcast program featuring several celebrities and public figures, including Jimmy Kimmel, Stephen Colbert, Jimmy Fallon, Lady Gaga, Paul McCartney, the Rolling Stones, Beyonce, Elton John, Stevie Wonder, David Beckham and former US First Ladies Michelle Obama and Laura Bush. These celebrities and public figures will be sharing music, comedy, and personal stories from their own homes.

10 April

- Africa has reported a total of nearly 11,000 cases and 562 deaths.
- Bangladesh reports a total of 27 deaths and 424 cases.
- Brazil reports a total of 19,638 cases and 1,056 deaths. Brazilian health authorities also report that the infected Yanomani teenager has died from the coronavirus.
- China reports 42 new cases (38 of them imported), bringing the total to 81,907. Chinese authorities also report 1 death, bringing the death toll to 3,336. Another 1,169 suspected cases or those who tested positive but were not showing symptoms are being monitored. More than 77,000 have recovered.
- Ecuador reports 2,196 new cases, bringing the total to 7,161. The country has also confirmed 297 deaths and another 311 likely deaths as the result of COVID-19.
- France reports 987 deaths, bringing the death toll to 13,917. The French Navy has reported 50 cases aboard the aircraft carrier Charles De Gaulle.

- Hungary reports 210 new cases, bringing the total to 1,190. The country has reported a total of 77 deaths.
- Iran reports 122 new deaths, bringing the total to 4,232. The country also reports 1,972 new cases, bringing the total to 68,912, with 3,969 in critical condition.
- Ireland confirmed 480 new cases and 25 deaths. This gave a total of 7,054 confirmed cases and 287 deaths. The Health Service Executive also acknowledges several other cases that have been confirmed by Germany, as previous tests had been sent to Germany, which brings the actual total to 8,089.
- Italy reports the death of 100 doctors.
- Japan reports a total of 6,003 cases and 99 deaths.
- Malaysia reports 118 new cases, bringing the total to 4,346 cases and 70 deaths. Malaysia authorities also reported that 222 patients have been discharged, bringing the total number of recoveries to 1,830 (or roughly 42% of patients).
- Mexico reports 2 new deaths, bringing the death toll to 194.
- The Netherlands reports 1,335 new cases, bringing the total to 23,907. The country reports 115 deaths, bringing the total to 2,511.
- New Zealand reports 44 new cases (23 confirmed and 21 probable), bringing the total to 1,283 (1,015 confirmed and 267 probable). NZ health authorities also report 56 new recoveries, bringing the total to 373. In addition, New Zealand reports its second death, a Christchurch woman in her 90s.
- Pakistan reports a total of 3,817 cases, 67 deaths, and 712 recoveries.

- The Philippines reports 119 new cases, bringing the total to 4,195. The country also reports 18 new deaths, bringing the total to 221.
- Russia reports 1,786 new cases, bringing the total number to 11,917. The country also reports 18 new deaths, bringing the death toll to 94.
- Singapore confirms 198 new cases, bringing the total number to 2,108. Another death is also confirmed, bringing the death toll to 7.
- South Korea reports 27 new cases, bringing the total to 10,450. The country has a total of 208 deaths. In addition, health authorities reported that 91 people who were thought to have recovered have shown symptoms of the coronavirus.
- Spain reports 4,566 new deaths, bringing the total to 15,843. The country reports 4,576 new cases, bringing the total to 157,022.
- Switzerland reports a total of 805 deaths and 24,308 infections.
- Taiwan reports 2 new cases, bringing the total to 382. Taiwanese authorities also report the country's sixth death.
- Thailand reports 50 new cases and 1 death, bringing the total number of cases to 2,473 and the death toll to 33.
- Timor Leste reports its second case. The country had reported its first case on 21 March, who has since recovered.
- Turkey reports 4,747 new cases, bringing the total to 47,029. The country reports 98 new deaths bringing the total to 1,006. Turkey also reports 281 recoveries, bringing the total number to 2,423.

- Ukraine reports 311 new cases and 12 new deaths, bringing the total numbers to 2,203 and 69, respectively.
- The United Kingdom reports 980 new deaths (886 in England), bringing the total to 8,958 (8,114 in England).
- The United States has reported over 16,500 deaths. Cook County Jail in Chicago reports 450 cases among staff and inmates.
- Yemen confirms its first case of coronavirus in Hadhramaut.
- According to Johns Hopkins University, there have been 1.6 million coronavirus cases, over 100,000 deaths, and 372,000 recoveries.
- Jonathan Van-Tam, England's deputy chief medical officer, tells the UK Government's daily briefing the lockdown is "beginning to pay off" but the UK is still in a "dangerous situation", and although cases in London have started to drop, they are still rising in Yorkshire and the North East.
- Matt Hancock tells the briefing a "Herculean effort" is being made to ensure daily deliveries of personal protective equipment (PPE) to frontline workers, including the establishment of a domestic manufacturing industry to produce the equipment. Fifteen drive-through testing centres have also been opened around the UK to test frontline workers.
- The Senegalese government bans companies from dismissing employees during the coronavirus pandemic except in cases of gross negligence, commencing 14 April.
- Zimbabwe's national carrier, Air Zimbabwe, which is facing a US$30 million debt, places all its workers on indefinite unpaid leave.

- The World Health Organization (WHO) Director-General Tedros Adhanom Ghebreyesus laid out six factors for consideration when lifting lockdowns, including that transmission, is controlled and sufficient public health and medical services are available.
- The Jordanian Armed Forces arrested the owner of Ro'ya TV and its news director for airing a news story showing a crowd of labourers complaining about their inability to work as a result of the country's coronavirus lockdown.
- Pakistan begins distributing Rs144 billion (US$863 million) in cash grants to low-income families across the country. In the first phase, the Government disbursed roughly US$300 million to banks, which distributed Rs12,000 (US$70) grants to low-income families.
- According to US Government figures, 16.8 million Americans have lost their jobs in the past three weeks as a result of the coronavirus.
- The US Centres for Disease Control extends their "No Sail Order" for cruise ships. There are approximately 100 cruise ships and nearly 80,000 crew off the East Coast, West Coast, and Gulf Coast of the United States. The order can only be rescinded under the following conditions: after the expiration of the US Secretary of Health and Human Services' declaration that COVID-19 constitutes a public health emergency; the CDC Director rescinds or modifies the order based on specific public health or other considerations; or 100 days after the date of publication in the Federal Register.
- The United States President Trump calls upon the US Congress to pass a US$251 billion bill providing emergency

funding for the business. He criticizes the Democratic Party for blocking the bill.

- Governor of California Gavin Newsom reports a 1.9% drop in intensive care unit admissions (roughly 1,132) in Californian hospitals.
- The New York City Department of Corrections reports that about two dozen unclaimed bodies are being buried each day at a mass grave on Hart Island. US immunologist Anthony Fauci warns that it is too early to roll back restrictions despite progress in combating the coronavirus pandemic in New York.
- The Secretary-General of the United Nations António Guterres warns the United Nations Security Council that the coronavirus pandemic is threatening international peace and security, "potentially leading to an increase in social unrest and violence that would greatly undermine our ability to fight the disease."
- The International Monetary Fund (IMF) approves disbursement of US$147 million under its Rapid Financing Instrument to help Gabon combat the impact of the coronavirus.
- Google and Apple Inc. announce that they will work together to develop an app for tracking coronavirus infections using existing Bluetooth and encryption technology.
- The International Monetary Fund announces that it will loan Albania US$190.5 million to deal with the impact of the coronavirus.
- German Foreign Minister Heiko Maas criticises the US' handling of the coronavirus pandemic as "too slow" during an interview with Der Spiegel.

- In Finland, Tomi Lounema, the head of the country's National Emergency Supply Centre, resigns over the purchase of the multi-million Euro purchase of Chinese face masks that proved unsuitable for local hospital usage.
- Hungarian Prime Minister Viktor Orbán makes a speech stating that the country's "tough measures" have slowed the spread of the coronavirus, but that country's "real test" still lies ahead. Orbán also stated that Hungary needed 8,000 ventilators and intensive care beds.
- Irish Taoiseach Leo Varadkar extends the country's stay-at-home restrictions until 5 May.
- The Italian Government bars entry to Italian ports by international rescue vessels ferrying migrants for the duration of the coronavirus pandemic. Italian Prime Minister Giuseppe Conte announces that the Italian government will be extending the nation's lockdown until 3 May.
- Kazakhstan extends its state of emergency until the end of April. The state of emergency allows the government to lock down all provinces and the capital and to shut down many businesses.
- The Swiss-based Cyclistes Professionnels Associé (CPA) issues a statement warning against pay cuts for cyclists during the coronavirus pandemic.
- The Russian Prosecutor General announces that it will be blocking access to "fake news" social media posts questioning Moscow's quarantine measures. Mayor of Moscow Sergei Sobyanin announces that the city will introduce a system of travel passes to monitor and regulate citizens' movements the following week.

- The Turkish Government imposes a 48-hour curfew on 31 cities, including Ankara and Istanbul.
- The English football club Arsenal announces that it will be providing 30,000 free meals and sanitary products to vulnerable people and join forces with a local church to deliver 15,000 tons of emergency supplies to Islington. The club also pledged to donate £100,000 ($124,000) to local organisations and another £50,000 pounds to a COVID-19 Crisis Fund.

11 April

- Armenia reports 966 total cases and 13 total deaths.
- Belarus reports a total of 23 deaths and 2,226 cases.
- Brazil reports a total of 1,056 deaths and 19,638 cases.
- Canada reports 1,316 new cases, bringing the total to 22,559. Canadian authorities also report 69 new deaths, bringing the total to 600.
- China reports 46 new cases (including 42 involving overseas travel), bringing the total to 81,953. Chinese authorities also report three new cases, bringing the death toll to 3,339. China also reports 34 new asymptomatic cases.
- France reports 353 hospital deaths and 290 nursing home deaths, bringing the death toll to 13,832.
- Indonesia reports 330 new cases, bringing the total to 3,842. Indonesian authorities also reported 21 deaths, bringing the death toll to 237.
- Iran reports 1,837 new cases, bringing the total to 70,029. Iranian authorities also report 125 new deaths, bringing the death toll to 4,357.

- Ireland confirmed 553 new cases and 33 deaths. This gave a total of 8,928 confirmed cases and 320 deaths, as 1 previously reported death was incorrectly attributed to COVID-19. These figures include results of tests sent to Germany.
- Israel reports a total of 101 deaths and 10,743 cases. Of the infected, 175 are in serious condition, 129 are on ventilators, 154 in moderate condition, and 7,000 are hospitalized at home. 1,341 have recovered from the coronavirus.
- Italy reports 619 new deaths, bringing the total to 19,468. The country has reported a total of over 150,000 cases.
- Kazakhstan reports 10 cases at the Tengiz oilfield.
- Malaysia reports 184 new cases, bringing the total to 4,530. Health authorities have also reported 3 new deaths, bringing the total to 73. According to Malaysian authorities, 44% of cases have recovered.
- The Netherlands reports 1,316 new cases, bringing the total to 24,413. Dutch authorities report 132 new deaths, bringing the death toll to 2,643.
- New Zealand reports 29 new cases (20 confirmed and 9 probable), bringing the total to 1,312 (1,035 confirmed and 276 probable). The country also reports 48 new recoveries, bringing the total to 422. In addition, authorities report 2 new deaths, bringing the total to 4.
- Pakistan reports 190 new cases, bringing the total to 4,788. Health authorities also reported 5 new deaths, bringing the total to 71. Pakistan has reported 50 patients in critical conditions and 762 recoveries.
- The Philippines reports 233 new cases, bringing the total to 4,428. 26 new deaths, bringing the total to 247. 17 patients

have recovered, bringing the total number of recoveries to 157.

- Russia reports 1,667 new cases, bringing the total to 13,584. Russian authorities also reported 12 new deaths, bringing the total to 106.
- Saba confirms its first case.
- Singapore reports 191 new cases, bringing the total number to 2,299. The country also reported 1 more death, bringing the death toll to 8.
- Spain reports 4,830 new cases, bringing the total to 161,852. Spanish authorities also reported 510 deaths, bringing the total to 16,353.
- Switzerland reports a total of 831 deaths and 24,900 cases.
- Thailand reports 2 new deaths, bringing the death toll to 35. Thai authorities also report 45 new cases, bringing the total to 2,518 and 1,135 recoveries.
- Ukraine reports 308 new cases and 4 new deaths, bringing the total numbers to 2,511 and 73, respectively. The number of recoveries (79) exceeded the number of lethal outcomes for the first time.
- The United Kingdom reports 917 deaths, bringing the death toll to 9,875. 269,598 have been tested, with 78,991 testing positive.
- The United States reports a total of 20,071 deaths and 522,000 cases. New York state reports 783 new deaths, bringing the death toll to 8,600.
- The global death toll is now over 107,000. Global infections number more than 1.7 million, and global recoveries number 396,000.

- Queen Elizabeth II makes her first-ever Easter message to the nation, in which she states, "coronavirus will not overcome us" and that "we need Easter as much as ever."
- After some NHS workers say they still do not have the correct personal protective equipment to treat patients, Home Secretary Priti Patel tells that day's Downing Street briefing she is "sorry if people feel there have been failings" in providing kit.
- The number of people in London hospitals for COVID-19 reaches its peak, according to week-on-week change data; elsewhere in the country, patient numbers continue to increase, although the rate of increase is slowing.
- Occupancy of critical care beds in England peaks at around 58% of capacity. Occupancy in the month of April for Scotland and Wales will only briefly exceed 40%, while Northern Ireland reported a peak of 51% early in the month.
- The UN Secretary-General called on religious leaders of all faiths to join forces and work for global peace and focus on the common battle to defeat COVID-19.
- In a joint appeal, the five UN envoys to the Middle East urged the region's warring parties to work towards an immediate end to hostilities, emphasizing the Secretary-General's recent call for a global ceasefire during the COVID-19 pandemic. In Iran, "low risk" businesses in most parts of the country except Tehran are allowed to reopen. However, President Hassan Rouhani urged Iranians to comply with social distancing and other health protocols.
- Armenian Prime Minister Nikol Pashinyan extends the country's state of emergency by 30 days. The country has closed all educational institutes, public transportation and

banned foreigners from entering. Armenia has also announced that it would postpone a referendum on changes to its Constitutional Court till after the emergency.

- The Austrian Federal Railways puts a quarter of its staff (10,000 workers) on short-time work in response to the coronavirus pandemic.
- In Belarus, many soccer fans boycotted matches in response to the Football Federation of Belarus' decision not to suspend matches on the grounds that the country had only reported a small number of cases. World Health Organization official Patrick O'Connor also calls upon Belarus to introduce new measures to combat the coronavirus.
- The Dutch Government calls for proposals to develop smartphone apps or software to battle the coronavirus, including conducting contact tracing.
- Pope Francis officiates over a memorial service honouring victims of the coronavirus pandemic, including medical personnel.
- US President Donald Trump orders top administration officials to take measures to aid Italy, including making US military personnel in the country available for telemedical services, setting up field hospitals, and transporting supplies.
- Ecuadorian President Lenin Moreno announces the creation of a humanitarian assistance fund that will be funded by citizens and companies to alleviate the economic effects of COVID-19.
- US public broadcaster Voice of America has rejected the Trump Administration's allegation that it is promoting Chinese propaganda by tweeting a video of celebrations at

the end of Wuhan's quarantine measures and observing the US had surpassed China's death toll.

- Mayor of New York Bill de Blasio announces that public schools will remain closed for the duration of the school year in order to combat the coronavirus pandemic. New York has reported the highest rate of infections and deaths in the United States.
- The United States Department of Defense announces that it will be invoking the Defense Production Act and investing US$133 million to increase US domestic N95 mask production by over 39 million over the next 90 days.
- The Uruguayan Government announces that it will be repatriating 16 New Zealanders and 96 Australians who had been stranded aboard the cruise ship Greg Mortimer in the La Plata River near Montevideo since 27 March. The passengers will be flown from Montevideo to Melbourne. The New Zealand Government has arranged to fly their nationals back to Auckland on a chartered flight.
- The United States Internal Revenue Service announces that the first coronavirus stimulus checks have been deposited in taxpayers' accounts. These economic relief payments are part of a US$2.2 trillion package passed by Congress to help people and businesses affected by the coronavirus pandemic. Most adults will get US$1,200, while parents will receive $500 for each qualifying child.
- US Commissioner of Food and Drugs Stephen Hahn announces that the Trump Administration is considering relaxing "stay-home" restrictions of 1 May.
- British Home Secretary Priti Patel has apologised for the shortage of PPE equipment among medical personnel and

has warned that paedophiles are seeking to exploit children online during the coronavirus pandemic. The British Government has also announced that it would invest more in domestic violence services, including online support services, hotlines and a national communications campaign in response to a surge in domestic violence cases. British vaccinologist Sarah Gilbert has expressed optimism that her team at the University of Oxford could develop a vaccine by September 2020.

12 April

- Canada reports 74 new deaths, bringing the total to 674. Canadian authorities report a total of 23,719 cases.
- China reports 99 new cases (97 overseas cases), bringing the total to 82,052. The death toll stands at 3,339.
- Hong Kong has reported a total of 4 deaths and 1,005 cases.
- France reports a death toll of 14,393.
- Guatemala reports 16 new cases, bringing the total to 153. The country has reported a total of 3 deaths.
- Indonesia reports 399 new cases, bringing the total to 4,241. Health authorities report 42 deaths, bringing the total to 373.
- Iran reports 117 deaths, bringing the total to 4,474. Iranian authorities report 71,686 cases.
- Ireland confirmed 430 new cases and 14 deaths. There are an additional 297 positive results from Germany, which were sent weeks ago. This gives a total of 9,655 confirmed cases and 334 deaths.

- Italy reports 431 deaths, bringing the death toll to 19,899. The country also reports 156,363 infections, of which 34,211 have recovered.
- Malaysia reports a total of 153 new cases, bringing the total to 4,683. 3 more deaths were reported, bringing the total to 76.
- The Netherlands reports 1,188 new cases, bringing the total to 25,587. Dutch authorities report 94 deaths, bringing the total to 2,737.
- New Zealand reports 18 new cases (14 confirmed and 4 probable), bringing the total to 1,330 (1,049 confirmed and 281 probable). Health authorities also reported 49 new recoveries, bringing the total to 471.
- The Philippines reports 50 new deaths, bringing the death toll to 297. Authorities also reported 220 new cases, bringing the total to 4,648. 40 patients recovered, bringing the total to 197.
- Russia reports 2,186 new cases, bringing the total to 17,770. Russian authorities report 23 deaths, bringing the total to 130.
- Singapore reports 233 new cases, bringing the total number to 2,532.
- Somalia reports its second death: Hirshabelle State Justice Minister Khalif Mumin Tohow.
- South Africa reports 145 new cases, bringing the total to 2,173.
- Spain reports 619 deaths, bringing the total to 16,972. Spanish authorities report a total of 166,019 cases.
- Thailand reports 33 new cases, bringing the total to 2,551. Thai authorities report 3 new deaths, bringing the total to 38.

- Turkey reports 4,789 new cases, bringing the total to 56,956. The country also reports 1,198 deaths and 3,446 recoveries.
- Ukraine reports 266 new cases and 10 new deaths, bringing the total numbers to 2,777 and 83, respectively. Additionally, 89 patients have recovered.
- The United Kingdom reports 737 new deaths, bringing the total to 10,612.
- There are about 1.7 million global cases and over 109,000 deaths.
- Prime Minister Boris Johnson is discharged from the hospital after being treated for coronavirus and will continue his recovery at Chequers.
- The number of people who died in hospital with coronavirus in the UK passes 10,000, after a daily rise of 737 to 10,612. Matt Hancock describes it as a "sombre day".
- The United States Internal Revenue Service announces that the first coronavirus stimulus checks have been deposited in taxpayers' accounts. These economic relief payments are part of a US$2.2 trillion package passed by Congress to help people and businesses affected by the coronavirus pandemic. Most adults will get US$1,200, while parents will receive $500 for each qualifying child.
- US Commissioner of Food and Drugs Stephen Hahn announces that the Trump Administration is considering relaxing "stay-home" restrictions of 1 May.
- The Egyptian Government postpones its bid to sell its stake in the state-owned Banque de Caire due to the spread of the coronavirus.
- The Jordanian Government extends a month-long lockdown until the end of April.

- Saudi Arabia orders an extension of the country's curfew until further notice.
- United Arab Emirates airliner Etihad Airways announces that it will operate special flights to Brussels, Dublin, London, Tokyo and Zurich between 14 and 22 April. This was in response to the UAE government stating that it would allow a number of limited outbound flights for those wishing to leave the country.
- The Organization of the Petroleum Exporting Countries, Russia and several oil-producing countries agree to reduce output by 9.7 million barrels per day (roughly 10%) in order to support oil prices amid the COVID-19 pandemic.

13 April

- The Africa Centres for Disease Control and Prevention (CDC) report 1,894 new cases, bringing the total in Africa to 14,744. 104 deaths have been recorded, bringing the African death toll to 793. The Africa CDC reports that 52 out of 55 African countries have been affected.
- Australia reports a total of 63 new cases, bringing the total to 6,366.
- Burundi reports its first death and a total of five cases.
- Canada reports a total of 734 deaths and 24,804 cases.
- China reports 108 new cases, with all but ten being imported cases.
- France reports 574 deaths, bringing the total to 14,967. 6,821 patients remain in intensive care.
- Germany reports 2,537 new cases and 126 deaths, bringing the total to 123,016 and 2,799, respectively.

- Indonesia reports 316 new cases, bringing the total to 4,557. Japanese authorities reported 26 deaths, bringing the total to 399.
- Iran reports 111 new deaths, bringing the total to 4,585. Iranian authorities reported 1,617 cases, bringing the total to 73,303. 3,877 remain in critical condition while 45,983.
- Ireland confirms 527 new cases reported by Irish labs and 465 more confirmed cases reported by German labs. 31 deaths reported. This gives a total of 10,647 confirmed cases and 365 deaths.
- Israel reports 11 deaths, bringing the death toll to 116. Israeli authorities report 11,586 cases, including 183 in serious condition and 132 on ventilators.
- Malaysia reports 134 new cases, bringing the total to 4,817. Malaysian authorities reported 1 new death, bringing the death toll to 77. 168 recovered, bringing the total to 2,276.
- New Zealand reports 19 new cases (15 confirmed and 4 probable), bringing the total to 1,349 (1,064 confirmed and 285 probable). Health authorities also reported 75 new recoveries, bringing the total to 546. NZ authorities also reported a new death, bringing the death toll to 5.
- Russia reports 2,258 new cases.
- Singapore reports 386 new cases, with many of these cases from dormitories, bringing the total to 2,918. Another death is confirmed, bringing the toll to 9.
- South Africa reports 99 new cases, taking the total to 2,272. South African authorities reported 2 deaths, bringing the death toll to 27.
- South Korea reports 25 new cases.

- Spain reports 517 deaths, bringing the death toll to 17,489. Spanish authorities report a total of 169,496 cases.
- Turkey reports 4,093 new cases, including 17 prisoners, bringing the total to 61,049. Turkish authorities report 98 new deaths, including three prisoners, bringing the total to 1,296. A total of 3,957 have recovered, and 34,456 tests have been carried out.
- Ukraine reports 325 new cases (the highest number to date) and 10 new deaths, bringing the total numbers to 3,102 and 93, respectively. Additionally, a total of 97 patients have recovered.
- The United Kingdom has reported 717 deaths, bringing the death toll 11,329. UK health authorities have reported 4,342 cases, bringing the total to 88,621. UK health authorities have conducted 18,000 tests in the last 24 hours.
- In the United States, the Associated Press reported that more than 3,600 deaths have been linked to coronavirus outbreaks in nursing homes and long-term care facilities. New York reports 671 new deaths, bringing the state's death toll to 10,056. According to figures released by Johns Hopkins University, there have been 23,070 fatalities, 572,169 confirmed cases, and 42,324 recoveries in the United States.
- According to data release by Johns Hopkins University, the number of global coronavirus cases exceeds 1.9 million, 118,500 deaths, and 500,000 recoveries. Johns Hopkins University later revised its figures to 1.918 million cases.
- Dominic Raab tells the Downing Street briefing the government does not expect to make any immediate

changes to the lockdown restrictions and that the UK's plan "is working, but we are still not past the peak of this virus".

- The Director-General of the World Health Organization (WHO) outlined the agency's latest advice, stressing a mix of social distancing, testing, contact tracing and isolation.
- The World Health Organization (WHO), the UN Children's Fund (UNICEF) and other health partners supporting the Measles & Rubella Initiative (M&RI) warned that over 117 million children in 37 countries risked missing out on a measles vaccine.
- The United Nations Children's Fund (UNICEF) warned that hundreds of thousands of children in detention were at "grave risk" of contracting COVID-19, calling for their urgent release.
- UNESCO warned of unreliable and false information about the COVID-19 pandemic, terming it a global 'disinfodemic'.
- Nigerian President Muhammadu Buhari announces that the Nigerian Government will extend lockdowns in the states of Lagos, Abuja and Ogun by another 14 days.
- South Africa evacuates 136 of its nationals from Nigeria on a chartered South African Airways flight.
- The British Government pledges US$284 million to the World Health Organization (WHO) and charities to help slow the spread of the coronavirus in vulnerable countries. The British Government has allocated 130 million to United Nations agencies, while 65 million was allocated to the WHO. British Prime Minister Boris Johnson is discharged from the hospital.
- Portugal's Sporting CP announces that it will cut players' salaries by 40% for three months in response to financial

losses caused by COVID-19. The sporting body's board of directors will also take a 50% pay cut.

- Turkish Interior Minister Süleyman Soylu resigns due to criticism of his decision to impose a weekend curfew in several major Turkish cities in response to COVID-19. Soylu's resignation was rejected by Turkish President Recep Tayyip Erdoğan.
- In the Vatican City, Pope Francis holds an Easter Sunday service where he offers prayers for the over 100,000 people who had perished during the coronavirus pandemic.
- French President Emmanuel Macron extends the nationwide lockdown until 11 May. Israeli Prime Minister Benjamin Netanyahu announces a nationwide lockdown during the Passover holiday and the Minouma festival. Between 5 pm on 14 April until 5 am on 16 April, Israelis will be barred from leaving their hometowns or, in the case of Jerusalem, the neighbourhoods where they live.
- Italian Football Federation President Gabriele Gravina expresses hope that players can be tested in early May for the coronavirus in order to prepare for the season to restart. The Kazakhstan government announces that 3.7 million Kazakhs have applied for financial aid. Of these, 1.8 million applications have been approved.
- Pope Francis calls on society to stand behind female victims of domestic violence while praising female doctors, nurses, police officers, prison guards, and sales staff involved in essential work.
- Russian President Vladimir Putin states that the coronavirus situation is getting worse in Russia and commits the Russian Defence Ministry's resources to deal with the crisis.

- Spanish authorities allow people living in regions of Spain where Easter Monday is not a holiday to resume work. Certain businesses like construction and manufacturing were allowed to reopen, but most shops, bars, and public places remain closed until 26 April.
- Turkish President Recep Tayyip Erdogan announces that Turkey will impose a new lockdown over the weekend to combat the spread of COVID-19.
- Ukrainian President Volodymyr Zelenskyy offers a US$1 million reward to Ukrainian scientists if they develop a vaccine for the coronavirus.
- The British Government's Chief Scientific Adviser Patrick Vallance forecasts that the number of coronavirus-related deaths will continue to rise this week before plateauing over the next two to three weeks. He thinks that the number of daily deaths should begin decreasing after that.
- During a media conference on Monday evening, World Health Organization Director-General Tedros Adhanom states that governments need to consider six criteria for lifting coronavirus lockdown restrictions: first, the transmission is controlled; second, systems are in place to detect, test, isolate and treat every case and trace their contacts; third, risks are minimised in care homes and other at-risk environments; fourth, preventive measures are in place in schools, offices and other places people need to go; fifth, importation risks can be managed; and sixth, communities are fully educated and able to deal with the "new norm."

- Ecuadorian police remove 800 bodies from homes in the Pacific port city of Guayaquil, the worst-hit locality in the country.
- United States President Donald Trump releases a campaign-style video during the daily White House Coronavirus Task Force briefing defending his Administration's response to the COVID-19 pandemic. US immunologist Anthony Fauci said that President Trump listened to his advice about the mitigation efforts needed to stop the spread of COVID-19.
- Top Democratic Congressional leaders Senate Minority Leader Chuck Schumer and Speaker of the United States House of Representatives Nancy Pelosi call on the Republican Party to work on new bipartisan legislation citing a lack of funding for the national testing needed to restart the US economy.
- The International Monetary Fund announces that it would provide immediate debt relief to 25 member countries under its "Catastrophe Containment and Relief Trust." The IMF is seeking to raise US$1.4 billion for that fund.
- In Yemen, Houthi–linked chief prosecutor announced that the group has released 2,361 prisoners since mid-March as part of precautionary measures against the spread of COVID-19.

14 April

- China confirms 89 new cases (86 of them imported) for 13 April, bringing the total to 82,249. No deaths have been reported. Of the new cases, 79 were reported in Heilongjiang, which borders Russia.
- France reports a total death toll of 15,729 and 6,370 in intensive care.
- Germany reports 2,082 new cases, bringing the total to 125,098. Germany reports a total of 98 deaths.
- Iran reports 98 deaths, bringing the death toll to 4,683.
- Ireland confirms 548 new cases reported by Irish labs and 284 more new cases reported by German labs. 11 new deaths are reported. This gives a total of 11,479 confirmed cases and 406 deaths.
- Italy reports 602 deaths, bringing the death toll to 21,067. Italian authorities report 2,972 new cases, bringing the total to 162,488. 3,186 remain in intensive care, while 37,130 have recovered.
- Malaysia reports 170 new cases, bringing the total to 2,427. Malaysian authorities report that 202 patients had recovered, bringing the total to 4,987. The country also reports five deaths, bringing the death toll to 82.
- The Netherlands reports 868 new cases, bringing the total to 27,914. Dutch authorities report 122 deaths, bringing the death toll to 2,945.
- New Zealand reports 17 new cases (8 confirmed and 9 probable), bringing the total to 1,366 (1,072 confirmed and 292 probable). NZ health authorities also report 82 new

recoveries, bringing the total to 628. NZ also report 4 new deaths, bringing the death toll to 9.

- Russia reports 2,774 new cases, bringing the total number to 21,012. Russian authorities report 22 deaths, bringing the total to 170. The country reports 224 recoveries, bringing the total to 1,694.
- Singapore reports 334 new cases, many of these cases from dormitories, bringing the total to 3,252. Another death is confirmed, bringing the toll to 10.
- South Korea reports 27 new cases.
- Spain reports 567 deaths, bringing the total to 18,056. Spanish authorities report 172,541 cases.
- Sweden reports a total of 1,033 deaths and 11,445 cases.
- Taiwan reports no new cases for the first time in a month. Taiwanese authorities have reported a total of 393 cases and six deaths.
- Turkey reports 4,093 new cases, bringing the total to 61,049. The country's death toll rises by 98 to 1,296. 3,957 people have recovered, and 34,456 have been tested in the past 24 hours.
- Ukraine reports 270 new cases and 5 new deaths, bringing the total numbers to 3,372 and 98, respectively. Overall, 119 patients have recovered.
- British nursing home company HC-One reports a total of 311 deaths among its residents in 232 of the firm's homes.
- The United States reports 2,228 deaths, bringing the total to above 28,300. The country has reported over 600,000 cases. The State Department reports its first death among staff members at its headquarters in Washington, bringing the death toll in its global workforce to five.

- According to figures released by Johns Hopkins University, there are about 1.93 million coronavirus cases, 120,000 deaths, and 450,000 recoveries worldwide.
- The Austrian Government allows the reopening of thousands of shops as part of a move to loosen lockdown restrictions.
- The European Commission limits restrictions on exporting coronavirus protective equipment to facemasks and exempts Western Balkan countries from such restrictions.
- Iceland announces that it is planning to lift movements restrictions on 4 May. As part of the relaxation, primary schools will fully open while high schools and universities will open with some limitations.
- British-Swedish company AstraZeneca announces that it will start a clinical trial to assess the potential of Calquence in treating coronavirus patients.
- The Office for National Statistics indicates that coronavirus was linked to 1 in five deaths during the week ending 3 April. More than 16,000 deaths in the UK were recorded for that week, 6,000 higher than would be the average for that time of year.
- Several UK charities, including Age UK and the Alzheimer's Society, express their concern that older people are being "airbrushed" out of official figures because they focus on hospital deaths and do not include those in care homes or a person's own home. Responding to these concerns, Therese Coffey, the Secretary of State for Work and Pensions, says that hospital figures are being used because "it's accurate and quick."
- Mobile operators report a further twenty attempted arson attacks on mobile phone masts over the previous weekend.

- The Ghana Education Service and Zoomlion Ghana Limited joined forces to launch an initiative to fumigate all senior high, special and technical schools in the country to curb the spread of the pandemic.
- President of Guinea Alpha Condé makes it compulsory for all citizens and residents to wear face masks, coming into effect on 18 April. Offenders face a civil disobedience tax of 30,000 Guinean francs (US$3.16, €2.8). Condéalso called upon all companies, ministries and NGOs to provide masks to their employees by Saturday and called for masks to be manufactured locally and sold cheaply.
- President of Uganda Yoweri Museveni extends the country's initial 14-day lockdown by an extra three weeks until 5 May in order to combat the spread of COVID-19.
- President of Zimbabwe Emmerson Mnangagwa threatens to jail the author of a statement, claiming that the nationwide lockdown had been extended for 20 years for posting "fake news."
- The first of the UN's World Food Programme (WFP) and World Health Organization (WHO) "Solidarity Flights" carried urgently needed medical equipment to Africa, part of a UN-wide initiative.
- The UN Secretary-General warned of "a dangerous epidemic of misinformation" during "the most challenging crisis we have faced since the Second World War", leaving millions scared and seeking clear advice.
- The UN Secretary-General urged unity and called for countries not to cut the resources of the World Health Organization (WHO), as US President Trump halted funding.

- Henrietta Fore, Executive Director of the UN Children's Fund (UNICEF), warned of online predators putting millions of children at risk during COVID-19 pandemic lockdowns.
- Forecasting the "worst economic downturn since the Great Depression", the International Monetary Fund reported that growth for 2020 was likely to be minus three per cent, a dramatic change since the previous World Economic Outlook report in January.
- Imran Riza, UN Resident and Humanitarian Coordinator for Syria warned of a major threat from the coronavirus threat, which had initiated a broad UN containment effort.
- The Ghana Education Service and Zoomlion Ghana Limited joined forces to launch an initiative to fumigate all senior high, special and technical schools in the country to curb the spread of the pandemic.
- President of Guinea Alpha Condé makes it compulsory for all citizens and residents to wear face masks, coming into effect on 18 April. Offenders face a civil disobedience tax of 30,000 Guinean francs (US$3.16, €2.8). Condéalso called upon all companies, ministries and NGOs to provide masks to their employees by Saturday and called for masks to be manufactured locally and sold cheaply.
- President of Uganda Yoweri Museveni extends the country's initial 14-day lockdown by an extra three weeks until 5 May in order to combat the spread of COVID-19.
- President of Zimbabwe Emmerson Mnangagwa threatens to jail the author of a statement, claiming that the nationwide lockdown had been extended for 20 years for posting "fake news."

15 April

- The International Monetary Fund approves a $115 million disbursement for Burkina Faso and another $114 million for Niger under its Rapid Credit Facility to help African states cope with the COVID-19 pandemic.
- In Malawi, the Minister of Health and Population Jappie Mhango announces that the Malawian Government will be imposing a three-week nationwide lockdown between 18 April and 9 May in a bit to combat the spread of the coronavirus.
- The Football Federation of Belarus postpones its Women's Premier League, which was scheduled to start on 16 April, after several players were found to have been in contact with suspected carriers of the coronavirus.
- Denmark begins reopening nurseries, kindergartens, and primary schools after a month-long closure on 12 March. However, classes are only resuming in about half of Denmark's municipalities and 35 per cent of Copenhagen's schools as others have requested more time to adjust to new health safety protocols.
- Finnish Prime Minister Sanna Marin lifts roadblocks and travel restrictions around the Uusimaa region which contains the capital Helsinki, easing a lockdown that began on 28 March.
- German Chancellor Angela Merkel announces that most shops up to 800sq metres (8,600 sq ft) will be allowed to reopen once they have "plans to maintain hygiene." However, schools will remain closed until 4 May. The German Government has also maintained a ban on large gatherings until 31 August.

- Portuguese President Marcelo Rebelo de Sousa states that Portugal has "flattened the curve" but is still too early to lift the nationwide lockdown. De Sousa extends Portugal's lockdown until 1 May.
- In Russia, veterans urge President Vladimir Putin to postpone a military parade to mark the 75th anniversary of World War Two, scheduled for 9 May, due to the risk posed by the coronavirus.
- The Turkish Interior Ministry imposes quarantines on 227 residential areas in 58 provinces, home to 250,000 people. The Ministry also announced that it was lifting restrictions on 41 residential areas in 14 provinces.
- UK luxury car manufacturer Aston Martin suspends manufacturing at two of its factories by another week in response to lockdown measures in the United Kingdom. First Minister of Northern Ireland Arlene Foster extends Northern Ireland's lockdown by three weeks in coordination with similar measures by the neighbouring Republic of Ireland, which are due to run until 5 May.
- The head of the World Health Organization (WHO) stated it was reviewing the impact of the United States (US) withholding funding and upheld the importance of international solidarity in tackling the COVID-19 pandemic one day after the US announced that it was cutting funding, pending a review of how the WHO responded to the initial outbreak in China.
- The World Health Organization (WHO) warned of a potential "second wave" of COVID-19 infections in an update to its strategic advice to governments, as some European countries began to relax lockdown measures.

- The International Organization for Migration expanded the scope of its Global Strategic Preparedness and Response Plan to include major interventions aiming to mitigate the severe health and socioeconomic impacts of the pandemic.
- Secretary-General António Guterres pledged that the UN would stand in solidarity with Africa in the face of the unprecedented economic, social and health impacts of the COVID-19 pandemic, from procuring test kits to promoting debt relief.
- David Boyd, UN Special Rapporteur on Human Rights and the Environment, appealed for countries not to respond to COVID-19 by lower environmental standards.
- In Brazil, the Governor of Rio de Janeiro, Wilson Witzel, tests positive for the coronavirus.
- Governor of New York Andrew Cuomo disputes President Donald Trump's claim of "total authority" to reopen the United States' economy, which has gone into lockdown as a result of COVID-19. In addition, American immunologist and head of the National Institute of Allergy and Infectious Diseases Anthony Fauci warns that it is too early for the US Government to consider reopening the economy due to the coronavirus pandemic.
- United States President Trump announces that the US will be withholding funding to the World Health Organization temporarily, alleging that the international organisation had neglected its duties and spread Chinese propaganda. Trump's decision was criticised by UN Secretary-General António Guterres, Dr Patrice Harris of the American Medical Association, infectious disease expert Dr Amesh Adalja of Johns Hopkins University, and Dr William Schaffner of

Vanderbilt University. Trump's decision was also criticised by the Chinese and German governments, the European Union, WHO Director-General Tedros Adhanom, and Speaker of the House Nancy Pelosi.

- United States Army General Mark A. Milley, the chairman of the Joint Chiefs of Staff, issues a statement that US intelligence services indicate that the coronavirus originated naturally rather than being created in a Chinese laboratory as suggested by various conspiracy theories.
- The International Monetary Fund's Chief Economist Gita Gopinath describes the economic fallout of the COVID-19 pandemic as the "worst recession" since the Great Depression in a foreword for the international organisation's World Economic Outlook. The IMF has also reported that it has loaned US$1 trillion to a hundred developing and under-developed countries affected by the coronavirus pandemic.
- Apple, Inc. launches a site to help public health authorities to track down people's travel movements to ensure they are complying with lockdown requirements. According to the company, the data is gathered by counting the number of routing requests from Apple Maps, which is installed on all iPhones and comparing it with past usage to detect changes in the volume of people driving, walking or taking public transit around the world.
- The Pakistani Government extends its lockdown to schools, shopping malls, public gatherings and non-essential work for two weeks but makes exceptions for certain economic sectors such as construction, cement and fertiliser plants, mines, glass manufacturers, veterinary services, bookshops and stationery stores, dry cleaners and some agriculture-related businesses.

- Turkey's Parliament announces that it has approved legislation to release 90,000 prisoners in a bid to ease overcrowding in prisons and prevent the spread of COVID-19.
- Canada reports a total of 27,540 cases and 903 deaths.
- France reports 1,438 new deaths (including hospital and rest home deaths), bringing the death toll to 17,167.
- Indonesia reports 297 new cases, bringing the total to 5,136. Indonesian health authorities report 10 new deaths, bringing the total to 469. 446 have recovered, and more than 36,000 people have been tested.
- Iran reports 94 new deaths, bringing the total to 4,777.
- Italy reports 578 deaths, bringing the death toll to 21,645. The country reports 2,667 new cases.
- Japan reports 457 new cases.
- Libya has reported a total of 36 cases and 1 death.
- Malaysia reports 85 new cases, bringing the total to 5,072. Malaysian health authorities also discharge 169 patients, bringing the total number of recoveries to 2,647. Malaysia also reports 1 new death, bringing the death toll to 83.
- The Maldives reports its first domestically-transmitted case. The country had previously reported 20 cases, which all involved overseas travellers.
- New Zealand reports 20 new cases (6 confirmed and 14 probable), bringing the total to 1,386 (1,078 confirmed and 306 probable). NZ health authorities also report 100 new recoveries, bringing the total to 728.
- Qatar reports 283 new cases, bringing the total to 3,711.
- Singapore reports 447 new cases, with many of these cases from dormitories, bringing the total to 3,699. In addition, a

person was later confirmed to have COVID-19 after he died, with the cause of death unrelated to COVID-19 complications.

- Spain reports 523 new deaths, bringing the death toll to 18,579.
- Switzerland reports a total of 973 deaths and 26,336 cases.
- Turkey reports 115 new cases, bringing the death toll to 1,518. The country has reported 4,281 new cases, bringing the total to 69,392.
- Ukraine reports 392 new cases and 10 new deaths, bringing the total numbers to 3,764 and 108, respectively; 143 patients have recovered overall.
- The United Kingdom reports 761 new deaths, bringing the death toll to 12,868. A total of 98,476 have tested positive for the coronavirus.
- Health Secretary Matt Hancock announces new guidelines that will allow close family members to see dying relatives in order to say goodbye to them. Hancock also launches a new network to provide personal protective equipment to care home staff.
- The 2020 Love Supreme Jazz Festival, scheduled for July, is cancelled.
- According to US Vice President Mike Pence, more than 3 million in the United States have been tested for the coronavirus. Pence has reported 619,000 cases, over 27,000 deaths, and 45,000 recoveries.
- Johns Hopkins University reports that the global number of coronavirus cases and deaths have reached 2,000,984 and 128,011, respectively.

- The Brazilian Health Secretary Wanderson de Oliveira resigns following disagreements between President Jair Bolsonaro and Health Minister Luiz Henrique Mandetta over Brazil's handling of the coronavirus pandemic.
- Colombian Justice Minister Margarita Cabello announces that 4,000 prisoners will be released from prison and placed under house arrest in a bid to combat the spread of COVID-19.
- Robert Redfield, the Director of the United States Centers for Disease Control and Prevention (CDC), suggests that 19-20 US states that have experienced "limited impact" from the coronavirus may be able to reopen by President Donald Trump's 1st May target date.
- The Omani Ministry of Finance orders all ministry and civilian government units to reduce approved liquidity for development budgets by ten per cent. It also ordered a halt to the creation of government companies performing the commercial activity in order to give priority to the private sector.
- Jordanian Prime Minister Omar Razzaz announces that the Jordanian Government will ease lockdown measures to allow more businesses and industries to resume work but will not yet live a curfew restricting movement.
- In Libya, the Tripoli-based Government of National Accord imposes a 24-hour curfew for ten days in order to combat the spread of the coronavirus.
- The Pakistani Government relaxes lockdown restrictions on key industries, including the lockdown sector, in order to minimise the economic damage caused by the lockdown.

- The Qatari Government expels several Nepalese workers for alleged "illegal, illicit activity." In response to criticism by Amnesty International, Qatar has defended the repatriation, claiming the workers had broken the law.
- At the G20 virtual summit hosted in Riyadh, Saudi Arabia, the G20 group of countries and private creditors agree to suspend debt repayments from developing countries for the duration of the coronavirus pandemic.
- The United Nations Economic and Social Commission for Western Asia reports that about 71 million people in the Arab world lack access to running water, increasing their risk of contracting the coronavirus.

16 April

- Africa has confirmed a total of 17,247 cases, 911 deaths, and over 3,500 recoveries.
- Bonaire reports its first case.
- China reports 46 new cases of the coronavirus (34 imported and 12 domestic). Of the 12 domestic cases, three are in Beijing, five in Guangdong province and four in Heilongjiang province.
- Eswatini/Swaziland reports its first death resulting from the coronavirus. The country has reported a total of 17 cases.
- France records 753 more deaths, bringing the total to 17,920. 6,248 remain in intensive care. The French Ministry of Armed Forces reports that 668 French marines have contracted the coronavirus.
- Germany reports 2,866 cases, bringing the total to 130,450. German authorities report 315 deaths, bringing the death toll to 3,569.

- Indonesia reports 380 new cases, bringing the total to 5,516. Indonesian authorities have reported 27 deaths, bringing the death toll to 496. 548 have recovered, and 11,000 tests have been conducted.
- Iran confirms 92 deaths, bringing the total to 4,869. Iranian authorities have confirmed 1,606 new cases, bringing the total to 77,995, with 3,594 in critical condition. 52,229 have recovered.
- Italy reports 525 deaths, bringing the death toll to 22,170. Italian authorities have also reported 3,76 cases, bringing the total to 168,941. 2,936 remain in intensive care, while 40,164 have recovered.
- Japan has reported a total of about 9,000 cases (including three cabinet officials) and nearly 200 deaths.
- Malaysia reports 110 new cases, bringing the total number of cases to 5,182. Malaysian authorities report 1 death, bringing the total to 84. 2,766 patients have recovered, while 2,332 are still being treated.
- The Netherlands reports 1,061 new cases, bringing the total to 29,214. Dutch authorities report 181 deaths, bringing the death toll to 3,315.
- New Zealand reports 15 new cases (six confirmed and nine probable), bringing the total to 1,401. 12 people remain in hospital, with three in intensive care and two in critical condition. 42 people have recovered, bringing the total number of recoveries to 770.
- The Philippines report 13 new deaths, bringing the total to 362. The country has reported a total of 207 cases, bringing the total to 5,660. 82 patients have recovered, bringing the total to 435.

- Russia has reported 3,448 cases, bringing the total to 27,938. 34 people have died, bringing the death toll to 232.
- Singapore reports 728 new cases, with many of these cases from dormitories, bringing the total to 4,427.
- Slovakia reports 114 new cases and 2 new deaths, bringing the total cases to 977.
- South Korea has reported a total of 229 deaths and 10,613 cases.
- Spain reports 551 new deaths as the death toll reaches 19,130. The country has reported a total of 182,816 cases.
- Thailand reports 29 new cases, bringing the total to 2,672. Thai authorities report 3 new deaths, bringing the total to 46.
- Timor Leste reports 10 more cases, bringing the total to 18.
- Turkey reports 125 deaths, bringing the country's death toll to 1,643. 4,801 new cases have been reported, bringing the total to 74,193. 7,089 have recovered while 1,854 patients remain in intensive care.
- Ukraine reports 397 new cases and 8 new deaths, bringing the total numbers to 4,161 and 116 respectively; a total of 186 patients have recovered.
- The United Kingdom reports 861 new deaths, bringing the total to 13,729. More than 100,000 have tested positive for the coronavirus.
- The United States reports a total of 31,002 deaths from the coronavirus, the highest in the world.
- The World Health Organization's Europe regional director Hans Kluge has reported over 1 million cases and 84,000 deaths in Europe.
- A 99-year-old war veteran, Tom Moore, completes 100 laps of his garden, eventually raising over £25 million for NHS

Charities Together, with over a million people donating via his JustGiving page.

- Foreign Secretary Dominic Raab announces a three-week extension to the nationwide lockdown measures as the number of confirmed COVID-19 cases in the UK surpasses 100,000.
- The NHS Nightingale Hospital Birmingham, at the National Exhibition Centre, is officially opened by Prince William.
- The UK stages a fourth round of applause for NHS staff and key workers at 8 pm.
- A spokesperson for Princess Beatrice of York and Edoardo Mapelli Mozzi confirms that their wedding, scheduled for 29 May, will be held on a later date.
- Dr John Nkengasong, Director of the Africa CDC, announces that the agency will distribute 1 million test kits across Africa with the goal of testing 15 million people over the next three months.
- In Kenya, Governor of Nairobi Mike Sonko draws media attention for distributing cognac and Hennessy to the poor, claiming it can cure the coronavirus. His claims have been rejected by the Kenyan Government and the liquor company LVMH.
- The Liberian Government announces that it will launch a radio schooling initiative for children whose education was disrupted after Liberia closed schools across the country on 16 March in response to the country's first coronavirus case.
- Nigeria's National Human Rights Commission reports there were eight documented incidents of extrajudicial killings by law security forces resulting in 18 deaths.

- South African Minister of Mineral Resources Gwede Mantashe announces that the South African Government will allow mines to operate at 50 per cent capacity in order to contain the spread of COVID-19.
- UN Secretary-General António Guterres launched a new UN report noting that the looming global recession due to the COVID-19 pandemic could cause hundreds of thousands of additional child deaths in 2020, reversing recent gains in reducing global infant mortality.
- Brazilian President Jair Bolsonaro dismisses Health Minister Luiz Henrique Mandetta due to disagreements over measures to combat the coronavirus. Bolsonaro appoints Nelson Teich as Brazil's new Health Minister.
- The Governors of New York and Maryland order residents to wear face masks in public spaces. The Governors of Connecticut and Pennsylvania are also recommending that residents wear face masks. Governor of New York Andrew Cuomo also extends his state's shutdown order until 15 May in order to combat the spread of the coronavirus.
- US President Donald Trump and Secretary of State Mike Pompeo have pressed China about to "come clean" about the origins of the coronavirus. Defense Secretary Mark Esper also accused the Chinese leadership of being "opaque and misleading" about the coronavirus outbreak. In response, Chinese Foreign Ministry spokesperson Zhao Lijian has asserted that the World Health Organization has found no evidence that the coronavirus was created in a laboratory.
- US President Trump has also released a roadmap for US governors to reopen the US economy in phases.

- The US Congress passes a coronavirus relief bill that will increase the federal budget deficit by US$1.8 trillion over the next cade. 17 Republican Members of Congress have also supported President Trump's decision to withhold aid to the World Health Organization. They propose demanding that WHO Director-General Tedros Adhanom resigns as a condition for resuming US contributions to the international organisation.
- The United States Government reports that 5.2 million American workers have become unemployed since last week.
- The Austrian Social Affairs and Health Minister Rudolf Anschober announces that the Austrian Government intends to test all rest-home residents, approximately 130,000 people.
- The Dutch Ministry of Social Affairs and Employment reports that the number of people applying for unemployment benefits had risen to 42% in March. The Ministry had also paid benefits to 37,800 newly unemployed, with the majority being former restaurant and bar workers as well as people under the age of 25 years. The Head of the Dutch National Institute for Health (RIVM), Jaap Van Dissel, presents a study to the Dutch Parliament suggesting that 3 per cent of the Dutch population have developed antibodies to combat the coronavirus.
- The European Commission advises member states using mobile apps to contain the spread of the coronavirus to ensure that such apps comply with the European Union's privacy rules and avoid using personalised location data.

- The German Federal Constitutional Court rules that Germans have the right to hold protests if they adhere to physical distancing rules.
- The Georgian Government bans the movement of all private vehicles until 21 April. Georgia has already imposed a state of emergency closing most businesses, schools, public transportation, and gatherings of more than three people until 10 May.
- The Hungarian Government announces that they intend to extend Hungary's lockdown by one week from Saturday (18 April) in order to combat the spread of COVID-19. Municipal authorities will be empowered to impose special restrictions over the weekend to ensure local communities are protected.
- The Polish Government announces that parks and forests will reopen to the public on Monday (20 April) and then revise the rules on the number of customers allowed in shops as part of efforts to loosen lockdown restrictions. The Polish Government also clarifies that the country's borders will remain closed until 3 May.
- Russian President Vladimir Putin announces that the Russian Government is postponing the country's annual World War II commemoration parade due to health risks associated with the coronavirus.
- Switzerland announces that it will ease restrictions in a three-stage process. First, hospitals will be allowed to perform all operations, including elective surgeries, while hair salons, massage parlours and cosmetic studies will be allowed to reopen on 27 April. Second, all primary schools, shops, and markets will be allowed to reopen from 11 May.

Third, the government will reopen secondary schools, vocational schools, and universities from 8 June.

- British Health Secretary Matt Hancock states that it is too early for the British Government to lift the coronavirus lockdown in order to prevent the spread of the coronavirus. At the advice of epidemiologist Neil Ferguson, the British Government maintains social distancing measures until a vaccine becomes available. Foreign Secretary Dominic Raab extends the UK's lockdown by another three weeks.
- The Gulf Cooperation Council approves Kuwait's proposal for a common network for food supply safety following an online meeting of trade and industry ministers.
- The Jordanian Prime Minister Omar Razzaz admits that his country's finances had been strained by the coronavirus pandemic, derailing the country's capital investment plan to boost sluggish growth and attract investment.
- Lebanese Prime Minister Hassan Diab states that 98% of Jordan's depositors will not be affected by an economic rescue plan which includes a proposal to fund some losses with a contribution from deposits.
- The Saudi Arabian Government announces that it will pledge US$500 million to support international efforts to combat the coronavirus pandemic and to help bridge a US$8 billion financing gap. This includes investing US$150m to the Coalition for Epidemic Preparedness and Innovation, US$150m to the Global Alliance for Vaccines and Immunisations, and US$200m to other health organisations and programmes.

17 April

- China reports 26 new cases, with 15 coming from abroad. Wuhan has also revised its official death toll from the coronavirus by 50% from 1,290 to 3,869, with local authorities citing incorrect reporting, delays, and omissions. This brings the country's death toll to at least 4,642.
- France reports 761 new deaths, bringing the total to 18,681. The French government also confirms that 1,081 crew members of the French aircraft carrier Charles De Gaulle have tested positive for the coronavirus. 524 sailors have also shown symptoms, while 24 remain in hospitals.
- Italy has reported 575 deaths, bringing the death toll to 22,745. The country has reported 3,493 new cases, bringing the total to 172,434.
- Malaysia has reported 69 new cases, bringing the total to 5,251. 2,967 patients have recovered, while 2,198 cases are receiving treatment at the country's health facilities. Malaysia also reports two new deaths, bringing the death toll to 86.
- The Netherlands reports 1,235 new cases, bringing the total to 30,449. The country has reported 144 deaths, bringing the death toll to 3,459.
- New Zealand has reported eight new cases (two confirmed and six probable), bringing the total to 1,409 (1,080 confirmed and 307 probable). NZ health authorities have reported 46 recoveries, bringing the total to 816. In addition, New Zealand authorities confirm two deaths, bringing the total to 11.
- Pakistan reports a total of 135 deaths and 7,025 cases.
- The Philippines have reported a total of 5,878 cases and 387 deaths.

- Qatar reports 560 new cases, bringing the total to 4,663. The country has also reported 49 recoveries that same day.
- Russia reports 4,069 new cases, bringing the total to 32,007. Russia also reports 41 deaths, bringing the total to 273.
- Singapore reports 623 new cases, with many of these cases from dormitories, bringing the total to 5,050. Another death was later confirmed, bringing the total to 11.
- South Korea reports 22 new cases, bringing the total to 10,635. The country has reported 230 deaths.
- Spain has reported a total of more than 20,000 deaths and 188,068 cases.
- In Syria, the Kurdish-administered northeast region reports its first death from the coronavirus.
- Turkey has reported 4,353 cases, bringing the total to 78,546. The country has reported a total of 1,769 deaths and 8,631 recoveries.
- Ukraine reports its record high number of new cases with 501 new cases, bringing the total to 4,662. Additionally, 9 deaths are reported, bringing the total number of lethal cases to 125, as well as a total of 246 recoveries.
- The United Arab Emirates has reported a total of 5,825 cases and 35 deaths.
- The United Kingdom reports a total of 14,576 deaths and 108,692 cases.
- According to Johns Hopkins University, the number of global deaths resulting from the coronavirus has reached 150,000.
- Matt Hancock confirms coronavirus tests will be rolled out to cover more public service staff such as police officers, firefighters and prison staff.

- Chancellor Rishi Sunak extends the subsidised wage scheme for furloughed workers for another month to the end of June.
- Later analysis of death registrations (all causes) in England and Wales by the Office for National Statistics finds the highest total this week, which at 21,805 is 207% of the five-year average for the same week. COVID-19 is mentioned in 8,730 cases.
- Michel Yao, the head of emergency operations for World Health Organization Africa, could rise to 10 million in three to six months based on computer modelling.
- The Malawian High Court issues a ruling temporarily barring the Malawian Government from imposing a 21-day lockdown following a petition by the human rights NGO Malawi Human Rights Defenders Coalition (HRDC) and protests by small-scale traders complaining that the lockdown would cause hardship and poverty.
- The head of the UN children's fund, UNICEF, warned that 250 million children globally living in the "waking nightmare" of conflict desperately needed warring parties to adopt the UN Secretary General's call for a global ceasefire as the COVID-19 pandemic spreads.
- Philip Alston, the UN Special Rapporteur on Extreme Poverty and Human Rights, warned that the United States must take urgent additional steps to prevent tens of millions of middle-class Americans impacted by the COVID-19 pandemic from being "plunged into poverty".
- UNWTO Secretary-General, Zurab Pololikashvili, warned that tourism, which accounts for 10 per cent of global GDP,

could lose millions of jobs but offered the potential for an economic recovery.

- Michelle Bachelet, the UN High Commissioner for Human Rights, issued new guidance setting out key actions to protect lesbian, gay, bisexual, trans and intersex (LGBTI) people against discrimination during the COVID-19 pandemic.
- Health ministers from six Balkan states, including Kosovar Health Minister Arben Tivia, agree to coordinate their responses to combat the spread of the coronavirus in the Western Balkans.
- The German Health Minister Jens Spahn states the coronavirus pandemic in Germany has become manageable again due to the higher rate of recoveries over infections.
- In the United Kingdom, Lord Mayor of London Sadiq Khan has called on the British Government to make it compulsory for people travelling or shopping around the capital to wear face masks.
- Saudi Minister of Finance Mohammed Al-Jadaan issues a statement that Saudi Arabia is in a good financial position to tackle the coronavirus pandemic due to its strong financial reserves and low national debt. The Grand Mufti Sheikh Abdulaziz al-Sheikh advises that Muslim evening prayers for Ramadan and the Eid al-Fitr feast should be performed at home for the duration of the coronavirus pandemic.
- The Emirate of Dubai extends a 24-hour curfew by one week.
- Canadian Prime Minister Justin Trudeau announces that Canada's border restrictions will remain in place "for a significant amount of time" in order to combat the spread of

the coronavirus. Deputy Prime Minister Freeland further elaborated and said, “Decisions about Canada’s border are taken by Canadians. Full stop.”

- The Guatemalan Government reports that 44 out of 76 Guatemalans deported on one flight from the United States have tested positive for the coronavirus. The Guatemalan Foreign Minister Pedro Brolo later announced that Guatemala had suspended deportation flights but neglected to mention whether it was linked to the coronavirus outbreak.
- The United States Navy’s Surgeon General Bruce Gillingham announces that sailors aboard the USS Theodore Roosevelt will be subject to a serology test that will test whether sailors have contracted the coronavirus and developed antibodies in response to it.
- US President Donald Trump has tweeted in support of anti-lockdown protests in the states of Minnesota, Michigan, and Virginia, protesting against state lockdown orders. In response, Washington Governor Jay Inslee has accused Trump of “fomenting domestic rebellion and spreading lies.”

18 April

- Algeria has reported a total of 364 deaths and 2,418 cases.
- Australia reports 3 new deaths, bringing the total to 68. Australian authorities have reported 36 new cases, bringing the total to 6,533.
- Bangladesh has reported a total of 2,144 and 84 deaths.
- Brazil has reported 2,917 new cases, bringing the total to 36,599. Brazil has reported 206 deaths, bringing the total to 2,347.

- China reports 27 new cases, with 20 originating from Heilongjiang province, bringing the total to 82,719. China has reported 77,029 recoveries. China has revised its death toll to 4,632 based on new figures from Wuhan.
- Croatia reports 18 new cases, bringing the total to 1,832. The country has also reported 39 deaths.
- Egypt reports 188 new cases, bringing the total to 3,032. The country has also reported 19 new deaths, bringing the total to 224.
- According to the Agence France-Presse, Europe has recorded a total of 100,510 cases, nearly two-thirds of the 157,163 fatalities worldwide.
- France has reported 642 deaths, bringing the death toll to 19,323. 5,833 remain in intensive care.
- Germany has reported 3,609 cases, bringing the total to 137,439. Germany has reported 242 new deaths, bringing the total to 4,110.
- Indonesia reports 325 new cases, bringing the total to 6,248. Indonesian health authorities report 15 new deaths, bringing the total to 535. However, the Indonesian Doctors Association have claimed that the figure is higher, citing that the official figures do not include the deaths of patients suspected of having the coronavirus but still awaiting tests.
- Iran reports 73 deaths, bringing the total to 5,031. Iran has reported a total of 80,868 cases.
- Japan has reported a total of over 200 deaths and 10,000 infections. Tokyo reports 181 new cases.
- Malaysia has reported 54 new cases, bringing the total number of cases to 5,305. Malaysian health authorities have discharged 135 patients, bringing the total number of

recoveries to 3,102. Malaysia has also reported two new deaths, bringing the death toll to 88.

- Mexico has reported 578 new cases, bringing the total to 6,875. Mexico has reported 60 new deaths, bringing the total to 546.
- Morocco reports 2,670 cases, 137 deaths, and 298 recoveries.
- Nepal has reported a total of 30 cases.
- The Netherlands has reported 1,140 new cases, bringing the total to 31,589. Dutch authorities have reported 142 new deaths, bringing the death toll to 3,601.
- New Zealand has reported 13 new cases (8 confirmed and 5 probable), bringing the total to 1,422 (1,094 confirmed and 328 probable). In addition, NZ health authorities report 51 new recoveries, bringing the total to 867.
- Palestinian officials report the first Palestinian death in disputed East Jerusalem.
- The Philippines has reported 10 new deaths, bringing the death toll to 397. Philippines health authorities have confirmed 209 new cases, bringing the total to 6,087. The Philippines has reported 29 recoveries, bringing the total to 516.
- Russia has reported 40 new deaths, bringing the death toll to 313. Russia also reports 4,785 new cases, bringing the total to 36,793. Moscow has reported 2,649 new cases and 21 new deaths.
- Singapore has reported 942 new cases (mainly foreign workers), bringing the total to 5,992. In addition, a person who had COVID-19 died, with the cause of death being a heart attack.

- South Korea has confirmed a total of 10,653 cases and 232 deaths.
- Spain has reported a total of 191,726 cases and 20,043 deaths.
- Switzerland reports a total of 1,111 deaths and 27,404 cases.
- Thailand has reported 33 new deaths, bringing the total to 2,733. Thai authorities have reported a total of 1,787 recoveries and 47 deaths.
- Turkey has reported 3,783 new cases, bringing the total to 82,239. 121 have died, bringing the death toll to 1,890. Turkey has reported 1,822 recoveries and 40,520 tests.
- Ukraine reports 444 new cases and 8 new deaths, bringing the total numbers to 5,106 and 133 respectively; a total of 275 patients have recovered.
- The United Kingdom reports 888 deaths in hospitals, bringing the death toll to 15,464. UK authorities have tested 357,023 people, with 114,217 testing positive.
- In the United States, the death toll has exceeded 31,000. New York state authorities have reported 540 deaths and over 2,000 hospital admissions in the last 24 hours.
- According to Johns Hopkins University, the number of global cases has reached 2.3 million while the global death toll has exceeded 159,000.
- Imran Ahmad-Khan, the MP for Wakefield, secures a shipment of 110,000 reusable face masks through his connections with charity Solidarités international and the Vietnamese Government for Mid Yorkshire Hospitals NHS Trust to help tackle the shortage of PPE.

- Unions representing doctors and nurses express their concern at a change in government guidelines advising medics to reuse gowns or wear other kits if stocks run low.
- Speaking at the Downing Street daily briefing, Robert Jenrick, the Communities Secretary, says a further 400,000 gowns will be arriving from Turkey the following day. (In the event, the shipment was delayed by several days and was said on 7 May to be unusable).
- Care England, the UK's largest care homes representative body, estimates that as many as 7,500 care home residents may have died because of coronavirus, compared to the official figure of 1,400 released a few days earlier.
- Jenrick announces a further £1.6bn of support for local authorities, on top of £1.6bn that was given to them on 19 March.
- Jenrick says that the virus appears to be having a "disproportionate impact" on the Black, Asian and minority ethnic (BAME) communities, while Stephen Powis says he has asked Public Health England to investigate what may be accounting for the increased risk within these groups.
- Jenrick says that parks and cemeteries must remain open during the lockdown.
- The Canadian Transportation Agency announces that all airline passengers will be required to wear a face mask or to cover to help combat the spread of the coronavirus.
- Guatemalan President Alejandro Giammattei suspends the flights of all deportees from the United States after tests indicated that several passengers aboard a flight from the US tested positive for the coronavirus.

- Mexican President Andres Manuel Lopez Obrador issues a Twitter message stating that US President Donald Trump had promised to help Mexico buy 1,000 ventilators and other intensive therapy equipment used for treating severe cases of the coronavirus.
- In the United States, there have been reports of protests against stay-at-home orders in Concord, New Hampshire; Annapolis, Maryland; and Austin, Texas. During his daily briefing, US President Donald Trump stated that China should face the consequences if they were "knowingly responsible" for the coronavirus pandemic.
- Amazon has started using thermal cameras to screen workers at its warehouses in order to detect cases of coronavirus.
- The Algerian Government extended its lockdown by 10 days, through 29 April.
- In Nigeria, Abba Kyari, the Chief of Staff to President Muhammadu Buhari, died from the coronavirus.
- The Iranian Government has allowed businesses in Tehran and some nearby towns to reopen on Saturday after weeks of lockdown. Gyms, restaurants, Tehran's grand bazaar, shrines and mosques remain closed while a ban on public gathering remains in force.
- The Moroccan Government extended the country's lockdown until 20 May.
- The Pakistani Government lifted restrictions on congregations at mosques, which allowed only three to five people for prayers.
- The United Arab Emirates Government announces that it will fine people up to 20,000 dirhams (US$5,500) if they

disseminate "fake news" about the coronavirus, including medical information that violates official advice about the coronavirus.

- The Croatian Government extended its lockdown by another 15 days, until 4 May.
- The Danish Government announces that it will invest 100 billion Danish Krones (US$14.6 billion) in direct economic aid, state-guaranteed loans and extended deadlines for tax payments to help businesses affected by the economic fallout of the coronavirus pandemic.
- The Greek Orthodox Church has conducted its Easter services in empty churches on Saturday night to comply with health restrictions to prevent the spread of the coronavirus.
- Israeli Prime Minister Benjamin Netanyahu announces that the Israeli Government will be relaxing lockdown restrictions by allowing some businesses to reopen and easing restrictions on movement.
- In response to a sharp spike in cases, Russian President Vladimir Putin orders the Russian government to provide a daily forecast of coronavirus cases.
- Spanish Prime Minister Pedro Sánchez announces that he would ask the Spanish Parliament to extend the national lockdown until 9 May. Sánchez has indicated that he wanted to relax restrictions on children, who will be allowed out of their homes after 27 April under restrictions.
- In the United Kingdom, Queen Elizabeth II announces that there will be no gun salutes to mark her birthday on 21 April, the first such request made in her 68-year reign. Housing Secretary Robert Jenrick announces that the UK

Government will do more to provide healthcare workers with personal protective equipment.

- Uzbekistan extended social distancing measures through 10 May.

19 April

- The Africa Centers for Disease Control and Prevention (Africa CDC) has reported 55 new deaths, bringing the death toll to 1,080. The continent has reported 1,047 new cases, bringing the total number of infections to 21,317.
- Canada has reported a total of 1,506 deaths and 33,922 cases.
- Chile has reported a total of over 10,000 cases and 133 deaths.
- China has reported 16 new cases (including nine imported cases), bringing the total to 82,735.
- France has reported 395 deaths, bringing the death toll to 19,718. 5,744 remain in intensive care.
- Germany has reported 2,458 new cases, bringing the total to 139,897. Germany also reports 184 new deaths, bringing the total to 4,294.
- Guinea has reported 518 cases and five deaths. The deceased include several senior government officials, including secretary-general Sekou Kourouma.
- Honduras has reported a total of 472 cases and 46 deaths.
- Indonesia has reported 327 new cases, bringing the total to 6,575. Indonesian health authorities also report 47 new deaths, bringing the total to 582.

- Israel has reported 97 new cases, bringing the total to 13,362, with 156 being in critical condition. Israel has also reported 7 deaths, bringing the death toll to 171.
- Italy has reported 433 new deaths and 3,047 new cases.
- Japan has reported 568 new cases, bringing the total to 10,361. If combined with the 712 cases reported on a cruise ship quarantined near Tokyo, the total figure rises to 11,073. Japan has also reported a total of 174 deaths.
- Malaysia has reported 84 new cases, bringing the total to 5,389. Malaysian health authorities have also reported 95 recoveries, bringing the total to 3,197. Malaysia also reports 1 new death, bringing the death toll to 89.
- Mexico has reported a total of 7,947 cases and 650 deaths.
- The Netherlands has reported 1,066 new cases, bringing the total to 32,655. Dutch authorities have also confirmed 83 deaths, bringing the death toll to 3,684.
- New Zealand has reported 9 new cases (4 confirmed and 5 probable), bringing the total to 1,431 (1,098 confirmed and 333 probable). Health authorities have also reported 45 new recoveries, bringing the total to 912. In addition, authorities confirm 1 death from the coronavirus during a post-morterm, bringing the total death toll to 12. Health authorities also confirm that three baby boys had contracted the coronavirus.
- Pakistan has reported 514 new cases, bringing the total to 7,993 cases. Pakistani authorities have reported 16 new deaths, bringing the death toll to 159.
- Panama has reported a total of 4,273 cases and 120 deaths.
- Peru has reported a total of 15,628 cases and 400 deaths.
- The Philippines has reported 172 new cases, bringing the total to 6,259. The country also reported 12 new deaths,

bringing the total to 409. 56 patients have recovered, bringing the total to 572.

- Poland reports 545 new cases, bringing the total to 9,287.
- Qatar has reported 440 new cases, bringing the total to 4,922. So far, the country has reported a total of eight deaths.
- Russia has reported 6,060 new cases, bringing the total to 42,853. Russia has reported 48 deaths, bringing the death toll to 361.
- Rwanda has reported a total of 44 cases.
- Singapore has reported 596 new cases, bringing the total to 6,588. Apart from 25 citizens and permanent residents, the majority of cases are in dormitories.
- South Korea has reported 15 new cases, bringing the total to 10,661 cases. There have also been a total of 234 deaths.
- Spain reports 410 new deaths, bringing the total to 20,453. Spain has reported a total of 195,944 cases.
- Taiwan has reported 22 new cases, bringing the total to 420. 21 of the newly infected cases had been Republic of China Navy sailors who had taken part in a goodwill mission to Palau. Taiwan has reported a total of six deaths.
- Ukraine reports 343 new cases and 8 new deaths, bringing the total numbers to 5,449 and 141 respectively; a total of 347 patients have recovered.
- The United Kingdom has reported 596 hospital deaths, bringing the death toll to 16,060.
- The number of recorded deaths increases by 596 to 16,060, a lower increase than in previous days. Dr Jenny Harries says the lower number of deaths is "very good news" but cautions against drawing conclusions from the figures.

- After a Sunday Times article suggests schools could reopen on 11 May, Gavin Williamson, the Secretary of State for Education, tells the Downing Street daily briefing he cannot give a date for when this will happen and that the focus will be on helping children to learn at home, with lessons made available online and free loans of laptops for disadvantaged children.
- BBC One airs a UK version of the Together at Home concert; a virtual global concert staged to celebrate healthcare workers and featuring musicians playing from home. The two-hour broadcast includes highlights of the US version and features stories of frontline workers along with extra footage of British artists.
- The United States reports 2,009 new cases, bringing the total to 735,336. The US has reported a total of 40,585 deaths, with almost half of them originating in New York State.
- Zimbabwe has reported a total of three deaths and 25 cases.
- According to figures released by Johns Hopkins University, more than 2.3 million people have been infected, and over 164,000 people have died.
- Rwanda and the Democratic Republic of Congo announce that they will mandate the wearing of face masks.
- President of Zimbabwe Emmerson Mnangagwa has extended the country's lockdown by two weeks.
- The head of the World Health Organization (WHO) urged the G20 leading global economies to plan to ease lockdowns against COVID-19 only as part of "a phased process".

- UN Secretary-General António Guterres sent a video message in support of the UN-supported 'One World: Together At Home' event.
- Croatian Interior Minister Davor Božinović lifts internal travel restrictions, allowing people to travel within their districts. However, the country's borders remain closed.
- Vice President of the European Commission for Values and Transparency Věra Jourová has criticised the European Union for what she described as its "morbid dependency" on China and India for medical supplies during a Czech television debate.
- French Health Minister Olivier Véran eases restrictions on visits to nursing and seniors' homes, which had been in place since 20 March20. Only two relatives may visit a senior or social care facility at the same time, while physical contact is prohibited.
- United Kingdom Minister for the Cabinet Office Michael Gove has rebuffed a BuzzFeed News report claiming that the British Government is considering a three-stage plan to start easing lockdown restrictions within weeks.
- Pakistani Prime Minister, Imran Khan, bows to pressure from religious scholars to keep mosques open for the duration of the Ramadan period. This decision came in response to threats by religious scholars to organise mass protests in defiance of the Pakistani Government's attempts to close mosques in response to the coronavirus pandemic. The Pakistani Consulate-General in Dubai announced that the first Pakistan International Airlines flight carrying 227 Pakistani nationals stranded in Dubai and the Northern

Emirates had departed for Pakistan that morning at 0700 local time.

- Tunisian Prime Minister Elyes Fakhfakh extends Tunisia's lockdown until 4 May.
- The Saudi Council of Senior Scholars advises Muslims to pray at home and avoid public gatherings during Ramadan if their countries require social distancing in order to prevent the spread of the coronavirus.
- In the United Arab Emirates, organisers of Dubai's Arabian Travel Market, which was scheduled to be held from 28 June to 1 July, have cancelled the event citing health and safety concerns.

20 April

- Canada has reported a total of 1,611 deaths and 33,922 cases.
- China has reported 12 new cases (eight of them imported) and 49 new asymptomatic cases but no deaths.
- Ecuador has reported a total of over 10,000 cases.
- France has reported a total of 20,265 deaths.
- Germany has reported 1,775 new cases, bringing the total to 141,672. Germany has reported 110 new deaths.
- Ghana has confirmed a total of 834 cases and nine deaths.
- Indonesia has reported 85 new cases, bringing the total number to 6,070. Indonesia has reported eight new deaths, bringing the death toll to 590. 747 people have recovered, while 49,700 tests have been conducted.
- Iran has reported 91 new deaths, bringing the death toll to 5,209. Iran has reported a total of 83,505 cases.

- Italy has reported that 108,237 were being treated at home or recovering in hospital, a drop by 20 from the total reported on Sunday.
- Malaysia has reported 36 new cases, bringing the country's total number of cases to 5,425. Malaysian authorities have discharged 98 patients, bringing the total number of recoveries to 3,295. Malaysia has reported no new deaths.
- The Netherlands has reported 750 new cases, bringing the total to 33,405. Dutch health authorities have also reported 67 new deaths, bringing the death toll to 3,751.
- New Zealand has reported 9 new cases (7 confirmed and 2 probable), bringing the total to 1,440 (1,105 confirmed and 335 probable). NZ health authorities have also recovered 62 new recoveries, bringing the total to 974. Fourteen people remain hospitalised.
- The Philippines has confirmed 19 new deaths, bringing the total to 428. The dead include former Senator and government minister Heherson Alvarez. The Philippines has also confirmed 200 new cases, bringing the total to 6,459. 41 patients have recovered, bringing the total to 613.
- Russia has confirmed 4,268 new cases, bringing the total to 47,121. 44 new deaths have been reported.
- Singapore has reported 1,426 new cases, bringing the total to 8,014.
- South Korea has reported 20 new cases (13 from overseas), bringing the total to 10,764.
- Spain has confirmed a total of 200,210 cases and 20,852 deaths.

- Switzerland has reported 204 new cases, bringing the total to 27,944. The country has also reported a total of 1,142 deaths.
- Thailand has reported 27 new cases, bringing the total to 2,792. Thailand has also reported 47 deaths and 1,999 recoveries.
- Turkey has reported 4,674 cases, bringing the total to 90,980. Turkey has also reported 123 deaths, bringing the death toll to 2,140. 13,430 people have recovered, while 39,703 people have been tested.
- Ukraine reports 261 new cases and 10 new deaths, bringing the total numbers to 5,710 and 151, respectively; 359 patients have recovered overall.
- Online applications for the Coronavirus Job Retention Scheme are opened, with 67,000 claims registered in the first 30 minutes.
- NHS Blood and Transplant asks those who have survived COVID-19 to donate blood for trials of a treatment that will involve giving the blood plasma of survivors to patients ill in hospital with the disease.
- Prof Dame Angela Maclean, the UK's deputy chief scientific adviser, says the number of confirmed cases is "flattening out". The number of people in hospital for COVID-19 has begun to fall in Scotland, Wales and every region of England, with significant falls in London and the Midlands.
- The United Nations General Assembly passed resolution A/RES/74/274: International cooperation to ensure global access to medicines, vaccines and medical equipment to face COVID-19, urging swift access to vaccines.

- The World Health Organization (WHO) reiterated its stance on the lifting of lockdown measures, stating, "We want to re-emphasise that easing restrictions is not the end of the epidemic in any country".
- The heads of multiple major UN humanitarian agencies and offices, including the World Health Organization (WHO), the World Food Programme (WFP), and the Office for Coordination of Humanitarian Affairs (OCHA), launched an urgent appeal for $350 million to support global aid hubs to help those vulnerable during the COVID-19 pandemic.
- Henrietta Fore, Executive Director of the United Nations Children's Fund (UNICEF) and UN High Commissioner for Refugees Filippo Grandi, issued a joint statement pledging to accelerate work to expand refugee children's access to protection, education, clean water, and sanitation.
- The UN's International Fund for Agricultural Development (IFAD) launched the Rural Poor Stimulus Facility, which aims to reduce the impact of COVID-19 on farmers and rural communities in developing countries.
- Gillian Triggs, Assistant High Commissioner for Protection at the Office of the UN High Commissioner for Refugees, warned of the urgent need to protect "refugee, displaced and stateless women and girls at the time of this pandemic".
- Brazilian President Jair Bolsonaro has called for Brazil's stay-at-home measures to end this week, claiming that the policy was killing jobs.
- United States Vice President Mike Pence has stated that the United States has sufficient testing capacity nationwide to allow any of the states to start lifting lockdown orders provided that they meet the other criteria for relaxation,

including 14 days of declining infections and having enough hospital capacity to treat the sick.

- Acting United States Secretary of Homeland Security Chad Wolf announced that the United States, Canada, and Mexico will be restricting non-essential travel across their borders in order to combat the spread of the coronavirus.
- Swiss pharmaceutical company Novartis gains approval from the United States Food and Drug Administration to conduct a randomised trial of the malaria drug hydroxychloroquine against the coronavirus.
- The New York State Nurses Association sues New York state and two hospitals, alleging that their members were exposed to hazardous working conditions, including nurses being forced to work when sick and insufficient PPE equipment.
- The United Nations Office for the Coordination of Humanitarian Affairs has issued an urgent call for US$350 million to support the global emergency supply system coordinated by the World Food Programme to ensure that supplies reach impoverished countries.
- Facebook has removed some posts by groups fomenting protests against stay-at-home orders in California, New Jersey and Nebraska after consulting with state officials.
- Ghana is using drones from Zipline to test people more quickly outside of the major cities. Zipline will fly samples collected from more than 1,000 health facilities in rural areas to laboratories in the capital Accra and Kumasi. The Ghanaian Government has also ended a three-week lockdown in Accra and Kumasi, the country's two major cities.

- A new study on food insecurity by an alliance of UN, governmental, and non-governmental agencies (Global Network Against Food Crises) warned that the COVID-19 pandemic was perpetuating a downward cycle of acute food insecurity for around 135 million people across 55 countries.
- Executive Director of the World Food Programme (WFP) David Beasley warned the UN Security Council to act fast in the face of famines of "biblical proportions" in what was not only "a global health pandemic but also a global humanitarian catastrophe".
- A UN ECLAC report warned that the COVID-19 pandemic would result in the worst economic contraction in the history of Latin American and the Caribbean since the Great Depression, with a projected -5.3 per cent drop in activity in 2020.
- New data from UNESCO and partners revealed extreme divides in digitally-based distance learning for most of the world's students now at home due to COVID-19, as half of all students currently out of the classroom (nearly 830 million learners globally) lacked access to a computer, with over 40 per cent having no home Internet.
- UN Secretary-General António Guterres pledged the UN's continued support to the Alliance of Small Island States on climate change and the socioeconomic effects of COVID-19.
- The Bahraini Government has announced that it will slash spending by government ministries and agencies by 30 per cent to help the country weather the coronavirus pandemic, including delaying some construction and consulting projects.

- The Iranian Government has begun reopening intercity highways and major shopping centres to stimulate its crippled economy. Shops in Tehran's Grand Bazaar have been allowed to reopen up to 6 pm local time.
- The Kuwaiti Government has extended the suspension of work in the public sector until 31 May and expanded the nationwide curfew to 16 hours (4 pm to 8 am) in order to combat the spread of the coronavirus.
- The Pakistani Government has announced that it will be shifting from a general lockdown to "smart lockdowns", focusing on coronavirus hotspots. The Government will use contact tracing and testing to identify such hotspots for "smart lockdowns."
- Saudi Arabia extends the suspension of praying in the Great Mosque and Al-Masjid an-Nabawi during Ramadan to combat the spread of COVID-19.
- The Belgian Government has indicated that it is planning to ease lockdown restrictions since the coronavirus pandemic in Belgium has peaked.
- The European Commissioner for Economic and Financial Affairs, Taxation and Customs Paolo Gentiloni stated during an interview that €1.5 trillion worth of aid would be needed to tackle the coronavirus pandemic.
- In Israel, demonstrators have protested against Prime Minister Benjamin Netanyahu's coronavirus restrictions while keeping two meters apart.
- The Lithuanian Finance Ministry has forecast that the Lithuanian economy will shrink by 7.8% this year if the coronavirus is contained by summer.

- Norway has begun reopening pre-school nurseries after a month-long lockdown. Norwegian Air has announced that four of its subsidiaries in Denmark and Sweden had filed for bankruptcy, affecting 4,700 jobs.
- The Polish Health Minister Łukasz Szumowski has issued a statement stating that the Polish Government may restore restrictions if there is a spike in cases. Earlier, the Polish Government had announced the reopening of parks and forests on Monday.
- Russian President Vladimir Putin has stated that Russia has managed to curb the spread of the coronavirus but that the outbreak had not yet peaked.
- Slovakian Prime Minister Igor Matovič has proposed a plan to reopen small shops of up to 300 square metres, outdoor sports grounds and takeaways from 23 April.
- Turkish President Recep Tayyip Erdogan announced that Turkey will impose a four-day lockdown on 31 cities commencing 24 April (Thursday) to combat the spread of the coronavirus.
- In the United Kingdom, NHS Blood and Transplant announced that they were planning to collect blood from coronavirus patients to investigate if convalescent plasma transfusion could speed up patients' rate of recovery. British Culture Secretary has also announced that the UK Government will review its approach to the coronavirus pandemic to identify areas for improvement in response to public criticism. Prince Philip has also issued a statement thanking health workers, scientists and other essential services for their work during the coronavirus pandemic. A spokesperson for British Prime Minister Boris Johnson has

also defended the Government's decision not to lift lockdown and social distancing measures, saying that the UK's main concern is to prevent a second wave of infections. British Chancellor of the Exchequer Rishi Sunak announced that over 140,000 companies, employing more than 1 million people, had applied for the Government's wage subsidy scheme.

- The International Monetary Fund's Managing Director Kristalina Georgieva has described the spread of the coronavirus as the worst crisis since the Great Depression during a media conference in Bulgaria.
- A new study on food insecurity by an alliance of UN, governmental, and non-governmental agencies (Global Network Against Food Crises) warned that the COVID-19 pandemic was perpetuating a downward cycle of acute food insecurity for around 135 million people across 55 countries.
- Executive Director of the World Food Programme (WFP) David Beasley warned the UN Security Council to act fast in the face of famines of "biblical proportions" in what was not only "a global health pandemic but also a global humanitarian catastrophe".
- A UN ECLAC report warned that the COVID-19 pandemic would result in the worst economic contraction in the history of Latin American and the Caribbean since the Great Depression, with a projected -5.3 per cent drop in activity in 2020.
- New data from UNESCO and partners revealed extreme divides in digitally-based distance learning for most of the world's students now at home due to COVID-19, as half of all students currently out of the classroom (nearly 830 million

learners globally) lacked access to a computer, with over 40 per cent having no home Internet.

- UN Secretary-General António Guterres pledged the UN's continued support to the Alliance of Small Island States on climate change and the socioeconomic effects of COVID-19.
- The Bahraini Government has announced that it will slash spending by government ministries and agencies by 30 percent to help the country weather the coronavirus pandemic, including delaying some construction and consulting projects.
- The Iranian Government has begun reopening intercity highways and major shopping centres to stimulate its crippled economy. Shops in Tehran's Grand Bazaar have been allowed to reopen up to 6 pm local time.
- The Kuwaiti Government has extended the suspension of work in the public sector until 31 May and expanded the nationwide curfew to 16 hours (4 pm to 8 am) in order to combat the spread of the coronavirus.
- The Pakistani Government has announced that it will be shifting from a general lockdown to "smart lockdowns," focusing on coronavirus hotspots. The Government will use contact tracing and testing to identify such hotspots for "smart lockdowns."
- Saudi Arabia extends the suspension of praying in the Great Mosque and Al-Masjid an-Nabawi during Ramadan to combat the spread of COVID-19.
- The Belgian Government has indicated that it is planning to ease lockdown restrictions since the coronavirus pandemic in Belgium has peaked.

- The European Commissioner for Economic and Financial Affairs, Taxation and Customs Paolo Gentiloni stated during an interview that €1.5 trillion worth of aid would be needed to tackle the coronavirus pandemic.
- In Israel, demonstrators have protested against Prime Minister Benjamin Netanyahu's coronavirus restrictions while keeping two meters apart.
- The Lithuanian Finance Ministry has forecast that the Lithuanian economy will shrink by 7.8% this year if the coronavirus is contained by summer.
- Norway has begun reopening pre-school nurseries after a month-long lockdown. Norwegian Air has announced that four of its subsidiaries in Denmark and Sweden had filed for bankruptcy, affecting 4,700 jobs.
- The Polish Health Minister Łukasz Szumowski has issued a statement stating that the Polish Government may restore restrictions if there is a spike in cases. Earlier, the Polish Government had announced the reopening of parks and forests on Monday.
- Russian President Vladimir Putin has stated that Russia has managed to curb the spread of the coronavirus but that the outbreak had not yet peaked.
- Slovakian Prime Minister Igor Matovič has proposed a plan to reopen small shops of up to 300 square metres, outdoor sports grounds, and takeaways from 23 April.
- Turkish President Recep Tayyip Erdogan announced that Turkey would impose a four-day lockdown on 31 cities commencing 24 April (Thursday) to combat the spread of the coronavirus.

- In the United Kingdom, NHS Blood and Transplant announced that they were planning to collect blood from coronavirus patients to investigate if convalescent plasma transfusion could speed up patients' rate of recovery. British Culture Secretary has also announced that the UK Government will review its approach to the coronavirus pandemic to identify areas for improvement in response to public criticism. Prince Philip has also issued a statement thanking health workers, scientists, and other essential services for their work during the coronavirus pandemic. A spokesperson for British Prime Minister Boris Johnson has also defended the Government's decision not to lift lockdown and social distancing measures, saying that the UK's main concern is to prevent a second wave of infections. British Chancellor of the Exchequer Rishi Sunak announced that over 140,000 companies, employing more than 1 million people, had applied for the Government's wage subsidy scheme.
- The International Monetary Fund's Managing Director Kristalina Georgieva has described the spread of the coronavirus as the worst crisis since the Great Depression during a media conference in Bulgaria.
- A new study on food insecurity by an alliance of UN, governmental, and non-governmental agencies (Global Network Against Food Crises) warned that the COVID-19 pandemic was perpetuating a downward cycle of acute food insecurity for around 135 million people across 55 countries.
- Executive Director of the World Food Programme (WFP) David Beasley warned the UN Security Council to act fast in the face of famines of "biblical proportions" in what was not

only “a global health pandemic but also a global humanitarian catastrophe.”

- A UN ECLAC report warned that the COVID-19 pandemic would result in the worst economic contraction in the history of Latin American and the Caribbean since the Great Depression, with a projected -5.3 percent drop in activity in 2020.
- New data from UNESCO and partners revealed extreme divides in digitally-based distance learning for most of the world's students now at home due to COVID-19, as half of all students currently out of the classroom (nearly 830 million learners globally) lacked access to a computer, with over 40 percent having no home Internet.
- UN Secretary-General António Guterres pledged the UN's continued support to the Alliance of Small Island States on climate change and the socioeconomic effects of COVID-19.

21 April

- Canada has reported a total of 37,382 cases and 1,728 deaths.
- China has reported 11 new cases and 37 asymptomatic cases but no new deaths.
- Indonesia reports 375 new cases, bringing the total to 7,135. Indonesian health authorities also report 26 new deaths, taking the death toll to 616.
- Italy has reported 534 new deaths, bringing the death toll to 24,648. Italy has reported over 180,000 cases, and almost 49,000 recovered people.

- In Japan, a crew member aboard Costa Atlantica in Nagasaki tested positive for the coronavirus. About 20 others are also down with a fever.
- Lebanon has reported a total of 677 cases and 21 deaths.
- Malaysia has reported 57 new cases, bringing the total to 5,482. 54 more patients have been discharged, bringing the number of recoveries to 3,349. Malaysia has recorded three more fatalities, bringing the death toll to 92.
- In Morocco, 68 people, mainly staff, have tested positive for the coronavirus in the southern city of Ouarzazate.
- The Netherlands has reported 729 new cases, bringing the total to 34,134. Dutch health authorities have reported 165 deaths, bringing the death toll to 3,916.
- New Zealand has reported 5 new cases (2 confirmed and 3 probable), bringing the total to 1,445 (1,107 confirmed and 338 probable). NZ authorities also report 32 new recoveries, bringing the total to 1,006. The country also reports a new death, bringing the death toll to 13. In addition, a New Zealand traveller in Peru died after missing a repatriation flight; however, this is not included in the Ministry of Health figures.
- Pakistan has confirmed 17 new deaths, bringing the death toll to 192. Pakistan also confirms 705 new cases, bringing the total to 9,214.
- The Philippines reports 9 new deaths, bringing the total to 437. The Philippines has reported 140 new cases, bringing the total to 6,599.
- Singapore has reported 1,111 new cases, bringing the total to 9,125.

- Spain has reported 430 new deaths, bringing the death toll to 21,282. Spain has reported nearly 4,000 new cases, bringing the total number of infections to 204,178.
- Turkey has reported 4,611 new cases, bringing the total to 95,591. Turkey reports 119 new deaths, bringing the death toll to 2,259.
- Ukraine reports 415 new cases and 10 new deaths, bringing the total numbers to 6,125 and 161 respectively; a total of 367 patients have recovered.
- In the UK, A further 823 deaths are recorded, taking the total to 17,337, a sharp rise on the previous day, but many of these relate to deaths that occurred in previous days and weeks, and some date back as far as March. Prof Sir David Spiegelhalter of the University of Cambridge says the figures suggest the UK is past the peak and in a "steadily" albeit slowly improving position.
- Figures released by the Office for National Statistics indicate deaths in England and Wales have reached a twenty-year high, with 18,500 deaths from all causes in the week up to 10 April, about 8,000 more than the average for that time of year. The deaths include those in care homes, where the 1,043 year-to-date deaths related to COVID-19 is a jump from the 217 reported a week ago.
- Matt Hancock says the government is "throwing everything" at developing a vaccine as he announces £42.5m for clinical trials being conducted by Imperial College London and the University of Oxford.
- Parliament reconvenes after the Easter recess with MPs approving a new arrangement with some in the House of Commons chamber and some attending via video link.

- Fundraiser Captain Tom Moore is the guest of honour at the opening of NHS Nightingale Hospital Yorkshire and the Humber in Harrogate.
- The United States has reported 2,721 new deaths and more than 40,000 new cases.
- Governor of Maryland Larry Hogan stated that his state had obtained 500,000 tests from South Korea following negotiations and criticized the federal government for not providing states with the resources to cope with the coronavirus pandemic. In response, US President Trump criticized Larry Hogan and other state governors, claiming that the US had sufficient resources for coronavirus testing.
- United States President Donald Trump announced that he would sign an executive order to temporarily suspend all immigration into the United States to combat the spread of the coronavirus, which he described as "the attack from the invisible enemy." This Executive Order will last for 90 days and deny entry to most work visa holders with the exception of healthcare and medical professionals and those working in the food industries. In addition, there will be a sixty-day ban on those seeking permanent residency status.
- The United States Senate has unanimously passed legislation establishing a US$484 billion program to support small businesses affected by the coronavirus pandemic, hospitals, and a national testing impetus.
- The United Nations General Assembly unanimously adopted a Mexican resolution backed by the United States calling for "equitable, efficient and timely access to any future vaccines developed to fight the coronavirus." That same day, the UNGA passed another resolution calling for global action to

develop and improve access to medicines, vaccines, and equipment to battle the pandemic and closer cooperation between the UN and World Health Organization.

- Austrian Chancellor Sebastian Kurz has announced that the Austrian Government will allow restaurants to reopen and religious services to resume from 15 May. Schools are scheduled to reopen for senior students in early May, while schools for younger pupils will reopen at a staggering pace from 15 May.
- The Danish Health Ministry announced that it would not allow public gatherings with over 500 people until at least 1 September, contradicting earlier reports that the Danish Government would not allow larger public gatherings until 10 May. A current limit on public gatherings of more than ten people remains in force until 10 May.
- German Food and Agriculture Minister Julia Klöckner stated during a G20 meeting that food exports should only be curbed during an emergency.
- Greek authorities have locked down a migrant hotel in Kranidi housing 470 migrants after a Somali woman tested positive for the coronavirus.
- Italian Prime Minister Giuseppe Conte has warned that easing lockdown restrictions may increase the spread of the coronavirus.
- The Spanish Government has announced that it will allow children under the age of 12 to leave their homes for 90 minutes with an accompanying adult due to concerns for the mental health of children.

- Turkish President Recep Tayyip Erdogan has described the coronavirus pandemic as the biggest global crisis since World War Two.
- In the United Kingdom, several engineering, aerospace, automotive, and Formula One companies have formed the VentilatorChallengeUK consortium in order to produce 1,500 ventilators per week.
- United Nations World Food Programme chief economist Arif Husain has warned that the number of people facing acute food insecurity could rise to 265 million as a result of the economic fallout of the coronavirus pandemic.
- World Health Organization spokesperson Fadela Chaib issued a statement during a Geneva media briefing that all available evidence suggests that the coronavirus originated in bats and was not created in a laboratory in response to US President Trump's statements that the US would investigate whether the ircoronavirus was manufactured in a lab.
- President of Afghanistan Ashraf Ghani and his wife Rula Ghani have tested negative for the coronavirus. At least forty presidential palace staff have tested positive for the coronavirus.
- The Iranian Government has temporarily released a thousand foreign prisoners, including British-Iranian woman Nazanin Zaghari-Ratcliffe in response to pressure from human rights groups.
- The Iraqi Government has announced that it will temporarily ease the 24-hour curfew ahead of Ramadan. The new curfew will be imposed mainly at night from 7 pm until 6 am

local time between 21 April and 11 May. However, a total ban will take place on Fridays and Saturdays.

- The Lebanese Parliament was relocated to a makeshift theatre to allow social distancing. Legislators were sprayed with disinfectant and had their temperatures taken.
- The Saudi Press Agency has announced that the Saudi Arabian Government intends to ease curfew restrictions it has imposed on several cities to allow more people to shop for essentials within their neighborhoods during the Ramadan period.
- Austrian Chancellor Sebastian Kurz has announced that the Austrian Government will allow restaurants to reopen and religious services to resume from 15 May. Schools are scheduled to reopen for senior students in early May, while schools for younger pupils will reopen at a staggering pace from 15 May.
- The Danish Health Ministry announced that it would not allow public gatherings with over 500 people until at least 1 September, contradicting earlier reports that the Danish Government would not allow larger public gatherings until 10 May. A current limit on public gatherings of more than ten people remains in force until 10 May.
- German Food and Agriculture Minister Julia Klöckner stated during a G20 meeting that food exports should only be curbed during an emergency.
- Greek authorities have locked down a migrant hotel in Kranidi housing 470 migrants after a Somali woman tested positive for the coronavirus.

- Italian Prime Minister Giuseppe Conte has warned that easing lockdown restrictions may increase the spread of the coronavirus.
- The Spanish Government has announced that it will allow children under the age of 12 to leave their homes for 90 minutes with an accompanying adult due to concerns for the mental health of children.
- Turkish President Recep Tayyip Erdogan has described the coronavirus pandemic as the biggest global crisis since World War Two.
- In the United Kingdom, several engineering, aerospace, automotive, and Formula One companies have formed the VentilatorChallengeUK consortium in order to produce 1,500 ventilators per week.
- United Nations World Food Programme chief economist Arif Husain has warned that the number of people facing acute food insecurity could rise to 265 million as a result of the economic fallout of the coronavirus pandemic.
- World Health Organization spokesperson Fadela Chaib issued a statement during a Geneva media briefing that all available evidence suggests that the coronavirus originated in bats and was not created in a laboratory in response to US President Trump's statements that the US would investigate whether the coronavirus was manufactured in a lab.
- Nigerian President Muhammadu Buhari has called for the release of prisoners awaiting trial, elderly, and terminally ill prisoners in an effort to ease overcrowding in Nigerian prisons.

- South African President Cyril Ramaphosa has announced a US$26 billion relief package to help businesses and people in need during the coronavirus pandemic.

22 April

- Bulgaria has reported a total number of 1,015 cases, 47 deaths, and 174 recoveries.
- Canada has reported a total of 1,871 deaths and 38,932 cases.
- China has reported 30 new cases (23 involving people returning from overseas) and 42 asymptomatic cases.
- Indonesia has reported 283 new cases, bringing the total to 7,418. Indonesia has also reported 19 deaths, bringing the death toll to 635. Indonesia has reported a total of 913 recoveries.
- Iran has reported 94 new deaths, bringing the death toll to 5,391. Iran has a total of 85,996 cases.
- Italy has reported 437 new deaths, bringing the death toll 25,085. Italian authorities have reported 3,370 cases, bringing the number of cases to 187,327.
- In Japan, Nagasaki authorities have confirmed 33 new cases aboard the Italian cruise ship Costa Atlantica based on contact tracing of an infected crew member, bringing the total to 34. The Costa Atlantica has remained in Nagasaki's shipyard since February. Eight babies and children at a Tokyo-based residential care facility have tested positive for the coronavirus.
- Jordan has reported a total of 435 cases, 297 recoveries, and seven deaths.

- Lebanon has reported the death of a Syrian Palestinian at Wavel refugee camp in the eastern Bekaa Valley.
- Malaysia has reported 50 new cases, bringing the total to 5,532. Malaysian health authorities have discharged 103 patients, bringing the total number of recoveries to 3,452. Malaysia reports one death, bringing the death toll to 93.
- The Netherlands has confirmed 708 new cases, bringing the total to 34,842. Dutch health authorities have confirmed 138 new deaths, bringing the death toll to 4,054.
- New Zealand has reported six new cases, bringing the total to 1,451 (1,113 confirmed and 338 probable). In addition, there have been 30 new recoveries, bringing the total to 1,036. Authorities have also reported another death, bringing the death toll to 14.
- The Philippines has reported 111 new cases, bringing the total number to 6,710. The Philippines has reported nine new deaths, bringing the total to 446. 39 patients have recovered, bringing the total number of recoveries to 693.
- Qatar has reported 608 new cases, bringing the total number of cases to 7,141. Qatar health authorities have confirmed 75 recoveries and one new death.
- Russia has reported 5,236 new cases, bringing the total to 57,999. Russia has reported 53 new deaths, bringing the death toll to 513.
- Singapore has reported 1,016 new cases, bringing the total to 10,141. Another death was confirmed later, bringing the death toll to 12.
- South Korea has reported 11 new cases (six involving overseas travel).

- Spain has reported 435 deaths, bringing the total to 21,717. The Spanish health ministry has reported 4,211 new cases, bringing the total to 208,389.
- Switzerland has reported a total of 1,217 deaths and 28,268 cases.
- Turkey has reported 3,083 new cases, bringing the total number of cases to 98,674. The country has reported 117 new deaths, bringing the total to 2,376; 16,477 people have recovered, and 37,535 people have been tested.
- Ukraine has reported a total of 6,592 cases, 174 deaths, and 424 recoveries.
- The United Kingdom has confirmed 763 new deaths, bringing the death toll to 18,100. The number of cases has reached 133,495. Foreign Secretary Dominic Raab has also confirmed the deaths of 69 National Health Service personnel as a result of the coronavirus pandemic.
- The United States has reported 1,738 new deaths, bringing the death toll to 46,583. Californian health authorities had also confirmed that two people in the state died from the coronavirus before the United States reported its first death in late February 2020.
- According to Johns Hopkins University, more than 2.5 million people globally have contracted the coronavirus, and at least 178,000 have died.
- The Health Protection (Coronavirus, Restrictions) (England) (Amendment) Regulations 2020 (SI 447) come into effect, correcting errors in the original lockdown regulations and allowing some visits to burial grounds and gardens of remembrance.

- Figures show that UK inflation fell to 1.5% in March, largely because of falls in the price of clothing and fuel ahead of the lockdown.
- United Kingdom Parliament holds the first virtual Prime Minister's Questions with Dominic Raab standing in for Boris Johnson, at which Raab confirms the target of 100,000 tests a day by the end of the month.
- In a Commons statement, Matt Hancock tells MPs, "we are at the peak" of the outbreak, but social distancing measures cannot be relaxed until the government's five tests have been met. Professor Chris Whitty, the government's chief medical adviser, tells the Downing Street briefing the UK will have to live with some social distancing measures for at least the rest of the year and that it is "wholly unrealistic" to expect life to suddenly return to normal in the short term.
- The German biotech company BioNTech has received approval from Germany's vaccine regulator to test a vaccine candidate, a project named BNT162, on 200 human test subjects.
- Spanish Prime Minister Pedro Sánchez has announced that Spain will be easing down coronavirus lockdown measures during the second half of May.
- Turkmenistan's Foreign Minister Raşit Meredow has insisted that his country has not reported any cases of the coronavirus.
- In the United Kingdom, Ed Davey, the acting leader of the Liberal Democrats, has called for an inquiry into the British Government's handling of the coronavirus, including the partial death toll, limited testing, and the lack of equipment at hospitals. British Foreign Secretary Dominic Raab confirmed

the deaths of 69 National Health Service personnel as a result of the coronavirus pandemic and announced that the Government had delivered 1 billion items of personal protective equipment as well as through the devolved administrations of Scotland, Wales, and Northern Ireland. Health Secretary Matt Hancock has confirmed that the British Government will implement large-scale contact tracing once they curb the number of new cases.

- Pope Francis has called for European unity in combating the coronavirus pandemic ahead of a European Union summit to discuss a contentious economic stimulation package.
- Mexican President Andres Manuel Lopez Obrador has announced that the Mexican Government will invest 622.6 billion Mexican pesos (US$25.6 billion) into social programmes and critical projects to combat the fallout of the coronavirus.
- Following a meeting between US President Donald Trump and New York Governor Andrew Cuomo, the President agreed that the federal government would help New York obtain enough chemical reagents to double the state's testing capacity to 40,000 tests a day. Cuomo has also announced plans to expand contact tracing in New York state in coordination with authorities in New Jersey and Connecticut and support from Bloomberg L.P...
- Robert R. Redfield, the Director of the Centers for Disease Control and Prevention (CDC), warned that a second wave of the coronavirus could be more destructive because it could collide with the flu season; he strongly encouraged people to get their flu jabs. The United States Agency for International Development's Acting-Administrator John Barsa

announces that the US Government will assess the way that the World Health Organization is being run.

- Missouri has filed a lawsuit against the Chinese Government over its handling of the coronavirus, claiming that China's response to the outbreak has brought devastating economic losses to the state. In response, the Chinese Foreign Ministry has dismissed the allegation as "nothing short of absurdity" and lacking legal or factual merit. In addition, United States Secretary of State Michael Pompeo has accused Beijing of delaying to report of human-to-human transmission of the coronavirus for a month until it had spread to every province in China.
- US medical company Indutex USA George Gianforcaro has protested the Federal Emergency Management Agency's decision to seize 400,000 N95 respirator masks meant for domestic customers.
- The Montreal-based International Civil Aviation Organization has estimated that global air travel could drop by as many as 1.2 billion travellers by September 2020.
- Streaming giant Netflix has reported that subscriptions have increased by 15.8 million between January and March 2020 due to people staying at home to comply with lockdown orders.
- The World Health Organization's Director-General Tedros Adhanom has expressed concern about the coronavirus' "upward trends" in parts of Africa, Central America, and South America and the management of international air travel. Adhanom has also urged Washington to reconsider its decision to suspend funding to the international organisation.

- The Israeli Defense Minister Naftali Bennett has cancelled an Israeli Army initiative to test coronavirus samples from the Hamas-controlled Gaza Strip.
- Lebanese authorities have placed the Wavel refugee camp in the eastern Bekaa valley under lockdown after a Syrian-Palestinian man tested positive for the coronavirus, becoming the first confirmed case in one of the country's refugee camps.
- Pakistani President Imran Khan has undergone testing for the coronavirus after he came into contact with infected philanthropist Faisal Edhi. Khan subsequently tested negative for the coronavirus.
- In Saudi Arabia, the Presidency of the Two Holy Mosques has announced that King Salman has approved performing the Tarawih at the two Holy Mosques. Still, that entry for pilgrims will remain suspended.
- The International Telecommunications Union (ITU) confirmed that 5G was in no way responsible for the spread of the COVID-19 virus.
- The Director-General of the World Health Organization (WHO) warned against 'complacency' as countries continued to battle COVID-19 and citizens grew weary of stay-at-home measures.
- On International Mother Earth Day, UN Secretary-General António Guterres flagged the COVID-19 pandemic as "an unprecedented wake-up call" and offered six ways to help the climate.
- The United States Agency for International Development's Acting-Administrator John Barsa announces that the US

Government will assess the way that the World Health Organization is being run.

- Missouri has filed a lawsuit against the Chinese Government over its handling of the coronavirus, claiming that China's response to the outbreak has brought devastating economic losses to the state. In response, the Chinese Foreign Ministry has dismissed the allegation as "nothing short of absurdity" and lacking legal or factual merit. In addition, United States Secretary of State Michael Pompeo has accused Beijing of delaying to report of human-to-human transmission of the coronavirus for a month until it had spread to every province in China.
- US medical company Indutex USA George Gianforcaro has protested the Federal Emergency Management Agency's decision to seize 400,000 N95 respirator masks meant for domestic customers.
- The Montreal-based International Civil Aviation Organization has estimated that global air travel could drop by as many as 1.2 billion travellers by September 2020.
- The World Health Organization's Director-General Tedros Adhanom has expressed concern about the coronavirus' "upward trends" in parts of Africa, Central America, and South America and the management of international air travel. Adhanom has also urged Washington to reconsider its decision to suspend funding to the international organisation.
- Police Minister Bheki Cele has confirmed the arrest of 131 government officials, including police officers, councillors, health officials, and corrections officers, for flouting the country's coronavirus regulations, including selling confiscated alcohol.

23 April

- China has reported ten new cases, bringing the total to 82,798. No new deaths have been reported.
- France has reported 516 new deaths, bringing the total to 21,856.
- Italy has reported 464 new cases, bringing the total to 189,973. The country has reported a total of 25,549.
- Japan has reported 14 new cases aboard the Italian cruise ship Costa Atlantica, bringing the total number of infected aboard the ship to 48. The Costa Atlantica is carrying 623 passengers.
- Malaysia has reported 71 new cases, bringing the total number of cases to 5,603. 3,542 have recovered. Malaysia also reports two new deaths, bringing the death toll to 95.
- New Zealand has reported three new cases (two confirmed and one probable). Three previous cases were also rescinded, keeping the total at 1,451. In addition, NZ authorities report 29 new recoveries, bringing the total to 1,065. Two further deaths are reported, bringing the death toll to 16.
- Pakistan has reported 765 new cases, bringing the total to 10,513.
- Singapore has reported 1,037 new cases, bringing the total to 11,178. In addition, a patient who had COVID-19 was found dead at a staircase landing, with the death caused by a fatal height injury.
- Spain has reported 440 new deaths, bringing the death toll to 22,157. The number of total cases has risen to 213,024.

- Turkey reports 115 new deaths, bringing the total to 2,941. The country has reported a total of 101,790 cases.
- Ukraine reports 578 new cases and 13 new deaths, bringing the total numbers to 7,170 and 187 respectively, as well as a total of 504 recoveries.
- The United Kingdom has reported 616 deaths in hospitals, bringing the death toll to 18,738. 16,786 of these deaths have occurred in England, which also reports 514 new deaths. UK health authorities have also tested 425,821 people, with 138,078 testing positive.
- In the United States, California reports 115 deaths in the past 24 hours.
- Venezuela has reported a total of 311 cases and 10 deaths.
- The Africa Centers for Disease Control and Prevention reports 26,000 cases across the continent, up from 16,000 a week ago. About 1,200 have died. Fewer than 500,000 tests have been conducted, some 325 per million population. Authorities are concerned that fragile health systems may soon be overwhelmed.
- The UN Secretary-General released a new policy brief on shaping an effective, inclusive response to the COVID-19 pandemic, echoed his February Call to Action to put human dignity and the Universal Declaration of Human Rights at the core of the UN's work, and warned that the coronavirus pandemic was "fast becoming a human rights crisis."
- In Canada, the Premier of Ontario Doug Ford and the Premier of Quebec Francois Legault have requested assistance from the Canadian Armed Forces in response to overstretched human resources at Canadian rest homes.

- United States President Donald Trump has criticized Georgian Governor Brian Kemp's decision to allow some non-essential businesses to reopen. In the United States, a total of 26 million people have applied for unemployment benefits in the last five weeks. According to the Fuller Project, two-thirds of unemployment claims were filed by women.
- The United States House of Representatives passes a US$484 billion coronavirus relief bill supporting small businesses and hospitals by 388–5. The House of Representatives, controlled by the Democratic Party, also approved the creation of a special advisory panel to investigate the federal government's response to the coronavirus pandemic.
- The U.S. Immigration and Customs Enforcement announces that it will test 2,000 immigration detainees for the coronavirus in response to a spate of outbreaks among deportees who had returned to Mexico and Guatemala.
- New York Governor Andrew Cuomo announced that a random screening of 3,000 residents found that 13.9% have tested positive for antibodies for the coronavirus, suggesting that about 2.7 million people in the state have been affected.
- United Nations Secretary-General António Guterres has released a report advocating that human rights should play a key role in guiding the response of states to the coronavirus pandemic. Guterres has also warned against the rise of hate speech, the targeting of vulnerable communities, and the danger of states adopting repressive measures in response to the coronavirus pandemic.

- The German investment bank KfW has delivered two mobile diagnostic laboratories to Uganda and Rwanda to help combat the coronavirus. More mobile laboratory units have been dispatched to the six-member states of the East African Community.
- The South African Competition Tribunal has launched an investigation of the pharmaceutical group Dis-Chem for increasing the price of face masks by 261%. South African President Cyril Ramaphosa has announced a partial reopening of the economy from 1 May, including easing travel restrictions and allowing some industries to operate under a five-level risk system.
- The Egyptian Government will maintain a nighttime curfew during the Ramadan period. Still, it will delay the start of the curfew from 8 pm to 9 pm to allow one extra hour of movement.
- Pakistani Prime Minister Imran Khan has confirmed that US President Donald Trump has offered to assist Pakistani efforts to combat the coronavirus, including providing ventilators and unspecified economic assistance. Khan also intends to launch a US$595 million appeal to fund Pakistan's "Preparedness and Response Plan to COVID-19", mainly lobbying international financial institutions and world powers.
- In the United Arab Emirates, Dubai has allowed cafes and restaurants to resume operations. Shopping malls will also be reopened from 12 pm to 10 pm but with a maximum capacity of 30 percent. Public transportation services, including the metro, will resume on 26 April.
- In Canada, the Premier of Ontario Doug Ford and the Premier of Quebec Francois Legault have requested

assistance from the Canadian Armed Forces in response to overstretched human resources at Canadian rest homes.

- United States President Donald Trump has criticized Georgian Governor Brian Kemp's decision to allow some non-essential businesses to reopen. In the United States, a total of 26 million people have applied for unemployment benefits in the last five weeks. According to the Fuller Project, two-thirds of unemployment claims were filed by women.
- The United States House of Representatives passes a US$484 billion coronavirus relief bill supporting small businesses and hospitals by 388–5. The House of Representatives, controlled by the Democratic Party, also approved the creation of a special advisory panel to investigate the federal government's response to the coronavirus pandemic.
- The U.S. Immigration and Customs Enforcement announces that it will test 2,000 immigration detainees for the coronavirus in response to a spate of outbreaks among deportees who had returned to Mexico and Guatemala.
- New York Governor Andrew Cuomo announced that a random screening of 3,000 residents found that 13.9% have tested positive for antibodies for the coronavirus, suggesting that about 2.7 million people in the state have been affected.
- United Nations Secretary-General António Guterres has released a report advocating that human rights should play a key role in guiding the response of states to the coronavirus pandemic. Guterres has also warned against the rise of hate speech, the targeting of vulnerable communities, and the danger of states adopting repressive measures in response to the coronavirus pandemic.

- The Czech Government announces that it will seek support from the Chamber of Deputies for an extension of the country's state of emergency until 25 May.
- Greece has extended lockdown measures by a week until 4 May, a move that will also delay the removal of hundreds of migrants from refugee camps. In addition, two asylum seekers on the island of Lesbos, one Iranian and one Afghan were shot and wounded after allegedly violating coronavirus quarantine restrictions.
- The Irish Health Minister Simon Harris has reported that hospital admissions in Ireland have fallen by 60% to about 40.
- The Swedish Government has limited online betting to 5,000 Swedish kronor (US$495) a week.
- The British Government's Chief Medical Officer Chris Whitty has recommended keeping social distancing measures in place for the rest of the year. The British Health Secretary Matthew Hancock has announced that coronavirus testing will be expanded to other "key workers" outside the medical and nursing home professions, including teachers, government servants, and delivery drivers. He also announced that the Government was launching a large-scale testing and tracking programme to keep the rate of coronavirus transmissions low.
- In the United Kingdom, a team of scientists at Oxford University has tested their first prototype vaccine, "ChAdOx1 nCoV-19," on their first batch of volunteers. Meanwhile, Italy's ReiThera, Germany's Leukocare, and Belgium's Univercell have confirmed they are working together on developing a trial vaccine within the next few months.

- The first human trials of a coronavirus vaccine in Europe begin in Oxford.
- A study involving 20,000 households in England, coordinated by the Office for National Statistics, will track the progress of COVID-19 and seek to better understand infection and immunity levels, with volunteers asked to provide nose and throat swabs on a regular basis to determine whether they have the virus.
- Matt Hancock states that daily test capacity has reached 51,000 and announces that all key workers and members of their households are now eligible for COVID-19 tests and will be able to book tests through the government website from the following day. Tests will be conducted at drive-through centres or using home testing kits. In contrast, mobile testing units operated by the armed forces would increase in number from the present eight to 92, with a further four operated by civilians in Northern Ireland.
- Hancock also announces preparations to reactivate contact tracing in a later phase of the outbreak, including the recruitment of 18,000 contact tracers to supplement Public Health England's staff.
- DIY chain B&Q confirms it has reopened 155 stores following a trial opening of a small number of outlets the previous weekend.
- BBC One airs The Big Night In, a first-of-its-kind joint broadcast with Children in Need and Comic Relief, featuring an evening of music and entertainment. The broadcast celebrates the acts of kindness, humour, and the spirit of hope and resilience keeping the nation going during the unprecedented COVID-19 pandemic, with viewers given a

chance to donate to a fund helping local charities and projects around the country. The event raises £27m for charity, with the government pledging to double that amount.

- At 8 pm, the UK stages a fifth round of applause for NHS staff and key workers.
- Oran Finnegan, the head of the International Committee of the Red Cross forensic unit, has advised international governments to prepare and plan for mass casualties resulting from the coronavirus, warning that the rising death toll could overwhelm the local capacity to handle the amount of dead bodies.
- The UEFA Champions League has postponed the UEFA Women's Euro 2021 to July 2022.
- The World Health Organization Europe Director Dr. Hans Kluge has reported that up to half of all coronavirus fatalities in Europe have occurred within nursing homes, showing that the pandemic has disproportionately affected the elderly. Kluge also called for healthcare workers in rest homes to be given more protective gear and support. The WHO also announced that it was launching a "landmark collaboration" to speed up the development, production, and distribution of drugs, tests, and vaccines to prevent, diagnose and treat COVID-19.
- According to the World Trade Organization (WTO), 80 countries have imposed bans or limited the export of face masks and other protective equipment. However, only 13 WTO members have notified the global trading organization as required by its regulations.

24 April

- Bangladesh has reported a total of 3,772 cases and 120 deaths. The Bangladesh Doctors Foundation also confirms that 251 doctors have tested positive for the coronavirus.
- Belarus has confirmed a total of 8,773 cases.
- China has reported six new cases (two involving overseas travel), bringing the total number of cases to 82,804.
- Djibouti has reported a total of 985 cases and two deaths.
- France has reported 389 new deaths, bringing the total to 22,245.
- Hong Kong has reported no new cases and deaths for the past two weeks. According to health authorities, the total number of cases stands at 1,036.
- India has reported 1,680 new cases (including 778 in Maharashtra state), bringing the total to 22,930.
- Indonesia has reported 436 new cases, bringing the total number to 8,211. 42 people have died, bringing the death toll to 689.
- Iran has reported 93 new deaths, bringing the death toll to 5,574. The country has a total of 88,194 cases, with 3,121 in serious condition.
- In Japan, Nagasaki authorities have reported that 91 crew members of the Italian cruise ship Costa Atlantica have tested positive for the coronavirus. Nagasaki authorities intend to test 260 of the 623 crew. The Japanese Government announced that those who test negative would be repatriated to their home countries.
- Lebanon has reported a total of 696 cases and 22 deaths.

- Malaysia has reported 88 new cases, bringing the total to 5,691. Malaysian authorities also report 121 new recoveries, bringing the total to 3,663. Malaysia also reports one new death, bringing the death toll to 96.
- The Netherlands has reported 806 new cases, bringing the total to 36,535. The country has reported 112 new deaths, bringing the death toll to 4,289.
- New Zealand has reported five new cases (2 confirmed and 3 probable), bringing the total to 1,456 (1,114 confirmed and 342 probable). Health authorities also report 30 recoveries, bringing the total to 1,095. In addition, another death was reported, bringing the total to 17.
- The Philippines has reported 211 new cases, bringing the total to 7,192. The country has also reported 15 deaths, bringing the total to 477. The Philippines also reports 40 new recoveries, bringing the total to 762.
- Portugal has reported a total of 22,797 cases and 854 fatalities.
- Qatar has reported 761 cases, bringing the total to 8,525. The country has reported ten new deaths.
- Singapore has reported 897 new cases, bringing the total to 12,075.
- Spain has reported 367 new deaths, bringing the death toll to 22,524. Spain has reported 219,764 cases.
- Switzerland has reported a total of 1,309 deaths and 28,677 cases.
- Thailand has reported 15 new cases, bringing the total to 2,854. Thailand reports no new deaths, with the death toll remaining at 50.

- Timor Leste has reported 24 cases and two recoveries. The infected include a nurse, who became the first confirmed health worker infected with the coronavirus.
- Turkey has reported 3,122 new cases, bringing the total to 104,912. The number of deaths rises by 109 to a total of 2,600.
- Ukraine reports 477 new cases and 6 new deaths, bringing the total numbers to 7,647 and 193 respectively; a total of 601 patients have recovered.
- In the United Kingdom, English hospitals report 587 deaths, bringing the death toll to 17,373.
- The United States has reported a total of 50,031 deaths and 870,648 cases, based on figures released by Johns Hopkins University. The USS Kidd has reported at least 18 cases aboard.
- Vietnam has reported two new cases, bringing the total to 270.
- The website for key workers to book a coronavirus test temporarily closes after a high demand for the tests; 5,000 test kits are ordered within its first two minutes online. The government says it will make more tests available.
- Transport Secretary Grant Shapps announces bilateral discussions with the Irish and French governments to safeguard freight routes and with Northern Ireland Executive regarding support for passenger flights. Funding is to be provided to support ferry routes to Northern Ireland, the Isle of Wight, and the Isles of Scilly.
- A version of "You'll Never Walk Alone" recorded by Captain Tom Moore and Michael Ball to raise money for the NHS

Charities Together fund reaches number one in the UK Singles Chart.

- In Belgium, Antwerp authorities announced that they will be testing virus bracelets to ensure that thousands of people employed in the city comply with social distancing rules. The Belgian Government has also announced that they will ease coronavirus restriction measures in May, allowing non-food businesses to reopen on 11 May and schools to reopen from 18 May.
- The French Health Ministry has restricted the sale of nicotine substitutes after some new research suggested that nicotine may offer some protection against the coronavirus.
- The Hungarian President Viktor Orban has announced that the Hungarian Government intends to replace the current lockdown, which imposes a blanket curfew over the population, with what he described as a more "fine-tuned plan."
- The Israeli government allows most businesses that are not in shopping malls and open markets to reopen as long as they adhere to standards of cleanliness, wearing protective gear, and social distancing. Hairdressers and beauty saloons can resume operations from Saturday midnight, while eateries can sell takeaways and provide home deliveries. The Israeli Government also increased fines for violating social distancing guidelines and maintained restrictions on non-essential travel.
- The Polish Education Minister Dariusz Piatkowski extends the closure of schools and early childhood education facilities from 26 April to 24 May.

- The Portuguese government announces that it intends to conduct 70,000 tests on residents and workers at care homes by the end of May 2020.
- Russian authorities announced that they will build a 1,000-bed hospital for coronavirus patients in St Petersburg in response to rising cases and deaths. The Defence Ministry is also building 16 hospitals across the country to cope with demand.
- UK Health Secretary Matt Hancock has defended the British Government's guidelines for personal protective equipment (PPE) in response to a lawsuit from two British doctors, who have expressed concern that existing PPE policies do not protect medical workers from the coronavirus. The opposition British Labour Party has announced a review into the impact of the coronavirus pandemic on the Black, Asian and other minority ethnic communities, who have been disproportionately affected by the pandemic. Transport for London has also announced that it would place 7,000 staff on furlough and access the British Government's job retention scheme.
- A spokesperson for the United States Mission in Geneva has confirmed that the United States will not be participating in the launch of a global initiative sponsored by French President Emmanuel Macron and German Chancellor Angela Merkel on Friday to speed up the development, production, and distribution of vaccines and drugs to combat the coronavirus pandemic.
- The World Health Organization's director-general Tedros Adhanom announced that the international organisation was partnering with world leaders and the private sector to speed up the development, production, and distribution of drugs

and vaccines to combat the coronavirus pandemic. The British and Spanish Governments have expressed support for the WHO's efforts.

- French pharmaceutical company Sanofi's CEO Paul Hudson has called for better European coordination to develop a vaccine for the coronavirus, criticizing what he regarded as Europe's slow response to the pandemic.
- Liberian President George Weah has extended the country's lockdown, which was first introduced on 8 April, by two weeks. Weah also added a new measure requiring people to wear face masks.
- The Legislative Assembly of El Salvador has been evacuated after the Interdisciplinary Epidemiological Control Team detected a "serious suspicion" of the coronavirus in the Assembly's "blue living room."
- Haiti has received 129 of its nationals on a deportation flight from the United States. The Haitian government requested that the United States test all deportees for the coronavirus, but US authorities only agreed to test those with symptoms. Returnees will be quarantined in a quarantine facility for two weeks.
- US President Donald Trump attracts controversy and criticism for remarks suggesting that the coronavirus could be treated by injecting disinfectant into the body. In response, Trump has said that his remarks were sarcastic. Trump and Vice President Mike Pence left a press conference early.
- William N. Bryan, the Acting Under Secretary of Homeland Security for Science and Technology, draws media attention

for claiming that sunlight, heat, and humidity weaken the coronavirus.

- The United States Department of Health and Human Services has announced that the Centers for Disease Control and Prevention (CDC) will be releasing US$631 million to state and local governments to assist with COVID-19 relief efforts.
- Mayor of San Francisco London Breed said the city orders for PPE from China were instead rerouted to France and FEMA. "We had isolation gowns on the way to San Francisco and then diverted to France," she said. Another order of equipment went through customs and then was "confiscated" by FEMA for other places. She later stated, "That at the height of this pandemic we are still having a conversation about PPE really does blow my mind. There has been nothing that has been more frustrating."
- The UN-backed the virtual launch of the G20 Access to COVID-19 Tools (ACT) Accelerator initiative to boost commitment and support for the production of COVID-19 diagnostics, therapeutics, and vaccines.
- UN High Commissioner for Human Rights, Michelle Bachelet, expressed alarm over press clampdowns stifling the free flow of information in some countries, vital in getting the COVID-19 under control.
- The UN Office for the Coordination of Humanitarian Affairs (OCHA), called for greater funding as it worked to set up basic handwashing stations, deliver clean drinking water and food, and launch public information campaigns on COVID-19 for 100 million people at risk.

- The UN Population Fund (UNFPA) and World Health Organization (WHO) reported that lessons learned during the Ebola outbreak in Liberia six years previously were helping it to confront COVID-19.
- The Lebanese High Defence Council has advised the Lebanese Government to extend the nationwide lockdown until 10 May but to ease restrictions over the coming weeks gradually. The Lebanese Government has extended the national lockdown until 10 May but has shortened the curfew by one hour from 8 pm to 5 am. Lebanon also announced a five-stage plan to reopen the country on 28 April, 4 May, 11 May, 25 May, and 6 June. Physical distancing and wearing masks will remain compulsory for the duration of the lockdown.
- Pakistani Prime Minister Imran Khan has confirmed that Pakistan is using a contact tracing system developed by the country's intelligence service Inter-Services Intelligence.
- United States Secretary of State Mike Pompeo has urged Egyptian Foreign Minister Sameh Shoukry to ensure that American nationals detained in Egyptian prisons are safe during the coronavirus pandemic.
- The Israeli government allows most businesses that are not in shopping malls and open markets to reopen as long as they adhere to standards of cleanliness, wearing protective gear, and social distancing. Hairdressers and beauty saloons can resume operations from Saturday midnight, while eateries can sell takeaways and provide home deliveries. The Israeli Government also increased fines for violating social distancing guidelines and maintained restrictions on non-essential travel.

- The Polish Education Minister Dariusz Piatkowski extends the closure of schools and early childhood education facilities from 26 April to 24 May.
- The Portuguese government announces that it intends to conduct 70,000 tests on residents and workers at care homes by the end of May 2020.
- Russian authorities announced that they will build a 1,000-bed hospital for coronavirus patients in St Petersburg in response to rising cases and deaths. The Defence Ministry is also building 16 hospitals across the country to cope with demand.
- UK Health Secretary Matt Hancock has defended the British Government's guidelines for personal protective equipment (PPE) in response to a lawsuit from two British doctors, who have expressed concern that existing PPE policies do not protect medical workers from the coronavirus. The opposition British Labour Party has announced a review into the impact of the coronavirus pandemic on the Black, Asian and other minority ethnic communities, who have been disproportionately affected by the pandemic. Transport for London has also announced that it would place 7,000 staff on furlough and access the British Government's job retention scheme.
- A spokesperson for the United States Mission in Geneva has confirmed that the United States will not be participating in the launch of a global initiative sponsored by French President Emmanuel Macron and German Chancellor Angela Merkel on Friday to speed up the development, production, and distribution of vaccines and drugs to combat the coronavirus pandemic.

- The World Health Organization's director-general Tedros Adhanom announced that the international organisation was partnering with world leaders and the private sector to speed up the development, production, and distribution of drugs and vaccines to combat the coronavirus pandemic. The British and Spanish Governments have expressed support for the WHO's efforts.
- French pharmaceutical company Sanofi's CEO Paul Hudson has called for better European coordination in efforts to develop a vaccine for the coronavirus, criticizing what he regarded as Europe's slow response to the pandemic.
- The Legislative Assembly of El Salvador has been evacuated after the Interdisciplinary Epidemiological Control Team detected a "serious suspicion" of the coronavirus in the Assembly's "blue living room."
- Haiti has received 129 of its nationals on a deportation flight from the United States. The Haitian government requested that the United States test all deportees for the coronavirus, but US authorities only agreed to test those with symptoms. Returnees will be quarantined in a quarantine facility for two weeks.
- US President Donald Trump attracts controversy and criticism for remarks suggesting that the coronavirus could be treated by injecting disinfectant into the body. In response, Trump has said that his remarks were sarcastic. Trump and Vice President Mike Pence left a press conference early.
- William N. Bryan, the Acting Under Secretary of Homeland Security for Science and Technology, draws media attention

for claiming that sunlight, heat, and humidity weaken the coronavirus.

- The United States Department of Health and Human Services has announced that the Centers for Disease Control and Prevention (CDC) will be releasing US$631 million to state and local governments to assist with COVID-19 relief efforts.
- Mayor of San Francisco London Breed said the city orders for PPE from China were instead rerouted to France and FEMA. "We had isolation gowns on the way to San Francisco and then diverted to France," she said. Another order of equipment went through customs and then was "confiscated" by FEMA for other places. She later stated, "That at the height of this pandemic we are still having a conversation about PPE really does blow my mind. There has been nothing that has been more frustrating."

25 April

- China has reported 12 new cases, bringing the total number of confirmed cases to 82,816. China has also reported 29 new asymptomatic cases. No new deaths have been reported, with the official death toll remaining at 4,632.
- France has reported 369 new deaths, bringing the death toll to 22,164. 124 patients have been admitted into intensive care in the previous 24 hours.
- Germany has reported 2,055 cases, bringing the total to 152,438. Germany has also reported 179 new deaths, bringing the cases to 5,500.

- Indonesia has reported 396 new cases, bringing the total to 8,607. Indonesia has reported 31 new deaths, bringing the death toll to 720.
- Iran has reported 76 new deaths, bringing the death toll to 5,650. Iran has also reported a total of 89,328 cases, with 3,096 in serious condition.
- Japan has reported a total of 12,800 cases and 345 deaths. Nagasaki authorities have reported 57 new cases among the crew of the cruise ship Costa Atlantica, bringing the total to 148. Tokyo has confirmed 103 new cases, bringing the total number of cases in Tokyo to 3,836.
- Malaysia has reported 51 new cases, bringing the total to 5,742. Malaysian authorities have also reported two deaths, bringing the death toll to 98.
- Mexico has reported a total of 12,872 cases and 1,221 deaths.
- The Netherlands has reported 655 cases, bringing the total to 37,190. The country has reported 120 new deaths, bringing the total to 4,409.
- New Zealand has reported five new cases (three confirmed and two probable), bringing the total to 1,461 (1,117 confirmed and 344 probable). NZ health authorities have reported 23 new recoveries, bringing the total to 1,118. One further death has also been reported, bringing the total to 18.
- The Philippines has reported 17 new deaths, bringing the death toll to 494. The Philippines has also reported 102 new cases, bringing the total to 7,294.
- Poland has reported a total of 11,067 cases and 499 deaths.

- Russia has reported 5,966 new cases, bringing the total to 74,588. Russia has reported 66 new deaths, bringing the death toll to 681.
- Singapore has reported 618 new cases, bringing the total to 12,693.
- Spain has reported 378 new deaths, bringing the total to 22,902. The country has reported a total of 223,759 cases.
- Sri Lanka has confirmed 60 new cases, bringing the total to 420. The country has also confirmed seven deaths.
- Thailand has reported 53 new cases, bringing the total to 2,907. Thailand has also reported one new death, bringing the death toll to 51. 2,547 patients have recovered.
- Turkey has reported 2,861 cases, bringing the total to 107,773. The country also reported 106 deaths, raising the death toll to 2,706. 25,582 have recovered, and 38,308 people have been tested in the last 24 hours.
- Ukraine reports 478 new cases and 8 new deaths, bringing the total numbers to 8,125 and 201, respectively; a total of 782 patients have recovered.
- The United Kingdom reports 813 new deaths, bringing the death toll to 20,319. UK authorities also reported 4,913 new cases, bringing the total to 148,377.
- The United States has reported a total of 895,766 cases. The US Centers for Disease Control and Prevention reported 1,623 new deaths, bringing the death toll to 50,439.
- Johns Hopkins University has reported that the global death toll now stands at 200,697.
- In Argentina, prisoners at Devoto prison in Buenos Aires have rioted to demand urgent health measures after a coronavirus case was confirmed at the facility

- Canadian Prime Minister Justin Trudeau clarified that plans to restart the economies of Canadian provinces do not hinge upon the presumption that people who have recovered from the coronavirus develop an immunity to it.
- The Maryland Emergency Management Agency has issued a Twitter alert advising residents that no disinfectant product should be administered through the body via "injection, ingestion or any other route." New York City had also reported 30 cases of disinfectant ingestion following Trump's remarks yesterday.
- The United States Department of the Treasury has disbursed US$9.5 billion in additional funds from the Payroll Support Program to US airliners, bringing the total amount of aid provided to the sector to US$12.4 million. 93 US air carriers have applied and received government financial assistance in response to the coronavirus pandemic.
- The UN World Health Organization (WHO) warned that there was no evidence that people who had recovered from COVID-19 and had antibodies were protected from a second infection.
- In Belarus, several people have tested positive for the coronavirus at an orphanage for 170 people.
- In France, the office of Prime Minister Edouard Philippe confirmed that he would present a plan to wind down the country's lockdown before the National Assembly on 28 April (Tuesday).
- Hundreds in Germany and Poland have gathered at the Polish border town of Zgorzelec against a mandatory coronavirus quarantine for those crossing the border. In Berlin, a thousand anti-lockdown protesters have staged a

rally, attended by both far-left and right-wing activists and groups. Police arrested several protesters for flouting lockdown measures.

- The Polish Health Minister Dr. Łukasz Szumowski has advised postponing the 2020 Polish presidential election, scheduled for 10 May. Despite pressure from the opposition, medical workers, the public, and allies and members of the ruling Law and Justice Party, the Polish government had refused to postpone the election.
- Spanish Prime Minister Pedro Sánchez has announced that people will be allowed to exercise from 2 May if the number of new coronavirus cases continues to drop.
- The United Kingdom has started trials to investigate whether plasma collected from donors who have recovered from the coronavirus can be used to treat patients who are severely unwell with it. Starship Technologies has announced that they will be using delivery robots to deliver groceries to National Health Service personnel. A 10 Downing Street spokesperson also confirmed that British Prime Minister Boris Johnson would return to work on Monday.
- The number of recorded deaths increases by 813, taking the total past 20,000 to 20,319. Thus the UK becomes the fifth country to pass the 20,000 mark along with the United States, Italy, Spain, and France.
- After figures show that A&E attendances are half their usual level, the health service urges people to seek healthcare if needed and not be put off by the coronavirus outbreak.
- COVID-19 tests for key workers are booked up within an hour.

- Guernsey partially lifts its lockdown restrictions, allowing gardeners, mechanics, estate agents, and builders to return to work.
- Air France–KLM's CEO Benjamin Smith, announces that the airline group will be implementing voluntary redundancies as part of its initial cost-cutting plans.
- The British budget airliner Wizz Air announces that it will resume flights from London's Luton Airport from 1 May, becoming one of the first European airliners to restore services.
- David Kaye, the United Nations special rapporteur on the Promotion and Protection of the Right to Freedom of Opinion and Expression, has released a summary of his report to the United Nations Human Rights Council on Twitter expressing concern that some policies meant to combat the coronavirus pandemic "may be failing to meet the standards of legality, necessity, and proportionality."
- The World Health Organization has issued a statement that there is no evidence that people who have recovered from the coronavirus and have antibodies are protected against a second coronavirus infection.
- The Algerian Government has allowed certain businesses, including those supplying building materials and public works, appliances, fabrics, jewellery, clothing, and shoes, cosmetics and perfumes, home and office furniture, pastries, hairdressers, and taxis, to resume business in order to reduce the economic and social impact of the coronavirus pandemic.

- The International Monetary Fund has disbursed US$309 million to help Mozambique to fight the coronavirus pandemic.
- Nigeria Governors' forum, representing the country's 36 governors, has petitioned Nigerian President Muhammadu Buhari to make it compulsory to wear face masks in public.
- South African Minister of Trade and Industry Ebrahim Patel announces plans to reopen South Africa's agricultural sector and allow some manufacturing and retail to resume.
- The Abu Dhabi airliner Etihad has suspended passenger flights until 15 May.
- 25 April
- In Argentina, prisoners at Devoto prison in Buenos Aires have rioted to demand urgent health measures after a coronavirus case was confirmed at the facility.
- Canadian Prime Minister Justin Trudeau clarified that plans to restart the economies of Canadian provinces do not hinge upon the presumption that people who have recovered from the coronavirus develop an immunity to it.
- The Maryland Emergency Management Agency has issued a Twitter alert advising residents that no disinfectant product should be administered through the body via "injection, ingestion or any other route." New York City has also reported 30 cases of disinfectant ingestion following Trump's remarks yesterday.
- The United States Department of the Treasury has disbursed US$9.5 billion in additional funds from the Payroll Support Program to US airliners, bringing the total amount of aid provided to the sector to US$12.4 million. 93 US air

carriers have applied and received government financial assistance in response to the coronavirus pandemic.

- The Algerian Government has allowed certain businesses, including those supplying building materials and public works, appliances, fabrics, jewellery, clothing, and shoes, cosmetics and perfumes, home and office furniture, pastries, hairdressers, and taxis, to resume business in order to reduce the economic and social impact of the coronavirus pandemic.
- The International Monetary Fund has disbursed US$309 million to help Mozambique to fight the coronavirus pandemic.
- Nigeria Governors' forum, representing the country's 36 governors, has petitioned Nigerian President Muhammadu Buhari to make it compulsory to wear face masks in public.
- South African Minister of Trade and Industry Ebrahim Patel announces plans to reopen South Africa's agricultural sector and allow some manufacturing and retail to resume.

26 April

- Belgium had reported 553 cases, including 127 admissions, the lowest level since 18 March when daily admissions reached a peak of 600.
- Canada has reported a total of 2,489 deaths. Canada has reported 1,427 new cases, bringing the total to 45,791.
- China has reported 11 new cases, bringing the total to 82,827. The National Health Commission also reported that all coronavirus patients in Wuhan had been discharged from the city's hospitals.

- France has reported 242 deaths, bringing the death toll to 22,856.
- Germany has reported 1,747 new cases, bringing the total to 154,175. The country's death toll rose by 140 to 5,640.
- India has reported a total of 26,496 cases and 824 deaths.
- Indonesia has reported 275 new cases, raising the total to 8,882. 23 people have died, bringing the death toll to 743.
- Iran has reported 60 new deaths, bringing the death toll to 5,710. Iran has reported a total of 90,481 cases.
- Japan has reported a total of 13,231 cases and 360 deaths. Tokyo has also reported 72 new cases, bringing the total in the capital to 3,900.
- Malaysia has reported 38 new cases, bringing the total to 5,870. 3,862 have recovered, while the death toll remains at 98.
- Mexico has reported 970 new cases, bringing the total to 13,842. Mexico has reported 84 deaths, bringing the death toll to 1,305.
- The Netherlands has reported 655 new cases, bringing the total to 37,845. The Netherlands has also reported 66 new deaths, bringing the death toll to 4,475.
- New Zealand has reported 9 new cases (4 confirmed and 5 probable), bringing the total to 1,470 (1,121 confirmed and 349 probable). NZ health authorities have reported 24 new recoveries, bringing the total to 1,142.
- The Philippines has reported seven new deaths, bringing the death toll to 501. The country has also reported 285 new cases, bringing the total to 7,579. 862 patients have recovered.

- Russia has reported 6,361 new cases, bringing the total to 80,949. 66 have died, bringing the death toll to 747.
- Singapore has reported 931 new cases (the majority foreign migrant workers and 15 permanent residents), bringing the total to 13,264. Among them include two imported cases, the first since 17 April.
- South Korea has reported 10 new cases (seven involving overseas travel and three in Daegu), bringing the total to 10,718. The death toll remains at 210.
- Spain has reported 288 new deaths, bringing the death toll to 23,190. Spain has reported a total of 207,634 cases.
- Thailand has reported 15 new cases, bringing the total to 2,922. 2,594 patients have recovered, and the death toll remains at 51.
- Turkey has reported 2,357 cases, bringing the total to 110,130. Turkey has reported 99 deaths, bringing the total to 2,805. Turkey has reported 29,140 recoveries.
- Ukraine has reported 492 new cases and 8 new deaths, bringing the total numbers to 8,617 and 209, respectively; a total of 840 patients have recovered.
- The United Kingdom has reported 413 new deaths, bringing the death toll to 20,732. The UK has reported 4,463 new cases, bringing the total to 152,840.
- According to a Reuters report, 96% of the 3,277 prisoners who tested positive for the coronavirus in the US states of Arkansas, North Carolina, Ohio, and Virginia were asymptomatic.
- The figure of 413 recorded deaths is the lowest daily total in April.

- Professor Stephen Powis tells the Downing Street daily briefing the benefit of social distancing is beginning to be felt, with the stabilisation of the number of new cases and a reduction of the number of people in hospital.
- Johns Hopkins University has reported over 200,000 deaths, 2.88 million cases, and 813,000 recoveries.
- The Prime Minister of Egypt, Mostafa Madbouly, has announced that Egypt plans to negotiate a one-year financial support programme with the International Monetary Fund.
- In his first public statement since returning to work, Boris Johnson says the UK is "at the moment of maximum risk," but "we are now beginning to turn the tide" as he urges people not to lose patience with the restrictions.
- The government announces that the families of NHS and care workers who die because of COVID-19 will be entitled to a payment of £60,000.
- The number of recorded deaths from COVID-19 rises by 360, taking the total to 21,092. This is the lowest daily rise for four weeks.
- Saudi Arabian King Salman has ordered a partial lifting of the curfew in all regions of the country except Mecca and previously quarantined neighborhoods. The curfew will be lifted between 9 am and 5 pm from Sunday onwards, while malls, wholesale and retail shops will be allowed to reopen from 29 April onwards for two weeks.
- At the start of World Immunization Week, UNICEF warned that millions of children were in danger of missing life-saving vaccines against measles, diphtheria, and polio due to disruptions in immunization as the world attempted to slow the transmission of COVID-19.

- The Cuban Government has sent 216 healthcare workers to South Africa to help with the coronavirus pandemic. Cuba has already sent 20 medical brigades, mainly to African and Caribbean countries but also Italy.
- The Honduras Government has extended a blanket curfew to contain the spread of the coronavirus by one week until 3 p.m. on 3 May.
- Governor of California Gavin Newsom has urged beachgoers in southern California to abide by social distancing guidelines.
- Italian Prime Minister Giuseppe Conte has announced that Italy will reopen its manufacturing industry from 4 May and schools from September. Companies will be required to introduce strict safety measures before resuming operations. Conte has also confirmed that professional sports teams can resume training on 18 May and individual sports teams on 4 May. As part of the plan, eateries will be allowed to provide takeaway and delivery services. People will be able to move within their home regions, and factories and construction sites will be allowed to resume work provided they adhere to social distancing. Museums and galleries will also reopen on 18 May.
- Dutch health authorities have quarantined two mink farms after several animals were found to be infected with the coronavirus.
- In Germany, car manufacturers Volkswagen and BWM have announced that they will reopen their factories on Monday in response to the relaxation of lockdown measures.
- The Spanish Government has allowed children to leave the house in order to exercise, play or go for a walk as part of

the relaxation of lockdown measures, which had previously only allowed adults to leave the house to buy groceries and medicine, walk the dog, and seek medical treatment. Children under the age of 14 are allowed one hour of supervised outdoor activity per day between 9 am and 9 pm local time but must remain within one kilometre of their home. However, children must be accompanied by adults and must adhere to social distancing policies, not using playgrounds, and not sharing toys. Schools also remain closed.

- President of Tajikistan Emomali Rahmon has ordered the closure of all schools, most businesses, and public gatherings, including sports gatherings.
- The Honduras Government has extended a blanket curfew to contain the spread of the coronavirus by one week until 3 p.m. on 3 May.
- Governor of California Gavin Newsom has urged beachgoers in southern California to abide by social distancing guidelines.

27 April

- Canada has reported a total of 2,617 deaths and 47,327 cases.
- China has reported three new cases (two overseas cases and one from Heilongjiang) and no new deaths.
- France has reported 437 deaths, bringing the total death toll to 23,293. 28,055 remain hospitalised, with 4,608 in intensive care.
- Germany has reported 1,018 new cases and 100 deaths.
- India has confirmed a total of 27,000 cases and 872 deaths.

- Iran has reported 700 deaths from ingested toxic methanol, mistakenly believing that it could cure the coronavirus.
- Italy has reported 333 deaths, bringing the death toll to 26,977. Italy has reported 1,739 cases, bringing the total number to 199,414.
- Malaysia has reported 40 new cases, bringing the total to 5,820. 95 patients have been discharged, bringing the number of recoveries to 3,957. Malaysia has also reported one new death, bringing the death toll to 99.
- The Netherlands has reported 400 new cases, bringing the total to 38,245. Dutch authorities have also confirmed 45 deaths, bringing the death toll to 4,518.
- New Zealand has reported five new cases (one confirmed and four probable). Six previous cases have also been rescinded, bringing the total to 1,469 (1,122 confirmed and 347 probable). NZ health authorities have also reported 38 new recoveries, bringing the total to 1,180. One further death has been reported, bringing the death toll to 19.
- Pakistan has reported 605 new cases and a total of 281 deaths.
- The Philippines has reported 198 new cases, bringing the total to 7,777. The country has reported ten new deaths, bringing the death toll to 511.
- Singapore has reported 799 new cases, bringing the total to 14,423. 2 deaths have been confirmed, bringing the total to 14.
- South Africa has reported a total of 4,546 cases and 87 deaths.
- Spain has reported 331 new deaths, bringing the death toll to 23,521.

- Thailand has reported 9 cases and 1 death, bringing the total to 2,931 cases and 52 deaths, respectively.
- Turkey has reported 2,131 new cases, bringing the total to 112,261. Turkey has reported 95 deaths, bringing the death toll to 2,900.
- Ukraine has reported 392 new cases and 11 new deaths, bringing the total numbers to 9,009 and 220 respectively; a total of 864 patients have recovered.
- The United Kingdom has reported 360 new deaths (including 82 medical workers), bringing the death toll to 21,092.
- In the United States, New York has recorded 337 new deaths.
- In the disputed territory of Gaza, the economy ministry has allowed restaurants to reopen in order to ease the economic hardship caused by the coronavirus pandemic. Restaurants must observe social distancing rules.
- The 2020 Formula One World Championship, scheduled to be held at Circuit Paul Ricard, Le Castellet on 28 June, has been cancelled by organisers in response to the coronavirus.
- The Norwegian Government has reopened primary schools to children aged six to ten years after six weeks of distance learning. To comply with health measures, classes will be limited to 15 kids.
- British Minister of State for Health Edward Argar has confirmed during a radio interview that the British Government will continue to test whether antibody tests can be used to combat the coronavirus pandemic. British Prime Minister Boris Johnson announces that he will meet with Labour Party leader Keir Starmer this week and the leaders of other parties the following week as part of efforts to build

consensus over plans to ease the coronavirus lockdown. A British court has also delayed the extradition hearing for journalist and activist Julian Assange since lockdown restrictions prevented his lawyers from attending court proceedings.

- The British Government has allowed members of the public to submit questions to government ministers, scientific, and medical officers during the daily briefing under Prime Minister Johnson's policy of "maximum possible transparency." The British Chancellor of the Exchequer, Rishi Sunak, has announced that the UK Government will provide state-backed loans to small businesses in order to protect the economy and workers during the lockdown.
- Turkish President Recep Tayyip Erdoğan announced that Turkey would send medical gear, including protective suits and masks, to the United States. He also imposed a three-day lockdown in 31 cities commencing 1 May and stated that weekend lockdowns would continue until Eid al-Fitr in late May 2020.
- The United Nations High Commissioner for Human Rights Michelle Bachelet has called Governments not to violate human rights under the pretext of "exceptional and emergency measures" during the coronavirus pandemic.
- Iranian President Hassan Rouhani has announced that Iran will be divided into green, red, and white zones based on the number of cases and deaths. Mosques located in the white zones will be allowed to reopen and resume Friday prayers.

- The Pakistan Civil Aviation Authority has extended a ban on all international flights in and out of the country until 15 May.

The only exceptions will be diplomatic, cargo flights, and special flights transporting stranded passengers.

- Brazilian Productivity and competition secretary Carlos da Costa has announced that the Brazilian Government is working on a plan to open up the Brazilian economy, including allowing professional football matches behind closed doors.
- The Mexican Government has confirmed that senior civil servant Irma Erendira Sandoval, the head of the country's public administration ministry, has tested positive for the coronavirus.
- United States President Donald Trump has dismissed media reports that he is planning to dismiss Health Secretary Alex Azar as "fake news" in a Tweet. White House Adviser and Director of the Office of Trade and Manufacturing Policy Peter Navarro has confirmed that the Trump Administration is exploring protocols for keeping factories open during the coronavirus pandemic, including social distancing, screening workers, and reconfiguring factories. Trump later attacked several Democratic–administered states and cities as being "poorly-run." His remarks coincided with a push by state governors seeking a US$500 million federal economic package. Trump also addressed a brief press conference focusing on how states could expand coronavirus testing and efforts to reopen the economy. He also announced that the US was investigating China's response to the coronavirus pandemic, the reopening of some schools, and North Korean leader Kim Jong Un.
- The United States Small Business Administration has lent an extra US$2 billion to small businesses through its Paycheck Protection Program after a number of borrowers in the first

round of funding for the coronavirus declined or returned their loans.

- US House Majority Leader Steny Hoyer announced that the United States House of Representatives would resume session on 4 May.
- Californian Governor Gavin Newsom announced that law enforcement authorities would step up the enforcement of coronavirus-related restrictions after crowds visited beaches over the weekend.
- New York Governor Andrew Cuomo has extended a stay-at-home order in much of the state until 15 May but indicated that restrictions could be waived in areas with sufficient hospital capacity. New York state officials also cancelled the 2020 New York Democratic primary due to health and safety concerns.
- Swedish Ambassador to the United States Karin Ulrika Olofsdotter also stated that Sweden could reach herd immunity by May during an interview with National Public Radio.
- The World Health Organization's top emergency expert Michael Ryan has described the US federal government's plan to combat the coronavirus pandemic as "very clearly-laid out" and "science-based," complimenting the cooperation between the federal and state governments.

28 April

- China has reported three new cases, bringing the total to 82,836. Chinese authorities have reported no new deaths.
- Egypt has reported a total of 4,782 cases.

- Germany has confirmed 1,114 new cases, bringing the total to 156,337. Germany has also reported 163 new deaths, bringing the death toll to 5,913.
- Indonesia has officially reported 415 new cases, bringing the total to 9,511. Indonesian health authorities have also reported eight new deaths, bringing the death toll to 773. Indonesia has also reported 1,254 recoveries. However, a Reuters report suggests that more than 2,000 Indonesians with acute symptoms of COVID-19 have died based on an analysis of data from 16 of Indonesia's 34 provinces.
- Iran has reported 71 deaths, raising the death toll to 5,877. Iran has reported a total of 92,584 cases.
- Italy has reported 382 deaths, causing the death toll to exceed 20,000. Italian authorities have reported 2,091 cases, bringing the total number to 201,505. 105,205 remain infected, while 68,941 have recovered. The Italian Civil Protection Department has reported that 1.275 million people have been tested.
- Malaysia has reported 31 new cases, bringing the total number to 5,851. Malaysia has reported 75 new recoveries, bringing the total number of recoveries to 4,032. Malaysia has reported one new death, bringing the total death toll to 100.
- The Netherlands has reported 171 cases, bringing the total to 38,416. Dutch authorities have also reported 48 new deaths, bringing the death toll to 4,566.
- New Zealand has reported three new cases (two confirmed and one probable), bringing the total to 1,472 (1,124 confirmed and 348 probable). NZ authorities have also reported 34 new recoveries, bringing the total to 1,214.

- Pakistan has reported at least 20 new deaths, bringing the death toll to 301. 751 new cases were reported, bringing the total number to 14,079.
- Peru has reported a total of 30,000 cases and 854 deaths.
- The Philippines has reported 181 new cases, bringing the total number to 7,958. Filipino authorities have also reported 43 recoveries, bringing the total number to 975. The Philippines has reported 19 more deaths, bringing the death toll to 530.
- Singapore has reported 528 new cases, bringing the total to 14,951.
- South Korea has reported 14 new cases, bringing the total to 10,752.
- Turkey has reported 92 deaths, bringing the death toll to 2,992. Turkey has also reported 2,392 cases, bringing the total to 114,653. 38,809 people have recovered, while 29,230 people have been tested in the past 24 hours.
- Ukraine has reported 401 new cases and 19 new deaths, bringing the total numbers to 9,410 and 239, respectively; a total of 992 patients have recovered.
- The United States has reported over 1 million cases and more than 57,000 deaths as a result of the coronavirus pandemic. Illinois has reported 142 deaths, bringing the total to 2,125. Illinois has also reported 2,219 cases, bringing the total to 48,102.
- Figures from the Office for National Statistics for the week ending 17 April show 22,351 deaths registered in England and Wales, nearly double the five-year average and the highest weekly total since comparable records began in 1993.

- The ONS report indicates that a third of coronavirus deaths in England and Wales are occurring in care homes, with 2,000 recorded in the week ending 17 April. The number of deaths from all causes in care homes is almost three times the number recorded three weeks ago.
- Matt Hancock announces that care home figures will be included in the daily death toll from the following day; official figures have previously included only hospital data.
- Testing capacity reaches 73,000 per day, although only 43,000 were carried out the previous day. Matt Hancock announces that testing will be expanded from the following day to include all care home workers and people (and their family members) with symptoms who must leave home for their job or are aged over 65.
- At 11 am the UK holds a minute's silence to remember key workers who have died from COVID-19.
- Egyptian President Abdel Fattah el-Sisi has renewed the country's national state of emergency by three months, citing health and security concerns. Egyptian has been in a state of emergency since the Palm Sunday church bombings in early April 2017.
- The United Nations Human Rights Commissioner Michelle Bachelet has called for the lifting of sanctions on Sudan to ease pressure on the country's health system during the coronavirus pandemic. The United Nations High Commissioner for Refugees has announced that it needs US$89.4 million to support refugee aid programs for Yemenis and other refugees in the midst of the coronavirus pandemic.

- Quebec Premier Francois Legault has announced plans to gradually reopen Quebec's economy in May while maintaining social distancing restrictions.
- Governor of New York Andrew Cuomo has announced that the number of hospital admissions has dropped to its lowest level in more than a month. He also clarified that regions in New York state wanting to reopen would need to have a hospital capacity rate below 70% and a transmission rate below 1.1%.
- United States President Donald Trump has announced that the US Government is considering testing passengers on international flights for the coronavirus.

29 April

- Azerbaijan has reported a total of 1,717 cases and 22 deaths.
- Bosnia has reported 93 new cases and two deaths, bringing the total to 1,677 and the death toll to 67. The surge in cases accompanied the easing of lockdown restrictions in the autonomous Federation of Bosnia and Herzegovina and the Republika Srpska.
- Brazil has reported 6,726 new cases, bringing the total number to 78,612. Brazil has reported a total of 5,466 deaths.
- China has reported 22 new cases, all involving overseas travel. Chinese authorities have reported no new deaths, with the official death toll remaining at 4,633.
- Germany has reported 1,304 new cases and 202 more deaths.

- India has reported 73 new deaths, bringing the death toll to 1,007. India has reported over 30,000 cases.
- Indonesia has reported 260 new cases, bringing the total number to 9,771. Indonesian health authorities have also reported 11 deaths, bringing the death toll to 784. 1,391 people have recovered, and more than 67,700 people have been tested.
- Iran has reported 80 new deaths, bringing the death toll to 5,957. Iran has reported a total of 93,657 cases.
- Malaysia has reported 94 new cases, bringing the total to 5,945. 55 patients have been discharged, bringing the number of recoveries to 4,087. The country's death toll remains at 100.
- The Netherlands has reported 386 cases, bringing the total number to 38,802. Dutch authorities have reported 145 deaths, bringing the death toll to 4,711.
- New Zealand has reported three new cases (one confirmed and two probable), bringing the total to 1,474 (1,126 confirmed and 348 probable). NZ health authorities have also reported 15 new recoveries, bringing the total to 1,229.
- Pakistan has reported 26 new deaths, bringing the death toll to 327. Pakistan has also reported 806 new cases, bringing the total to 14,885. A total of at least 3,245 patients have recovered.
- Poland has reported a total of 12,415 cases and 606 deaths.
- Russia has reported 5,841 new cases, bringing the total number to 99,399. Russia has reported 108 new deaths, bringing the death toll to 972.
- Serbia has reported a total of 8,724 cases and 173 deaths.

- Singapore has reported 690 new cases, bringing the total to 15,641.
- South Africa has reported 354 new cases, bringing the total to 5,350. South Africa has reported ten new deaths, bringing the death toll to 103. South African authorities have conducted a total of 197,127 tests, with 11,630 being done in the last 24 hours.
- Spain has reported 325 deaths, bringing the death toll to 24,275. Spain has reported 2,144 cases, bringing the total to 212,917.
- Turkey has reported a total of nearly 115,000 cases and nearly 3,000 deaths.
- Ukraine has reported 456 new cases and 11 new deaths, bringing the total numbers to 9,866 and 250, respectively; a total of 1,103 patients have recovered.
- Speaking to the House of Commons Education Select Committee, Gavin Williamson, the Secretary of State for Education, says that the reopening of schools will take place in a "phased manner."
- Official figures begin including deaths in care homes and the community, resulting in the number of recorded deaths increasing by 4,419 to 26,097. Dominic Raab tells the Downing Street daily briefing the figures have been included retrospectively and account for care home and community deaths between 2 March and 28 April. In the most recent 24-hour period, there have been 765 deaths.
- A pug named Winston became the first pet dog in the United States to test positive for COVID-19. Winston's family had taken part in Duke University's Molecular and

Epidemiological Study of Suspected Infection research study.

- The United States Department of Commerce has reported that the United States' gross domestic product declined by a 4.8% in the period between January and March 2020.
- During a State Department press conference, the United States Secretary of State Mike Pompeo claimed that Chinese laboratories lack adequate security to prevent future pandemics.
- Alphabet Inc.'s Chief Financial Officer Ruth Porat has reported a decline in advertising revenue due to a drop in Google users searching for commercial topics on the search engine.
- Boeing CEO David Calhoun has announced that it plans to lay off ten percent of its workforce and reduce the production of its main commercial planes after reporting a first-quarter US$641 million loss as a result of the economic impact of the coronavirus on the airline sector.
- Gilead Sciences has announced that its experimental anti-virus drug remdesivir has helped COVID-19 patients during a clinical trial. US President Donald Trump has welcomed the news while immunologist and White House Coronavirus Task Force member Anthony Fauci has advised caution.
- Iranian President Hassan Rouhani has allowed the reopening of businesses despite the persistent coronavirus pandemic.
- The Emir of Qatar Tamim bin Hamad Al Thani has dispatched medical supplies to Iran and Algeria to aid their efforts to combat the coronavirus pandemic.

- The Tunisian Government has announced that it will ease lockdown restrictions to allow the reopening of the food, industry, construction, and half the civil service sectors in early May. Clothing shops, shopping malls, and some public transportation will resume from 11 May.
- The Abu Dhabi airline Eithad has delayed the resumption of passenger flights from 16 May until 16 June.

30 April

- Bosnia-Herzegovina has reported a total of 1,757 cases and 69 deaths.
- Brazil has reported 7,218 new cases, bringing the total to 85,380. Brazil also reported 435 new deaths, bringing the death toll to 5,901.
- China has reported four new cases, bringing the total number to 82,862, of which 1,664 are imported.
- Comoros has reported its first case, a 50-year old Franco-Comorian man.
- Indonesia has reported 347 new cases, bringing the total to 10,118. Indonesian health authorities have reported 8 new deaths, bringing the death toll to 792. A total of 1,522 people have recovered, and 72,300 have been tested.
- Iran has confirmed 71 new deaths, bringing the death toll above 6,028.
- Italy has reported 285 deaths, bringing the death toll to 27,967. Italy has reported 1,872 cases, bringing the total number to 205,463. The total number of infected declined from 104,657 on 28 April to 101,551 on 1st May.
- Malaysia has reported 57 new cases, bringing the total number to 6,002. Malaysian health authorities have

discharged 84 patients, bringing the total number of recoveries to 4,171. Malaysia has reported two deaths, bringing the death toll to 102.

- The Maldives has reported its first death. The country has reported a total of 280 cases, the majority among its migrant workforce.
- The Netherlands has reported 514 cases, bringing the total to 39,316. The Dutch have reported 84 deaths, bringing the death toll to 4,795.
- New Zealand has reported three new cases, and one rescinded probable case, bringing the total to 1,476 (1,129 confirmed and 347 probable). NZ authorities have also reported 12 new recoveries, bringing the total to 1,241.
- Pakistan has reported 874 new cases, bringing the total to 15,759. Pakistan has reported a total of 4,052 recoveries. Pakistan has also reported 19 deaths, bringing the death toll to 346.
- Peru has reported 3,045 cases, bringing the number of cases to 36,976. Peru has reported a total of 1,051 deaths.
- The Philippines has reported 276 new cases, bringing the total number to 8,488. The Philippines has also reported 10 new deaths, bringing the death toll to 568. The Philippines has also reported 20 new recoveries, bringing the total number to 1,043.
- Russia has reported 7,099 new cases, bringing the total to 106,498. Russia has reported 101 new deaths, bringing the total to 1,073.
- Singapore has reported 528 new cases, taking the total number to 16,169. Another death was later confirmed, bringing the total to 15.

- South Korea has reported one new death, bringing the death toll to 247. South Korea has reported no new cases, keeping the national tally at 10,765.
- Spain has reported 268 new deaths, bringing the death toll to 24,543. Spain has reported a total of 213,435 cases.
- Sri Lanka has reported a total of 630 cases and seven deaths.
- Tajikistan has reported its first 15 cases.
- Thailand has reported seven new cases, bringing the total number to 2,954. No new deaths have been reported, with the death toll remaining at 54.
- Turkey has confirmed 2,615 new cases, bringing the total to 120,204. Turkey has reported 203 deaths, bringing the death toll to 3,174.
- Ukraine has reported 540 new cases and 11 new deaths, bringing the total numbers to 10,406 and 261 respectively; a total of 1,238 patients have recovered.
- The United Kingdom has reported 674 deaths, bringing the death toll to 26,711. English authorities have reported 391 new deaths, bringing the hospital death toll in England to 20,137.
- Prime Minister Boris Johnson says the UK is "past the peak" of the COVID-19 outbreak but that the country must not "risk a second spike," and announces that he will set out a "comprehensive plan" for easing the lockdown "next week." He also stresses the importance of keeping down the reproductive rate, which "is going to be vital to our recovery."
- Captain Tom Moore celebrates his 100th birthday and is made an honorary colonel by the Queen. His appeal to raise money for the NHS reaches £32m.

- At 8 pm, the UK stages its weekly round of applause for NHS staff and key workers.
- ITV announces plans to resume filming live studio-based shows such as Britain's Got Talent and The Masked Singer, but without the presence of an audience.
- The British Library is to archive hundreds of essays submitted to BBC Radio 4's PM programme by listeners detailing their coronavirus experiences. The Covid Chronicles, launched in March, has seen listeners submit their accounts of their lives during the lockdown restrictions, some of which have been broadcast.
- Yemen has reported its first two deaths and five new cases.
- Sub-Saharan Africa has confirmed around 238,00 cases and 900 deaths.
- According to Johns Hopkins University, the global number of recoveries has reached 1,004,483 people.
- Kuwaiti airlines Jazeera Airways has laid off 320 employees, or roughly 37% of its workforce. This includes cabin crew, ground staff, and support staff.
- The Qatari Government has announced that it will be producing artificial respiratory machines to cope with domestic and international health demands in response to the coronavirus pandemic.
- United States President Donald Trump claimed that he had seen evidence that the coronavirus originated in the Wuhan Institute of Virology. That same day, US intelligence agencies concluded that the coronavirus was neither "man-made or genetically modified" but that they were still investigating whether the pandemic originated with infected animals or an accident at the Wuhan laboratory.

- Californian Governor Gavin Newsom has ordered the closure of the state's beaches and parks from 1 May after large crowds visited them the previous weekend, violating social distancing rules.
- New York Governor Andrew Cuomo issued a statement that he would need between 6,400 and 17,000 people to trace people who had contracted the coronavirus.
- The United States Department of Labor reported an additional 3.8 million unemployment claims last week, bringing the total unemployed to more than 30 million.
- The International Monetary Fund has approved US$650 million in emergency assistance to the Dominican Republic.
- Médecins Sans Frontières has criticized the United States Government for threatening trade sanctions against several countries that Washington has accused of not protecting intellectual properties in the pharmaceutical sector, including India, Brazil, China, Chile, and Canada.
- NASCAR executive vice-president Steve O'Donnell announcing that NASCAR's racing season will resume on 17 May at Darlington Raceway in Darlington, South Carolina.
- US pharmaceutical company Pfizer's vaccines head Nanette Cocero has announced that the company aims to produce 10-20 million doses of a coronavirus vaccine that it is developing with the German company BioNTech for possible emergency use depending on the vaccine trial results.
- The United Nations Secretary-General António Guterres issued a statement criticizing the lack of leadership by world powers and raising concern about the inadequate support for the fight against the coronavirus in developing countries.

Conclusion

The world began to alter in full force at the start of 2020. We would never be able to return to the lives we had known before, forcing us to modify our ways of living.

Everyone has been equally affected by the Covid-19 pandemic. People have lost loved ones, their jobs, and their homes. While businesses and governments fell, individuals began to realise they needed to take safeguards to preserve themselves. Governments advocated policies for social distancing and lockdowns.

Most of the year was spent in terror. They knew the virus was here to stay, and all they could do was take the appropriate measures and protect themselves and their loved ones.

For the Record is written as a memory of the harrowing year we have all experienced. This book takes its readers on a chronological trip starting on January 1st till April 30th, detailing what transpired throughout the world on each date of the year 2020.

The story of Covid-19 continues in Volume 2: Fact Not Fiction and Volume 3: The Virus and The Vaccine, mapping May 2020 – December 2020.

References

Responses to the COVID-19 pandemic in April 2020 (2021) Wikipedia. Available at: https://en.wikipedia.org/wiki/Responses_to_the_COVID-19_pandemic_in_April_2020 (Accessed: 2 May 2021).

Responses to the COVID-19 pandemic in January 2020 (2021a) Wikipedia. Available at: https://en.wikipedia.org/wiki/Responses_to_the_COVID-19_pandemic_in_January_2020 (Accessed: 22 May 2021).

Responses to the COVID-19 pandemic in January 2020 (2021b) Wikipedia. Available at: https://en.wikipedia.org/wiki/Responses_to_the_COVID-19_pandemic_in_January_2020 (Accessed: 22 May 2021).

Responses to the COVID-19 pandemic in February 2020 (2021) Wikipedia. Available at: https://en.wikipedia.org/wiki/Responses_to_the_COVID-19_pandemic_in_February_2020 (Accessed: 2 May 2021).

Responses to the COVID-19 pandemic in March 2020 (2021) Wikipedia. Available at: https://en.wikipedia.org/wiki/Responses_to_the_COVID-19_pandemic_in_March_2020 (Accessed: 2 May 2021).

Timeline of the COVID-19 pandemic (2021) Wikipedia. Available at: https://en.wikipedia.org/wiki/Timeline_of_the_COVID-19_pandemic (Accessed: 20 April 2021).

Timeline of the COVID-19 pandemic in Afghanistan (2021) Wikipedia. Available at:

https://en.wikipedia.org/wiki/Timeline_of_the_COVID-19_pandemic_in_Afghanistan (Accessed: 20 April 2021).

Timeline of the COVID-19 pandemic in April 2020 (2021) Wikipedia. Available at: https://en.wikipedia.org/wiki/Timeline_of_the_COVID-19_pandemic_in_April_2020 (Accessed: 20 April 2021).

Timeline of the COVID-19 pandemic in Argentina (2021) Wikipedia. Available at: https://en.wikipedia.org/wiki/Timeline_of_the_COVID-19_pandemic_in_Argentina (Accessed: 20 April 2021).

Timeline of the COVID-19 pandemic in Australia (2021) Wikipedia. Available at: https://en.wikipedia.org/wiki/Timeline_of_the_COVID-19_pandemic_in_Australia (Accessed: 20 April 2021).

Timeline of the COVID-19 pandemic in Bangladesh (2021) Wikipedia. Available at: https://en.wikipedia.org/wiki/Timeline_of_the_COVID-19_pandemic_in_Bangladesh (Accessed: 20 April 2021).

Timeline of the COVID-19 pandemic in Belarus (2021) Wikipedia. Available at: https://en.wikipedia.org/wiki/Timeline_of_the_COVID-19_pandemic_in_Belarus (Accessed: 20 April 2021).

Timeline of the COVID-19 pandemic in Brazil (2021) Wikipedia. Available at: https://en.wikipedia.org/wiki/Timeline_of_the_COVID-19_pandemic_in_Brazil (Accessed: 7 May 2021).

Timeline of the COVID-19 pandemic in Canada (2021) Wikipedia. Available at:

https://en.wikipedia.org/wiki/Timeline_of_the_COVID-19_pandemic_in_Canada (Accessed: 7 May 2021).

Timeline of the COVID-19 pandemic in Croatia (2021) Wikipedia. Available at: https://en.wikipedia.org/wiki/Timeline_of_the_COVID-19_pandemic_in_Croatia (Accessed: 7 May 2021).

Timeline of the COVID-19 pandemic in England (January–June 2020) (2021) Wikipedia. Available at: https://en.wikipedia.org/wiki/Timeline_of_the_COVID-19_pandemic_in_England_(January–June_2020) (Accessed: 10 March 2021).

Timeline of the COVID-19 pandemic in England (July–December 2020) (2021) Wikipedia. Available at: https://en.wikipedia.org/wiki/Timeline_of_the_COVID-19_pandemic_in_England_(July–December_2020) (Accessed: 20 May 2021).

Timeline of the COVID-19 pandemic in February 2020 (2021) Wikipedia. Available at: https://en.wikipedia.org/wiki/Timeline_of_the_COVID-19_pandemic_in_February_2020 (Accessed: 20 May 2021).

Timeline of the COVID-19 pandemic in Fiji (2021) Wikipedia. Available at: https://en.wikipedia.org/wiki/Timeline_of_the_COVID-19_pandemic_in_Fiji (Accessed: 10 March 2021).

Timeline of the COVID-19 pandemic in Ghana (2021) Wikipedia. Available at: https://en.wikipedia.org/wiki/Timeline_of_the_COVID-19_pandemic_in_Ghana (Accessed: 10 March 2021).

Timeline of the COVID-19 pandemic in India (2021) Wikipedia. Available at: https://en.wikipedia.org/wiki/Timeline_of_the_COVID-19_pandemic_in_India (Accessed: 5 June 2021).

Timeline of the COVID-19 pandemic in Indonesia (2021) Wikipedia. Available at: https://en.wikipedia.org/wiki/Timeline_of_the_COVID-19_pandemic_in_Indonesia (Accessed: 5 June 2021).

Timeline of the COVID-19 pandemic in January 2020 (2021) Wikipedia. Available at: https://en.wikipedia.org/wiki/Timeline_of_the_COVID-19_pandemic_in_January_2020 (Accessed: 22 February 2021).

Timeline of the COVID-19 pandemic in Japan (2021) Wikipedia. Available at: https://en.wikipedia.org/wiki/Timeline_of_the_COVID-19_pandemic_in_Japan (Accessed: 22 February 2021).

Timeline of the COVID-19 pandemic in Malaysia (2021) Wikipedia. Available at: https://en.wikipedia.org/wiki/Timeline_of_the_COVID-19_pandemic_in_Malaysia (Accessed: 15 January 2021).

Timeline of the COVID-19 pandemic in March 2020 (2021) Wikipedia. Available at: https://en.wikipedia.org/wiki/Timeline_of_the_COVID-19_pandemic_in_March_2020 (Accessed: 22 February 2021).

Timeline of the COVID-19 pandemic in Mexico (2021) Wikipedia. Available at: https://en.wikipedia.org/wiki/Timeline_of_the_COVID-19_pandemic_in_Mexico (Accessed: 18 April 2021).

Timeline of the COVID-19 pandemic in Nepal (2021) Wikipedia. Available at: https://en.wikipedia.org/wiki/Timeline_of_the_COVID-19_pandemic_in_Nepal (Accessed: 22 February 2021).

Timeline of the COVID-19 pandemic in New Zealand (2021) Wikipedia. Available at: https://en.wikipedia.org/wiki/Timeline_of_the_COVID-19_pandemic_in_New_Zealand (Accessed: 23 March 2021).

Timeline of the COVID-19 pandemic in Nigeria (2021) Wikipedia. Available at: https://en.wikipedia.org/wiki/Timeline_of_the_COVID-19_pandemic_in_Nigeria (Accessed: 20 May 2021).

Timeline of the COVID-19 pandemic in Pakistan (2021) Wikipedia. Available at: https://en.wikipedia.org/wiki/Timeline_of_the_COVID-19_pandemic_in_Pakistan (Accessed: 10 January 2021).

Timeline of the COVID-19 pandemic in Romania (2021) Wikipedia. Available at: https://en.wikipedia.org/wiki/Timeline_of_the_COVID-19_pandemic_in_Romania (Accessed: 10 February 2021).

Timeline of the COVID-19 pandemic in Russia (2021) Wikipedia. Available at: https://en.wikipedia.org/wiki/Timeline_of_the_COVID-19_pandemic_in_Russia (Accessed: 23 February 2021).

Timeline of the COVID-19 pandemic in Singapore (2021) Wikipedia. Available at: https://en.wikipedia.org/wiki/Timeline_of_the_COVID-19_pandemic_in_Singapore (Accessed: 23 February 2021).

Timeline of the COVID-19 pandemic in Spain (2021) Wikipedia. Available at: https://en.wikipedia.org/wiki/Timeline_of_the_COVID-19_pandemic_in_Spain (Accessed: 23 February 2021).

Timeline of the COVID-19 pandemic in Sweden (2021) Wikipedia. Available at: https://en.wikipedia.org/wiki/Timeline_of_the_COVID-19_pandemic_in_Sweden (Accessed: 16 May 2021).

Timeline of the COVID-19 pandemic in Thailand (2021) Wikipedia. Available at: https://en.wikipedia.org/wiki/Timeline_of_the_COVID-19_pandemic_in_Thailand (Accessed: 16 May 2021).

Timeline of the COVID-19 pandemic in the Philippines (2021) Wikipedia. Available at: https://en.wikipedia.org/wiki/Timeline_of_the_COVID-19_pandemic_in_the_Philippines (Accessed: 20 May 2021).

Timeline of the COVID-19 pandemic in the Republic of Ireland (2021) Wikipedia. Available at: https://en.wikipedia.org/wiki/Timeline_of_the_COVID-19_pandemic_in_the_Republic_of_Ireland (Accessed: 23 February 2021).

Timeline of the COVID-19 pandemic in the United Kingdom (January–June 2020) (2021) Wikipedia. Available at: https://en.wikipedia.org/wiki/Timeline_of_the_COVID-19_pandemic_in_the_United_Kingdom_(January–June_2020) (Accessed: 23 March 2021).

Timeline of the COVID-19 pandemic in the United Kingdom (July–December 2020) (2021) Wikipedia. Available at:

https://en.wikipedia.org/wiki/Timeline_of_the_COVID-19_pandemic_in_the_United_Kingdom_(July–December_2020) (Accessed: 23 February 2021).

Timeline of the COVID-19 pandemic in the United States (2020) (2021) Wikipedia. Available at: https://en.wikipedia.org/wiki/Timeline_of_the_COVID-19_pandemic_in_the_United_States_(2020) (Accessed: 10 march 2021).

Timeline of the COVID-19 pandemic in Trinidad and Tobago (2021) Wikipedia. Available at: https://en.wikipedia.org/wiki/Timeline_of_the_COVID-19_pandemic_in_Trinidad_and_Tobago (Accessed: 19 May 2021).

Timeline of the COVID-19 pandemic in Turkey (2021) Wikipedia. Available at: https://en.wikipedia.org/wiki/Timeline_of_the_COVID-19_pandemic_in_Turkey (Accessed: 19 May 2021).

Timeline of the COVID-19 pandemic in Uruguay (2021) Wikipedia. Available at: https://en.wikipedia.org/wiki/Timeline_of_the_COVID-19_pandemic_in_Uruguay (Accessed: 23 February 2021).

Timeline of the COVID-19 pandemic in Vietnam (2021) Wikipedia. Available at: https://en.wikipedia.org/wiki/Timeline_of_the_COVID-19_pandemic_in_Vietnam (Accessed: 15 January 2021).

World Health Organization's response to the COVID-19 pandemic (2021) Wikipedia. Available at: https://en.wikipedia.org/wiki/World_Health_Organization%27s_re

sponse_to_the_COVID-19_pandemic (Accessed: 10 January 2021).

https://www.telegraph.co.uk/global-health/science-and-disease/wuhan-officials-identified-huanan-market-pandemic-risk-least/

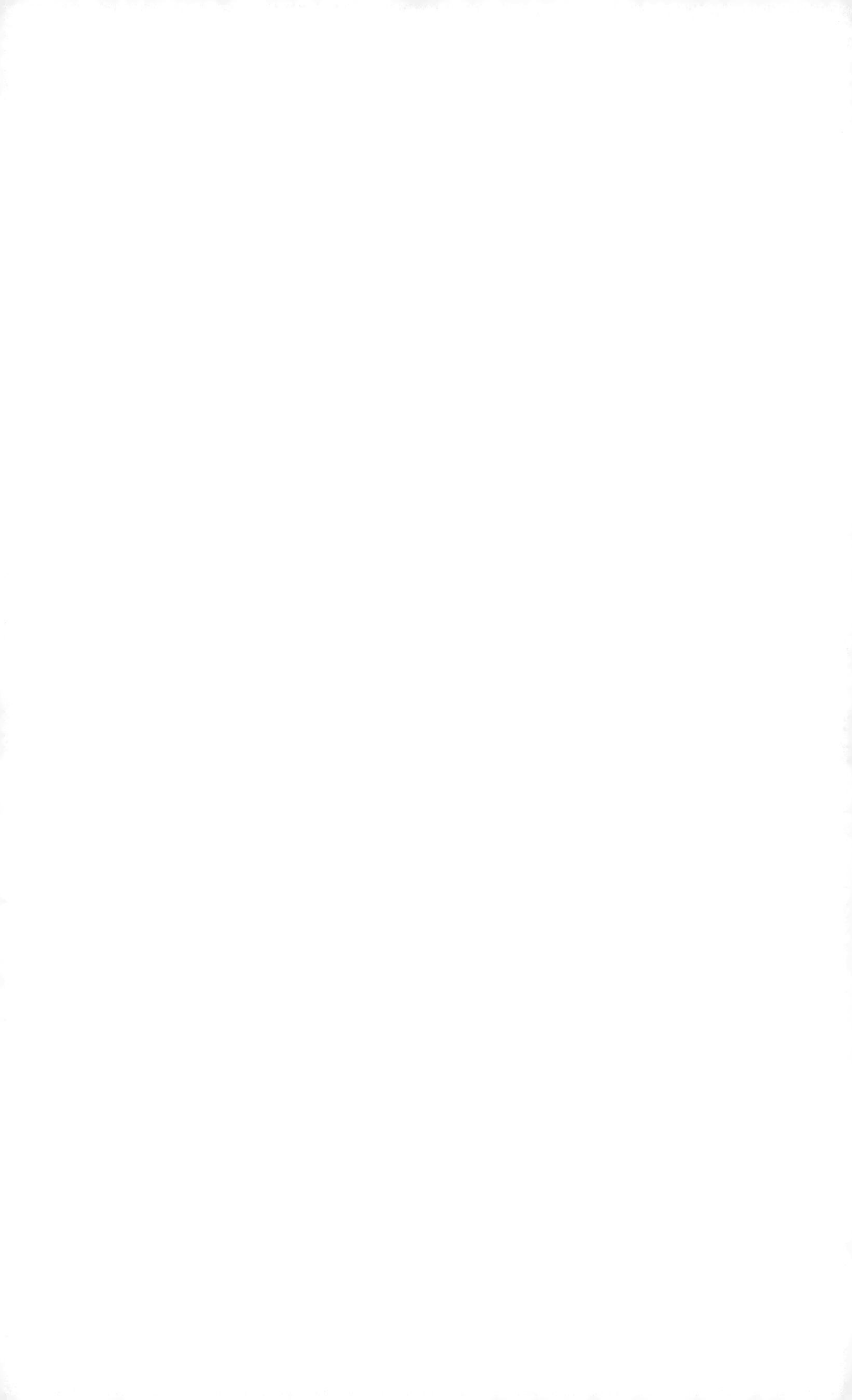

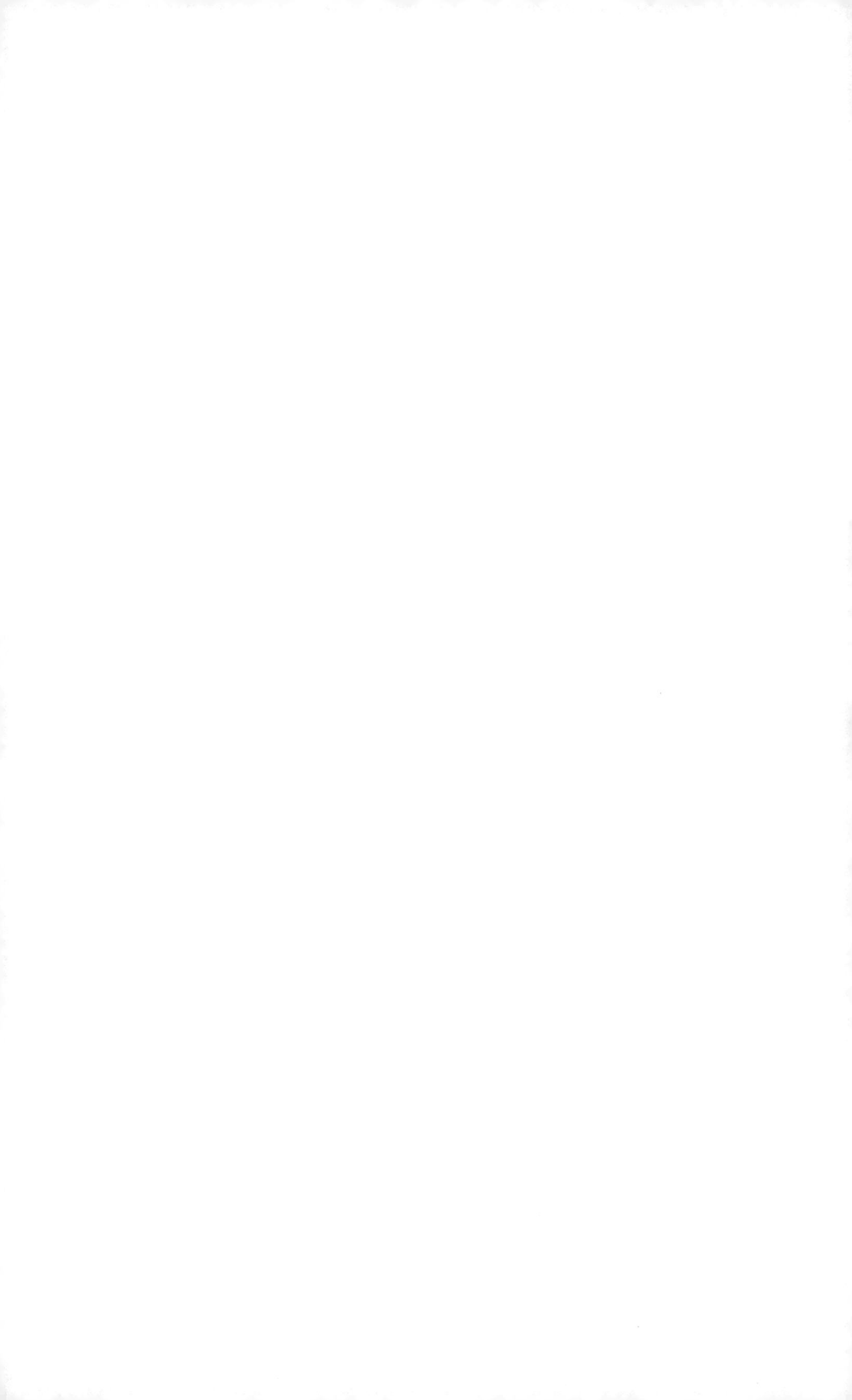

www.ingramcontent.com/pod-product-compliance
Ingram Content Group UK Ltd.
Pitfield, Milton Keynes, MK11 3LW, UK
UKHW020145250726
13967UKWH00002B/880